New Trends in Allergy II

Edited by
J. Ring and G. Burg

With a Foreword by O. Braun-Falco

With 105 Figures and 71 Tables

Springer-Verlag
Berlin Heidelberg New York
London Paris Tokyo

Professor Dr. Dr. Johannes Ring
Professor Dr. Günter Burg

Dermatologische Klinik und Poliklinik der
Ludwig-Maximilians-Universität München
(Head: Prof. Dr. Dr. hc. O. Braun-Falco),
Frauenlobstraße 9–11, 8000 Munich,
Federal Republic of Germany

The abstracts of the papers have already been published in the journal *Allergologie*, volume 8/7, 1985, pp. 293–310 and are reprinted with kind permission by Dustri-Verlag, Deisenhofen, Federal Republic of Germany

ISBN-13:978-3-642-71318-7 e-ISBN-13:978-3-642-71316-3
DOI: 10.1007/978-3-642-71316-3

Library of Congress Cataloging in Publication Data.
New trends in allergy II. Papers given at an international symposium held on 26–28 July 1985 in Munich.
Bibliography: p. Includes index.
1. Allergy–Congresses. I. Ring, Johannes, 1945– .
II. Burg, Günter. RC583.2.N482 1986 616.97 86-13083
ISBN-13:978-3-642-71318-7 (U.S.)

Softcover reprint of the hardcover 1st edition 1986

2127/3145-543210

Foreword

Allergic reactions and allergic diseases are found in many fields of medicine. As well as affecting the skin, allergic diseases occur in internal organs such as the lungs and the kidneys and in the vascular and nervous systems.

Interdisciplinary understanding and cooperation thus seem necessary to get a better insight into allergic reactions in the different fields of medicine in order that we may give our patients the best diagnostic and therapeutic care.

Allergic diseases are on the increase. Studies from Sweden show that 15% of the population there are atopic, and some people speculate that in Germany about 10%–15% of all adults suffer from one of the many different allergic conditions. We in our clinic also have the impression that the incidence of atopic reactions has increased in recent years. The figure of 15% would mean something like 200 000 people in Munich alone!

We all know that a wide variety of environmental factors can induce allergic reactions in the skin, the respiratory system, or internal organs. The most important allergens in our environment are pollen, molds, animal dander, housedust mite, food or food additives, various insects, industrial compounds and drugs.

The direct costs of hospital and community medical care, other services, and drugs to help patients with asthma, hay fever, and skin allergies have increased considerably in the last 10 years. The figures should make it clear to everybody that we are dealing with a health and environmental problem of great practical importance.

This volume contains the invitation papers given at an international symposium held on 26–28 July 1985 in Munich, at which a wide spectrum of allergological problems was covered. Some chapters deal with basic research in allergy, for example the important questions of mediators of allergic reactions, regulation of IgE synthesis, and contact sensitization. Other papers describe advances in clinical allergology, e.g., in asthma, atopic eczema, food allergy, drug reactions, and contact allergy. Therapeutic aspects are considered in the sections on hyposensitization and pharmacotherapy.

Of course, a printed book never can truly reflect the lively atmosphere of an international symposium such as this. Over 500 participants from all over the world gathered in an extremely friendly spirit, highlighted by the unforgettable Bavarian evening with King Ludwig II!

I would like to thank all those at the Dermatology Clinic of the University of Munich who did so much to ensure the success of the symposium. I am also grateful to Springer-Verlag for publishing the book so rapidly. May it find a wide audience and thus improve the understanding of allergic diseases to the benefit of our patients!

Munich, June 1986

O. BRAUN-FALCO

Table of Contents

Mediators

Atopic Eczema and Food Allergy

List of Contributors

ALLEN, D. H., M.B., Ph.D., F.R.A.C.P.
Department of Thoracic Medicine, Royal North Shore Hospital, Sydney, Australia

BAKER, G., M.B., BSc., F.R.A.C.P.
Department of Thoracic Medicine, Royal North Shore Hospital, Sydney, Australia

BAUR, X., Priv. Doz. Dr. med.
Pneumologische Abteilung, I. Medizinische Klinik der Universität München, Klinikum Großhadern, Marchioninistraße 15, 8000 München 70, Federal Republic of Germany

BENEZRA, C., Prof. Dr. med.
Laboratoire de Dermatochimie, Associé au CNRS, Université Louis Pasteur, Clinique Dermatologique, CHU, 67091 Strasbourg, France

BENVENISTE, J., M.D.
INSERM U.200, Université Paris-Sud, 32 rue des Carnets, 92140 Clamart, France

BIRCH, R. E., Ph.D.,
Division of Allergy and Immunology, Department of Pediatrics, Washington University School of Medicine, 660 South Euclid Avenue, St. Louis, MO 63178, USA

BOGNER, J., Dr. med.
Dermatologische Klinik und Poliklinik der Universität München, Frauenlobstraße 9–11, 8000 München 2, Federal Republic of Germany

BONNLÄNDER, A.-R., cand. med.
Dermatologische Klinik und Poliklinik der Universität München, Frauenlobstraße 9–11, 8000 München 2, Federal Republic of Germany

BRAUN-FALCO, O., Prof. Dr. med. Dr. h.c.
Dermatologische Klinik und Poliklinik der Universität München, Frauenlobstraße 9–11, 8000 München 2, Federal Republic of Germany

BURG, G., Prof. Dr. med.
Dermatologische Klinik und Poliklinik der Universität München,
Frauenlobstraße 9–11, 8000 München 2, Federal Republic of Germany

CZARNETZKI, BEATE M., Prof. Dr. med.
Universitäts-Hautklinik Münster, Von-Esmarch-Straße 56, 4400 Münster,
Federal Republic of Germany

DELOHERY, J., M.B., F.R.A.C.P.
Department of Thoracic Medicine, Royal North Shore Hospital, Sydney,
Australia

DORN, M., Priv. Doz. Dr. med.
Dermatologische Klinik und Poliklinik der Universität München,
Frauenlobstraße 9–11, 8000 München 2, Federal Republic of Germany

DORSCH, W., Priv. Doz. Dr. med.
Kinderpoliklinik der Universität München, Pettenkoferstraße 8 a,
8000 München 2, Federal Republic of Germany

DREBORG, S., M.D.
Department of Pediatrics, University Hospital, 581 85 Linköping, Sweden

FLEISCHER, B., Priv. Doz. Dr. med.
Abteilung Medizinische Mikrobiologie und Immunologie, Universität Ulm,
Oberer Eselsberg, 7900 Ulm, Federal Republic of Germany

FLOHÉ, L., Prof. Dr. med.
Grünenthal GmbH, 5100 Aachen, Federal Republic of Germany

FUCHS, E., Prof. Dr. med.
Deutsche Klinik für Diagnostik, Fachbereich Allergologie, Aukammallee 33,
6200 Wiesbaden, Federal Republic of Germany

GALOSI, A., Dr. med.
Hauptplatz 2, 8068 Pfaffenhofen, Federal Republic of Germany

HÄGERMARK, Ö., Prof. Dr. med.
Department of Dermatology, Karolinska Sjukhuset, 104 01 Stockholm, Sweden

VON DER HELM, DOROTHEA, Dr. med.
Dermatologische Klinik und Poliklinik der Universität München,
Frauenlobstraße 9–11, 8000 München 2, Federal Republic of Germany

IBEL, H., Dr. med.
Dermatologische Klinik und Poliklinik der Universität München,
Frauenlobstraße 9–11, 8000 München 2, Federal Republic of Germany

Johansson, S. G. O., Prof. Dr. med.
Department of Clinical Immunology, Karolinska Sjukhuset, 104 01 Stockholm, Sweden

Kligman, A. M., M.D., Ph.D.
Department of Dermatology, University of Pennsylvania, Medical Educational Building, 36th & Hamilton Walk, Philadelphia, PA 19104, USA

Knop, J., Prof. Dr. med.
Hautklinik der Universität Münster, Von-Esmarch-Straße 56, 4400 Münster, Federal Republic of Germany

Knutti-Müller, J., Dr. med.
Institut für klinische Immunologie, Inselspital, 3000 Bern, Switzerland

Kulczycki, Jr., A., M.D.
Washington University School of Medicine, 660 South Euclid Avenue, Saint Louis, MO 63110, USA

Lewin, J., Dr. med.
II. Medizinische Klinik des Klinikums Rechts der Isar der Technischen Universität München, 8000 München, Federal Republic of Germany

Løwenstein, H., Prof. Dr. med.
The Protein Laboratory, University of Copenhagen, Sigurdsgade 34, 2200 Copenhagen, Denmark

Maasch, H.-J., Dr. rer. nat.
Allergopharma, Herrengraben 10, 2057 Reinbeck b. Hamburg, Federal Republic of Germany

Mathison, D. A., M.D.
Division of Allergy and Immunology and Department of Basic and Clinical Research, Scripps Clinic and Research Foundation, 10666 North Torrey Pines Road, La Jolla, CA 92037, USA

Mayr, T., Dr. med.
Dermatologische Klinik und Poliklinik der Universität München, Frauenlobstraße 9–11, 8000 München 2, Federal Republic of Germany

Meurer, M., Priv. Doz. Dr. med.
Dermatologische Klinik und Poliklinik der Universität München, Frauenlobstraße 9–11, 8000 München 2, Federal Republic of Germany

Overell, B. G., M.D., Ph.D.
Bencard Pharmaceuticals, Yew Tree Bottom Road, Epsom, Surrey KT18 5XQ, Great Britain

PARKER, C. W., M.D.
Howard Hughes Medical Institute Laboratory, Department of Internal Medicine, Division of Allergy and Immunology, Washington University School of Medicine, 660 South Euclid Avenue, St. Louis, MO 63110, USA

POLMAR, S. H., Ph.D., M.D.
Division of Allergy and Immunology, Department of Pediatrics, Washington University School of Medicine, 660 South Euclid Avenue, St. Louis, MO 63178, USA

PRZYBILLA, B., Dr. med.
Dermatologische Klinik und Poliklinik der Universität München, Frauenlobstraße 9–11, 8000 München 2, Federal Republic of Germany

REIMANN, H. J., Priv. Doz. Dr. med.
II. Medizinische Klinik des Klinikums Rechts der Isar der Technischen Universität München, 8000 München, Federal Republic of Germany

RICHTER, A. W., Prof. Dr. med.
Department of Biomedical Research, Pharmacia AB, 751 82 Uppsala, Sweden

RING, J., Prof. Dr. med. Dr. phil.
Dermatologische Klinik und Poliklinik der Universität München, Frauenlobstraße 9–11, 8000 München 2, Federal Republic of Germany

RUZICKA, T., Priv. Doz. Dr. med.
Dermatologische Klinik und Poliklinik der Universität München, Frauenlobstraße 9–11, 8000 München 2, Federal Republic of Germany

SCHMIDT, U., Dr. med.
II. Medizinische Klinik des Klinikums Rechts der Isar der Technischen Universität München, 8000 München, Federal Republic of Germany

SCHWAB, ULRIKE, Dr. med.
Dermatologische Klinik und Poliklinik der Universität München, Frauenlobstraße 9–11, 8000 München 2, Federal Republic of Germany

SEDLMEIER, FRANZISKA
Dermatologische Klinik und Poliklinik der Universität München, Frauenlobstraße 9–11, 8000 München 2, Federal Republic of Germany

SIMMET, T., Dr. med.
Institut für Pharmakologie und Toxikologie, Ruhr-Universität Bochum, Im Lottental, 4630 Bochum 1, Federal Republic of Germany

SIMON, R. A., M.D.
Division of Allergy and Immunology and Department of Basic and Clinical Research, Scripps Clinic and Research Foundation, 1066 North Torrey Pines Road, La Jolla, CA 92037, USA

SOOTHILL, J. F., Prof. Dr. med.
Department of Immunology, Institute of Child Health, University of London, 30 Guilford Street, London WC1N 1EH, Great Britain

SPIEGELBERG, H. L., M. D.
Department of Immunology, Scripps Clinic and Research Foundation, 10666 North Torrey Pines Road, La Jolla, CA 92037, USA

STADLER, B., Dr. med.
Institut für klinische Immunologie, Inselspital, 3000 Bern, Switzerland

STEVENSON, D. D., M. D.
Division of Allergy and Immunology and Department of Basic and Clinical Research, Scripps Clinic and Research Foundation, 10666 North Torrey Pines Road, La Jolla, CA 92037, USA

THIEL, CLAUDIA, Dr. med.
Deutsche Klinik für Diagnostik, Fachbereich Allergologie, Aukammallee 33, 6200 Wiesbaden, Federal Republic of Germany

UEHARA, M., M.D.
Department of Dermatology, Shiga University of Medical Science, Seta, Otsu 520-21, Japan

WAHL, R., Dr. med.
Allergopharm, Herrengraben 10, 2057 Reinbeck b. Hamburg, Federal Republic of Germany

WAHN, U., Prof. Dr. med.
Universitäts-Kinderklinik, Klinikum Charlottenburg, 1000 Berlin 19/West

WALZ, ULRIKE, Dr. med.
Dermatologische Klinik und Poliklinik der Universität München, Frauenlobstraße 9–11, 8000 München 2, Federal Republic of Germany

DE WECK, A. L., Prof. Dr. med.
Institut für klinische Immunologie, Inselspital, 3000 Bern, Switzerland

WEDNER, H. J., M.D.
Division of Immunology, Department of Medicine, Washington University School of Medicine, St. Louis, MO 63110, USA

WHEELER, A. W., M.D.
Bencard Pharmaceuticals, Yew Tree Bottom Road, Epsom, Surrey KT18 5XQ, Great Britain

WINZER, M., Dr. med.
Klinik für Dermatologie und Venerologie, Medizinische Universität zu Lübeck, Ratzeburger Allee 160, 2400 Lübeck, Federal Republic of Germany

WOLFF, H. H., Prof. Dr. med.
Klinik für Dermatologie und Venerologie, Medizinische Universität zu Lübeck, Ratzeburger Allee 160, 2400 Lübeck, Federal Republic of Germany

ZELLMER, A., Dr. med.
II. Medizinische Klinik des Klinikums Rechts der Isar der Technischen Universität München, 8000 München, Federal Republic of Germany

ZINKERNAGEL, R. M., Prof. Dr. med.
Institut für Pathologie der Universität Zürich, Universitätsspital, Sternartstraße 2, 8091 Zürich, Switzerland

List of Chairmen

BANDMANN, H.-J., Prof. Dr. med. †
Dermatologische und allergologische Abteilung, Städtisches Krankenhaus München-Schwabing, Kölner Platz 1, 8000 München 40, Federal Republic of Germany

FORCK, G., Prof. Dr. med.
Abteilung für Allergologie und Gewebedermatologie, Hautklinik der Universität Münster, Von-Esmarch-Straße 56, 4400 Münster, Federal Republic of Germany

FRITSCH, P., Prof. Dr. med.
Universitätsklinik für Dermatologie und Venerologie, Anichstraße 35, 6020 Innsbruck, Austria

FRUHMANN, G., Prof. Dr. med.
Pneumologische Abteilung, I. Medizinische Klinik der Universität München, Klinikum Großhadern, Marchioninistraße 15, 8000 München 70, Federal Republic of Germany

FUCHS, E., Prof. Dr. med.
Deutsche Klinik für Diagnostik, Fachbereich Allergologie, Aukammallee 33, 6200 Wiesbaden, Federal Republic of Germany

GIANETTI, A., Prof. Dr. med.
Department of Dermatology, University of Modena, Modena, Italy

GREAVES, M. W., Prof. Dr. med.
Department of Dermatology, St. John's Hospital, London, Great Britain

JUHLIN, L., Prof. Dr. med.
Department of Dermatology, University Hospital of Uppsala, Uppsala, Sweden

KALDEN, J. R., Prof. Dr. med.
Institut und Poliklinik für Klinische Immunologie und Rheumatologie, Universität Erlangen-Nürnberg, Krankenhausstraße 12, 8520 Erlangen, Federal Republic of Germany

König, W., Prof. Dr. med.
Arbeitsgruppe für Abwehrmechanismen, Institut für Medizinische Mikrobiologie, Ruhr-Universität Bochum, 4630 Bochum 1,
Federal Republic of Germany

Kownatzki, E., Prof. Dr. med.
Abteilung Experimentelle Dermatologie, Hautklinik der Universität Freiburg, Hauptstraße 7, 7800 Freiburg i. Br., Federal Republic of Germany

Kraft, D., Prof. Dr. med.
Institut für allgemeine und experimentelle Pathologie der Universität Wien, Schwarzspanierstraße 17, 1000 Wien, Austria

Marghescu, S., Prof. Dr. med.
Hautklinik Linden der Medizinschen Hochschule Hannover, Ricklinger Straße 5, 3000 Hannover 91, Federal Republic of Germany

Nolte, D., Prof. Dr. med.
Städtisches Krankenhaus, 8230 Bad Reichenhall, Federal Republic of Germany

Plewig, G., Prof. Dr. med.
Hautklinik der Universität Düsseldorf, Moorenstraße 5, 4000 Düsseldorf 1, Federal Republic of Germany

Rajka, G., Prof. Dr. med.
Department of Dermatology, Rikshospitalet, Oslo, Norway

Rieber, P., Prof. Dr. med.
Institut für Immunologie der Universität München, Goethestraße 31, 8000 München 2, Federal Republic of Germany

Riethmüller, G., Prof. Dr. med.
Institut für Immunologie der Universität München, Goethestraße 31, 8000 München 2, Federal Republic of Germany

Saurat, J. H., Prof. Dr. med.
Departmet of Dermatology, University of Genève, Genève, Switzerland

Schmutzler, W., Prof. Dr. med.
Abteilung Pharmakologie, Rheinisch-Westfälische Technische Hochschule Aachen, 5100 Aachen, Federal Republic of Germany

Schöpf, E., Prof. Dr. med.
Hautklinik der Universität Freiburg, Hauptstraße 7, 7800 Freiburg i. Br., Federal Republic of Germany

Schulz, K.-H., Prof. Dr. med.
Universitäts-Hautklinik und Poliklinik, Universitäts-Krankenhaus Eppendorf, Martinistraße 52, 2000 Hamburg 20, Federal Republic of Germany

Steigleder, G. K., Prof. Dr. med.
Hautklinik der Universität Köln, Joseph-Stelzmann-Straße 9, 5000 Köln 41, Federal Republic of Germany

Stüttgen, G., Prof. Dr. med.
Hautklinik und Poliklinik, Rudolf-Virchow-Krankenhaus, Freie Universität Berlin, Augustenburger Platz 1, 1000 Berlin 65/West

Basic Immunology

Biological Role of Major Transplantation Antigens in T Cell Self-recognition: Possible Consequences in Clinical Medicine

R. M. Zinkernagel
Institut für Pathologie, Universitäts-Spital Zürich, 8091 Zürich, Switzerland

Abstract

During the past years, our ideas on immunity have changed fundamentally: Thymus derived lymphocytes (T cells) express two specificities, one for foreign antigenic determinants and one for a cell-surface self-determinant coded by the major histocompatibility gene complex (MHC) i.e. T cells are restricted. These findings have been influencing basic immunology and are relevant to our understanding of immune phenomena in infectious disease:

1. T cell restriction determines what antigens are immunogenic.
2. T cell restriction has to be taken into account for *in vitro* testing of cell-mediated immunity.
3. The specificity for self-MHC of T cells is determined during maturation in the thymus; therefore reconstitution of immunodeficiency depends on thymus grafts and bone marrow stem cells sharing MHC determinants.
4. T cell restriction may well give us one key to understand why some disease susceptibilities may be linked to the MHC (HLA in human, H-2 in mice).

Diseases whose susceptibility is associated with certain alleles of MHC reflect (a) immuno-pathologic effects of T cells, (b) T cell effector function determined by the restricting MHC products and (c) an intimate link between MHC polymorphism and size of the T cell receptor repertoire. Immunopathological T cell-dependent diseases therefore are likely to be associated with the MHC, and MHC association signals T cell-mediated immunopathology. Since the balance between infectious agents and immune reactivity determines disease outcome it is of great importance to understand the parameters of the infectious agents and of the host influencing this equilibrium before attempting to manipulate immunopathological disease with immunostimulant or immunosuppressive treatments.

Introduction

Major transplantation antigens play a crucial role in lymphocyte interactions amongst themselves as well as with other somatic cells [18, 21, 24, 27]. That this is their real biological function and not to make transplantation surgery or tumor research more difficult was first signaled by the finding that susceptibility to certain diseases is linked, albeit weakly, to the major transplantation antigens coded by the major histocompatibility gene complex (MHC, HLA in humans, H-2 in mice) [9, 10, 12]. Any list of the more clear-cut HLA-disease associations immediatetely suggests that they are all caused by immune-mediated pathogenesis. How can these two phenomena, HLA-disease associations and their immune pathogenesis, be explained? And can we understand why HLA-disease associations are often rather weak?

Immunity 1985

The function of the immune system is to maintain homeostasis in higher vertebrates; its two main arms, cellular and humoral immunity, very efficiently defend the host against acute cytopathic infectious agents. The main targets of T cells are intracellular agents, while those of antibodies are primarily extracellular ones. However, this immune defense does not cover all viruses and bacteria with the same efficiency and many other causes of disease, such as protozoan or metazoan infections and tumors, are more or less out of the reach of efficient immune surveillance.

T cell immunity is at its best when dealing with acute intracellular agents, such as cytopathic viruses. This T cell activity is easily measured in a classical ^{51}Cr release cytotoxicity assay in vitro [6, 27, 28]. T cell-mediated lysis of virus-infected target cells is virus specific, since only target cells infected with the proper virus are lysed. But in addition, target cell lysis of virus-infected cells depends upon T cells and target cells sharing classical transplantation antigens. Many experiments over the past 12 years have clearly documented that the following general rules govern lymphocyte–lymphocyte and lymphocyte–somatic cell interactions [18, 21, 27]:

- T cells recognize self-transplantation antigens together with foreign antigenic determinants exclusively on cell surfaces.
- T cell specificity for self-transplantation antigens (a) is specific for polymorphic determinants, (b) is selected during differentiation in the thymus, (c) determines the effector function of T cells [cytotoxic T cells recognize class I, i.e., the classical transplantation antigens HLA-A, B, C or H-2K, D, L, whereas differentiation-promoting T cells (helper or DTH T cells) are specific for class II, HLA-D or H-2I] and (d) regulates T cell responsiveness (i.e., the quality and quantity of cytotoxic T cell response are regulated by HLA-A, B, C or H-2K, D, L, those of differentiation-promoting T cell response by HLA-D or H-2I gene products).

Role of Cytotoxic T Cells

One may question the physiological role of cytolytic T cells: Why should T cells mediate cell and tissue destruction to combat intracellular infectious agents [15, 26, 27]? There is good evidence that cytotoxic T cells destroy virus-infected cells before viral progeny are assembled, thus eliminating virus during the eclipse phase of virus replication. Virus elimination via immunological host cell destruction is, in the case of cytopathic viruses, an efficient way of preventing virus spread and the resulting more extensive virus-mediated cell and tissue damage [26]. In the case of noncytopathic viruses, this immunological defense mechanism becomes less attractive, because host cells are not destroyed by virus but only by the T cell immune response [5, 10, 12, 27]. Because T cells apparently can not distinguish cytopathic from noncytopathic viruses, immune-mediated cell and tissue damage results, in the latter infections, in immune disease.

Lymphocytic Choriomeningitis: a T Cell-Mediated Immune Disease

Examples of infections with noncytopathic viruses are lymphocytic choriomeningitis (LCM) in mice [10, 12, 14, 22, 23, 27] and hepatitis B in humans [13, 15]. LCM in mice develops after intracerebral injection of LCMV only in immunocompetent mice. Mice lacking T cells or those immunosuppressed by irradiation or cytostatic drugs do not develop inflammatory reactions and thus no LCM disease; but they fail to eliminate virus and as a result become LCMV carriers [12, 14]. LCM disease has been carefully analyzed and has been clearly shown to be T cell mediated [8, 10]. Lethal LCM disease apparently depends upon effector T cells being preferentially recruited to the acutely infected leptomeninges. This notion is supported by the finding that high doses of LCMV simultaneously injected i.c. and i.v. often do not cause fatal LCM disease, because effector T cells are recruited to infected cells all over the organism and therefore are diluted out.

Disease depends in both LCM and hepatitis B upon the balance between virus spread and immune response. Efficient T cell-mediated immune response leads to rapid elimination of the virus, limited cell and tissue damage, and therefore limited disease. Absence of an immune response results in unchecked growth of virus and in a virus carrier state. Slow and low immune responsiveness allows extended spread of virus with chronic T cell-mediated tissue destruction, a classical immunopathological conflict situation.

Since major transplantation antigens are recognized as self by T cells and define their function and regulate their responsiveness, they may drastically influence the balance between virus and immune-mediated tissue damage.

Among many other variables characteristic for the virus or the host [2, 3, 11, 17], severity of disease has in fact been shown to be determined also by major transplantation antigens in both hepatitis B virus [13, 15] infections in humans and in LCM virus infections in mice [1, 22].

Factors Influencing Susceptibility to LCM Disease

Various LCMV isolates [21, 22] that by conventional serology are indistinguishable have been tested recently and were found to vary greatly with respect to the disease they induce. It is unclear how these differences come about, but it seems that included among various other possibilities such as susceptibility to interferons, macrophage activation, natural killer cells, etc., it is their antigenic quality that appears to vary [2, 27]. There are at least two types of host factors that regulate disease susceptibility to LCM in mice. First there is a very important general genetic influence that is independent of the MHC (H-2) [27]. Dependent upon this genetic background, the two LCMV strains used induce all four possible disease susceptibility patterns summarized in Table 1. Second, in one inbred mouse strain tested in detail (B 10) the major transplantation antigens coded by the H-2D region determine whether B 10 mice are susceptible or not to one of the LCMV isolates (Table 2). Since the H-2D class I transplan-

Table 1. Patterns of susceptibility to LCM disease in various inbred strains of mice

	SJL	C57BL/10	CBA	DBA/2
LCMV-A	++	++	–	–
LCMV-D	++	–	++	–

++ Indicates susceptibility, i. e., mice die
– Indicates resistance, i. e., mice survive after intracerebral injection of about 10^3 replicating LCMV particles within 6–10 days after initiation of infection

Table 2. Influences of H-2 loci on susceptibility to LCMV disease and LCMV-specific cytotoxic T cell activity in meningeal infiltrates of B10 mice

H-2 of B10 mice K I D[a]	% of mice susceptible to LCMV-D	Relative LCMV-specific cytotoxic T cell activity restricted to H-2D[b]
$K^kI^kD^k$	0	1
$K^kI^kD^q$	100	10– 50
$K^qI^qD^q$	100	20–100

[a] H-2K,D corresponds to HLA-A,B in humans, H-2I, to HLA-D
[b] See [28]

tation antigens mediate cytotoxic T cell function and regulate antiviral cytotoxic T cells, it was obviously important to evaluate whether these H-2D-regulated differences in susceptibility to LCM correlated with T cell-mediated immunopathology caused by LCMV-specific cytotoxic T cells: the result was that high and early cytotoxic LCMV-specific and H-2D-restricted T cell activity correlated positively with susceptibility to LCM disease [27] (Table 2).

Conclusion

In a model infection with a noncytopathic virus (LCMV) in mice a clear-cut influence of the MHC on disease susceptibility could be shown [1, 27]. This influence was only seen if the right cloned virus isolate was used to infect the correct mouse strain. Susceptibility to LCMV correlated well with the capacity of mice to generate LCMV-specific cytotoxic T cells. MHC genes regulating both susceptibility to disease and cytotoxic T cell activity mapped to the same H-2D MHC locus. The q allele conferred susceptibility and early and high cytotoxic T cell activity, while the k (or b, d not shown) allele(s) conferred resistance and slow and low cytotoxic T cell activity.

Therefore, in this model LCMV-triggered cytotoxic T cell-mediated immunopathology that is regulated by H-2D is responsible for the linkage of LCM disease susceptibility to the MHC. These findings support the notion that many diseases, susceptibility to which is linked to the MHC, may be caused by T cell-mediated immunopathological mechanisms triggered by noncytopathic infectious agents. Admittedly, in very few HLA-linked diseases do we know of a causative infectious agent and one may therefore prefer to use other explanations for MHC-disease associations [reviewed in 9]. However, our findings suggest that variants of quite common infectious agents may cause some of the HLA-linked diseases, whereas as yet unknown agents that do not usually cause acute infections may be the cause of others. These explanations are supported by the evidence [2, 22, 25] that LCMV isolates that are indistinguishable by classical serology differ greatly with respect to their recognition by T cells (and possibly by other factors) and therefore may cause differing diseases. Under the well-defined conditions used here with inbred mice and cloned virus isolates, MHC-disease association could be shown to be absolute. This is quite in contrast to all of the HLA-disease associations found in humans, which, as stated earlier, are usually weak [9]. Several explanations for this finding can now be offered. First, as already discussed, various isolates of infectious agents may differ despite the fact that they are serologically indistinguishable; the cloned virus used in our experiments obviously renders this parameter constant. Second, HLA typing based on serology has similar limitations. Recent experiments using T cells or genetic probes for typing clearly show that serologically defined HLA-A or HLA-D antigens comprise a variety of subtypes [4, 7]; in our experiments this variability is excluded by using inbred strains of mice. Third, the general genetic background of humans differs between individuals, families, and races as much as it clearly differs between inbred strains of mice (Table 1). HLA-disease associations therefore can only become visible if, as in mice, the right virus isolate infects humans of the correct general genetic background so that HLA regulation of the T cell response becomes recognizable.

The results and interpretations presented lead to another important consequence with respect to application of immune-modulating therapeutic protocols during immunpathologically mediated disease. Unless one knows the precise balance, kinetics, and actual relationship between the parasite and the host response, it is equally likely that one will influence the host-parasite balance in a detrimental direction as in a beneficial one.

In conclusion, the proposal is made, illustrated, and supported by experimental evidence that T cell-mediated immunopathology triggered initially by low- or noncytopathic infectious agents may cause diseases that are linked to the MHC. It is obvious that not all MHC-disease associations are explained by this pathophysiological mechanism, but a reasonable guess would be that many such linkages may follow the rules outlined. Conversely, the proposal implies that MHC-disease associations quite generally signal T cell-mediated pathophysiology of the disease.

References

1. Allen JE, Doherty PC (1985) Consequences of a single Ir-gene defect for the pathogenesis of lymphocytic choriomeningitis. Immunogenetics 21:581–588
2. Ahmed R, Salmi A, Butler LD, Chiller JM, Oldstone MBA (1984) Selection of genetic variants of lymphocytic choriomeningitis virus in spleens of persistently infected mice. J Exp Med 60:521–540
3. Bang FB (1973) Genetics of resistance of animals to viruses. Adv Virus Res 23:269–346
4. Biddison WE, Ward FE, Shearer GM, Shaw S (1980) The self determinants recognized by human virus-immune T cells can be distinguished from the serologically defined HLA antigens. J Immunol 124:548–563
5. Byrne JA, Oldstone MBA (1974) Biology of cloned cytotoxic T lymphocytes specific for lymphocytic choriomeningitis virus: clearance of virus in vivo. J Virol 51:682–686
6. Cerottini JC, Brunner KT (1974) Cell mediated cytotoxicity, allograft rejection and tumor immunity. Adv Immunol 19:67–127
7. Cohen D, Dausset J (1973) HLA-gene polymorphism. Progr Immunol 5:1–12
8. Cole GA, Nathanson N, Prendergast RA (1972) Requirement for θ-bearing cells in lymphocytic choriomeningitis virus-infected central nervous system disease. Nature 238:335–337
9. Dausset J, Svejgaard A (eds) (1977) HLA and disease. Munksgaard, Copenhagen, pp 1–310
10. Doherty PC, Zinkernagel RM (1974) T cell mediated immunopathology in viral infections. Transplant Rev 19:89–120
11. Friedman RM, Vogel SN (1983) Interferons with special emphasis on the immune system. Adv Immunol 34:97–140
12. Hotchin J (1971) Persistent and slow virus infections. Monogr Virol 3:1–110
13. Jeannet M, Farquet JJ (1974) HLA antigens in asymptomatic chronic HBAg carriers. Lancet 2:1383–1384
14. Lehmann-Grube F (1971) Lymphocytic choriomeningitis virus. Monogr Virol 10:2–171
15. Mackay IR (1976) The concept of autoimmune liver disease. Bull NY Acad Med Sci 52:433–447

16. McDevitt HO, Bodmer WF (1974) HLA immune response genes and disease. Lancet 1:1269–1275
17. Mims CA (1982) Pathogenesis of infectious disease, 2nd edn. Academic, London, pp 1–297
18. Möller G (ed) (1977) Ir genes and T lymphocytes. Immunol Rev 38:1–162
19. Möller G (ed) (1983) HLA and disease susceptibility. Immunol Rev 70:1–180
20. Moskophidis D, Lehmann-Grube F (1983) The immune response of the mouse to lymphocytic choriomeningitis virus. III. Differences of numbers of cytotoxic T lymphocytes in spleens of mice of different strains. Cell Immunol 77:279–293
21. Paul WE, Benacerraf B (1977) Functional specificity of thymus dependent lymphocytes. Science 195:1293–1299
22. Pfau CJ, Valenti JK, Pevear DC, Hunt KD (1982) Lymphocytic choriomeningitis virus killer T cells are lethal only in weakly disseminated infections. J Exp Med 156:79–90
23. Rowe WR (1954) Studies on pathogenesis and immunity in lymphocytic choriomeningitis infection of the mouse. Res Rep Nav Med Res Inst 12:167–222
24. Townsend ARM, McMichael AJ (1984) The specificity of cytotoxic T lymphocytes stimulated with influenza virus; studies in mice and humans. Progr Allergy 36:10–97
25. Wiktor TJ, Koprowski H (1978) Monoclonal antibodies against rabies virus produced by somatic cell hybridisation, detection of antigenic variants. Proc Natl Acad Sci USA 75:3938–3943
26. Zinkernagel RM, Althage A (1977) Antiviral protection by virus-immune cytotoxic T cells: infected target cells are lysed before infectious virus progeny is assembled. J Exp Med 145:644–651
27. Zinkernagel RM, Doherty PC (1979) MHC-restricted cytotoxic T cells: studies on the biological role of polymorphic major transplantation antigens determining T cell restriction-specificity, function, and responsiveness. Adv Immunol 27:51–177
28. Zinkernagel RM, Pfau CJ, Hengartner H, Althage A (1985) A model for MHC-disease associations: susceptibility to murine lymphocytic choriomeningitis maps to class I MHC genes and correlates with LCMV-specific cytotoxic T cell-activity. Nature (in press)

Interleukins

B. Fleischer

Abteilung Medizinische Mikrobiologie und Immunologie, Universität Ulm, 7900 Ulm, Federal Republic of Germany

Abstract

Interleukins comprise a large heterogenous group of molecules produced by various types of leukocytes, predominantly T lymphocytes, that regulate growth and differentiation of lymphoid and hemopoetic cells. Many interleukins have been purified to homogeneity, some of them can already be produced by recombinant DNA techniques. Although the use of such reagents has helped to clarify the role of interleukins in the course of lymphocyte activation and maturation, many questions as to the physiological role of these components are still open. As an example, the role of various signals given by antigen and interleukins in the sequence of activation and maturation of cytotoxic T lymphocytes from resting precursor cells will be described. A similar lymphokine-regulated sequence is the growth and differentiation of B lymphocytes to plasma cells. The possible therapeutic significance of interleukins will be discussed.

Introduction

Interleukins comprise a heterogeneous group of proteins and glycoproteins which are produced by various types of leukocytes (predominantly T-lymphocytes), and which regulate the growth, differentiation, and function of lymphoid and hematopoietic cells. This definition, however, is likely to be too narrow since several such factors can be produced by cells other than leukocytes and have effects outside of the immune system; therefore the term cytokines would be more appropriate.

The term "interleukin" was created in 1979 [1], when it became obvious that several functional activities could be attributed to a single molecularly defined protein. This had been a long and difficult task since traditionally these cytokines were defined on the basis of the biological activity of a crude supernatant in a particular assay system rather than on definitive biochemical *and* functional criteria. Although in theory it is almost impossible to exclude definitively the possibility that two functional activities copurifying during biochemical characterization are not due to a mixture of two molecular species, results from a large number of independent and collaborative studies have indicated that several activities of certain factor preparations are actually different biological facets of a single biochemical entity. Indeed, the recent success in producing several cytokines by recombinant DNA technology has unequivocally resolved this issue for some factors.

Interleukin-1

Interleukin-1 (Il-1) is a hormone-like protein with a molecular weight (MW) of 14000 (murine) or 15000 (human) that is involved in many different aspects of immunity and inflammation [2, 3]. It was originally described as a factor produced by activated macrophages, but in recent years it has been found to be released by a variety of cell types into the culture supernatant, including endothelial cells, large granular lymphocytes, keratinocytes, astrocytes, and fibroblasts. Although initially its role in inflammatory responses was mainly attributed to its effects on cells of the immune system, it is clear from recent results from a number of laboratories that Il-1 is a general mediator of inflammation.

Induction of fever produced by an action in the central nervous system was the first effect of Il-1 described [4]. Other actions include local catabolic effects on muscle, bone, and cartilage and the local release of inflammatory mediators from neutrophils, macrophages, fibroblasts, and synovial and endothelial cells. Although it is possible that all these effects are caused by Il-1, the final proof is still missing and will await the use of Il-1 produced by gene cloning.

Immunologically relevant is the involvement of Il-1 in the activation of several cell types participating in an immune response – T-lymphocytes, B-lymphocytes, natural killer cells, and macrophages. The requirement for Il-1 in the mitogenic activation of thymocytes was the first immunological effect of Il-1 described [5] and still serves as the most sensitive assay for Il-1. Similarly, peripheral mature T cells apparently require Il-1 or Il-1-like factors produced by adherent accessory cells to respond to antigens or mitogens. Whereas complete removal of accessory cells leads to lymphocyte unresponsiveness to mitogens even in the presence of Il-1 [6], Il-1 can restore T cell activation when accessory cells are either largely depleted or metabolically impaired. There is evidence – although so far indirect – that the release of Il-1 from accessory cells is controlled by T inducer cells. B-lymphocytes can likewise respond to Il-1; in synergy with other lymphokines it is required for B cell activation and maturation in vitro. Il-1 also acts on certain macrophage subsets, activating them to produce mediators.

The many targets and actions of Il-1 make different receptors plausible; however, a receptor for Il-1 has so far not been demonstrated. An interesting finding is the detection of Il-1 in normal serum or urine, making a role of this mediator in physiological states likely. The multitude of different actions and effects on different systems of the organism as well as the many diverse tissues capable of producing Il-1 demonstrate a bidirectional connection of the immune system and other parts of the body.

Interleukin-2 and T Cell Activation

Interleukin-2 (Il-2), formerly termed T cell growth factor due to its ability to promote the growth of activated T cells, plays an essential and central role in the activation and differentiation of T-lymphocytes [7–9]. Murine Il-2 is a non-covalently linked dimer with an MW of 30000, while human Il-2 is a single variably glycosylated polypeptide with an MW of 15000. Il-2 is usually assayed by its ability to sustain the proliferation of Il-2 dependent T cells, although the recent availability of monoclonal antibodies to Il-2 allows for the use of sensitive immunoassays.

The major source of Il-2 is the helper T-lymphocyte population, although other T cell subsets also contain cells capable of producing the factor. Il-2 is released by T cells in response to two signals provided by the antigen-presenting accessory cell: (a) antigen in the context of gene products of the major histocompatibility complex (MHC) and (b) Il-1.

Il-2 acts on its target cell by binding to a 55000-dalton specific cell-surface receptor of particularly high affinity. Resting T cells do not express significant numbers of the Il-2 receptor, while after activation by antigen recognition or mitogen binding T cell blasts display about 10000–20000 binding sites for Il-2. Thus, the immune specificity of T cell growth is generated by the Il-2 receptor expression only on antigen-activated T cells. Both Il-2 production and Il-2 receptor expression are transient after T cell activation, thus contributing to the conservation of specificity and self-limitation of the Il-2 driven immune response.

Target cells for Il-2 are primarily T-lymphocytes, both T helper cells that use their own Il-2 as well as precursor cells for cytotoxic T-lymphocytes (CTLs). Recent evidence suggests that, depending on the system, additional factors can be required that regulate the differentiation of CTL precursors into functionally competent CTLs. Besides this central effect on T cells, Il-2 has direct growth- as well as differentiation-promoting effects for certain B-lymphocytes. In addition, natural killer cells and the so-called lymphokine-activated killer cells seem to be directly activated by Il-2, beyond the activation via immune interferon (IFN-γ), the production of which is increased by Il-2. Il-2 has also been shown to stimulate the production of other lymphokines, such as B cell-stimulating factors or IFN-γ. Obviously, Il-2 is a central regulatory molecule affecting many stages of cellular and humoral immune responses.

Interleukin-3

This designation was introduced by Ihle and co-workers [10] to describe a factor that induced maturation in lymphomyeloid precursors of athymic nude mice. Although it was initially believed that Il-3 dependent cells were T cell in nature, it is now clear that Il-3 is a hemopoietic colony-stimulating factor (CSF) stimulating a wide range of colony-forming cells and it therefore has many synonyms (e.g., burst-promoting activity, mast cell growth factor, P cell-stimulating factor). Murine Il-3 is a single glycosylated polypeptide of 24000 daltons. Producer cells so far identified are activated T-lymphocytes and the myeloid leukemia cell line WEHI-3. If the term Il-3 is accepted for this multi-CSF, other CSFs may also be added to the growing list of interleukins. Besides Il-3, three other CSFs have been purified and characterized. All are glycoproteins that stimulate granulocyte and/or macrophage colony formation in bone marrow cultures and are active at picomolar concentrations in vitro [11]. In addition, some of the CSFs have been shown to stimulate mature macrophages, mast cells, and granulocytes. CSFs can be produced by a variety of cell types, including fibroblasts, T cells, endothelial cells, and macrophages; there appear, however, to be different sources for different CSFs.

Immune Interferon

Immune interferon (IFN-γ) was discovered by its antiviral activity but its complex activities and pleiotropic effects make it one of the most interesting lymphokines [12]. It is produced by helper as well as cytotoxic T-lymphocytes upon stimulation with specific antigen or mitogen, and also by natural killer cells. IFN-γ is a single glycoprotein of 20000–25000 daltons due to variable glycosylation.

A remarkable property of IFN-γ is its ability to potentiate the effects of other lymphokines. Therefore some activities initially ascribed to IFN-γ may be due to its synergistic effects with other mediators. Several effects, however, are probably due to IFN-γ itself, as has been demonstrated in some instances by the use of recombinant IFN-γ. IFN-γ enhances cytotoxicity by natural killer cells and activates several macrophage functions, including tumoricidal activity, antigen presentation, and destruction of intracellular pathogens. Most or all of the previously described activities of a macrophage-activating factor in lymphocyte-conditioned medium are probably caused by IFN-γ. The growth inhibitory effect of IFN-γ on a variety of transformed and normal (e.g., hemopietic) cells in vitro may be due to the marked synergistic action with lymphotoxin. IFN-γ directly induces the expression of MHC antigens, in particular class II antigens, on a variety of cell types, including endothelial cells, Langerhans cells, astrocytes, and epithelial and certain tumor cells, providing such cells with the ability to present antigens to immune helper T cells. This new appearance of class II antigens on the surface of normally class II-negative cells has been implicated as a possible pathogenetic mechanism in autoimmune disorders [13]. Furthermore, IFN-γ induces the differentiation of several myeloid and monocytic cell types to the mature diffentiated phenotype both in normal bone marrow and in leukemia cells, including the expression of high affinity Fc-receptors. In the differentiation of B-lymphocytes to plasma cells, IFN-γ has been reported to substitute to some extent for late-acting T cell-derived helper factors.

In conclusion, IFN-γ has regulatory and potentiating effects in several phases of an antigen-specific immune response and also activates effector cells of nonspecific resistance and inflammation.

Therapeutic Considerations

Since several interleukins and lymphokines can now be produced by recombinant DNA technology in bacteria, their in vivo application for therapeutic purposes can be envisaged. The optimal condition for a clinical application would be a deficiency state with a defect in the production of a given interleukin but with the preserved activity to respond to it. Unfortunately, no such defect is yet known.

Since Il-2 is the best characterized lymphokine, preliminary studies have been performed with it both in animal models and in humans. In athymic nude mice Il-2 induces CTLs and helper T cells in vivo [14], while in tumor-bearing mice tumor growth is reduced by simultaneous application of Il-2 and T-lymphocytes. As might be expected, some T cell functions of some patients with inherited or acquired immunodeficiency can be improved or even corrected in vitro. In the few patients with immunodeficiency who have been treated with Il-2, only a weak and short-lasting effect was observed.

The in vivo application of interleukins (e.g., Il-2) has some limitations of which one should be aware. Pharmacokinetic studies have shown that Il-2 is rapidly (within minutes) cleared from the circulation; only after frequent low dose injections could a prolonged serum level be achieved [15]. Serum and tissue may contain inhibitors of Il-2 action [16]. On the other hand, since in vitro a short pulse with Il-2 leads to T cell growth for more than 48 h, the short half-life of Il-2 in vivo does not exclude a long-lasting effect.

More delicate is our still limited knowledge about the physiological mechanisms in vivo in which Il-2 is involved. Requirement for additional signals – as required in vitro – may limit the in vivo effect of interleukins; on the other hand unphysiologically high concentrations of Il-2 could lead to a pathological state of autoreactivity or break self-tolerance. Indeed, it has recently been reported that tolerance induction in newborn mice is blocked by simultaneous injection of Il-2 [17].

Nevertheless, it can be hoped that the increasing availability of cDNA probes for interleukins and of pure bacteria-produced mediators will finally allow exact characterization and selective manipulation of defined steps in an interleukin-driven immune response.

References

1. Aarden LA, Brunner TK, Cerottini JC et al. (1979) Revised nomenclature for antigen-nonspecific T cell proliferation and helper factors. J Immunol 127:2928

2. Durum SK, Schmidt JA, Oppenheim JJ (1985) Interleukin 1: an immunological perspective. Ann Rev Immunol 3:263
3. Mizel SB (1982) Interleukin 1 and T cell activation. Immunol Rev 63:51
4. Beeson PB (1984) Temperature elevating effect of a substance obtained from polymorphonuclear leukocytes. J Clin Invest 27:524
5. Gery I, Gershon RK, Waksman BH (1972) Potentiating of the T-lymphocyte response to mitogens. J Exp Med 136:128
6. Thiele DL, Kurosaka M, Lipsky PE (1983) Phenotype of the accessory cell necessary for mitogen-stimulated T and B cell responses in human peripheral blood: delineation by its sensibility to the lysosomotropic agent L-leucin-methylester. J Immunol 131:2282
7. Wagner H, Röllinghoff M (eds) (1980) Interleukin 2. Behring Inst Mitt 67
8. Möller G (ed) (1982) Interleukins and lymphocyte activation. Immunol Rev 63
9. Smith KA (1984) Interleukin 2. Ann Rev Immunol 2:319
10. Ihle JN, Rebar L, Keller J et al. (1982) Interleukin 3: possible roles in the regulation of lymphocyte differentiation and growth. Immunol Rev 63:5
11. Nicola NA, Vardas M (1984) Hemopoietic colony-stimulating factors. Immunol Today 5:76
12. Trinchieri G, Perussia B (1985) Immune interferon: a pleiotropic lymphokine with multiple effects. Immunol Today 6:131
13. Bottazo GF, Pujol-Borell R, Hanafusa T, Feldmann M (1983) Role of aberrant HLA-DR expression and antigen presentation in induction of endocrine autoimmunity. Lancet 2:1115
14. Wagner H, Hardt C, Heeg K, Pfizenmaier K, Röllinghoff M (1980) T cell derived helper factor allows in vivo induction of cytotoxic T cells in nu/nu mice. Nature 284:278
15. Cheever MA, Thompson JA, Kern DE, Greenberg PD (1985) Interleukin 2 administered in vivo: influence of Il-2 route and timing on T cell growth. J Immunol 134:3895
16. Hardt C, Röllinghoff M, Pfizenmaier K, Mosmann H, Wagner H (1981) Lyt-23+ cyclophosphamide-sensitive T cells regulate the activity of an interleukin 2 inhibitor in vivo. J Exp Med 154:262
17. Malkovsky M, Medawar PB, Thatcher DR et al. (1985) Acquired immunological tolerance of foreign cells is impaired by recombinant interleukin 2 or vitamin A acetate. Proc Nat Acad Sci USA 82:536

Immunoglobulin E

Regulation of IgE by Lymphoid Cell-Derived Factors

A. L. de Weck, B. Stadler, and J. Knutti-Müller
Institut für Klinische Immunologie, Inselspital, 3000 Bern, Switzerland

Abstract

Both experiments in rodents and experiments of nature in man suggest that isotypic regulation of the IgE response and its suppression represent a normal state of regulation. Accordingly, the abnormally elevated production of IgE to ubiquitous allergens, as observed in atopic people, might represent to some extent a breakdown of suppression and the expression of a state of partial immunodeficiency. Recent studies by several groups suggest that the isotypic regulation of IgE production is operated at several levels:

a) a network of T/B cell interactions in which non IgE-binding factors are produced by T and B cells (D. H. Katz);
b) IgE-binding molecules produced by T cells controlling the production/secretion of IgE by IgE-bearing B cells (several groups);
c) glycosylation-regulating factors which influence the enhancing or suppressing activity of IgE binding factors (K. Ishizaka).

The development of a sensitive IgE-binding assay on nitrocellulose membranes with the help of monoclonal anti-IgE antibodies has enabled us to follow the appearance of IgE binding factors in the supernatants of human T cell clones and of T-T hybridomas, as well as in the serum of atopic patients. Various purification procedures enable to assess the molecular characteristics of these factors, which appear to be heterogeneous (60, 30, 15 and lower Kds). Besides their biophysical characteristics, these factors may also be assessed by their functional effect on an IgE producing B cell line and by their interaction with various antisera directed against Fc receptors. Perspectives for the clinical use of IgE regulating factors will be discussed.

The IgE response

Immunoglobulin E (IgE) plays a major role in the pathogenesis of widespread allergic diseases, such as rhinitis and asthma. Hyperproduction of IgE antibodies is also one of the main features of the genetically determined atopic state, which includes patients predisposed to rhinitis, asthma, and atopic dermatitis [1]. Hyperproduction of IgE has also been described in the hyper-IgE syndrome [2, 3] and in some immunodeficient states [4, 5].

Table 1. Evidence for suppressive factors in IgE responses

In rodents, conversion of poor IgE responders to high IgE responders by:
- Low dose X-rays
- Pretreatment with cyclophosphamide
- Anti-T suppressor serum
- Thymectomy

In man, experiments of nature:
- High IgE levels in some T cell immunodeficient states (Wiskott-Aldrich syndrome, transient hypogammaglobulinemia, Hodgkin's disease)
- Diminished T suppressor cell activity in hyper-IgE syndrome and atopic state
- IgE formation with some adjuvants (aluminum hydroxide)
- Elevation of IgE levels following viral infections
- IgE formation in response to drugs administered together with X-ray therapy or T cell suppression

Experimentally:
- Depressing effect of normal T cells on IgE synthesis in vitro from atopic and hyper-IgE leukocytes
- Depressing effect of normal serum (factors) on IgE synthesis in vitro from atopic and hyper-IgE leukocytes

Although the hyperproduction of IgE associated with allergic diseases has long been considered a peculiar form of hyperimmunization, experiments by Tada and his colleagues at the beginning of the 1970s [6, 7], soon followed by several other groups [8], have shown that the hyperproduction of IgE is in fact the consequence of a selective lack of suppression, in other words of a selective immunodeficiency in which the normally IgE-suppressive mechanisms are impaired or lacking.

The defect in normal IgE suppression which appears to be genetically conditioned in atopic individuals and in some inbred strains of mice [9] may also be brought about by external events, such as viral infections [10] or immunosuppressive agents [11]. With regard to such cases, D. Katz has proposed the concept of "allergic breakthrough", meaning the breakdown of the damping mechanism which suppresses IgE formation in normal individuals.

In recent years, evidence has accumulated for such suppressive mechanisms both in animals and in man (Table 1). The nature and mode of operation of these immunosuppressive mechanisms have also been largely clarified, at least in rodents [12–14]. It would, however, be erroneous to attribute all IgE hyperproduction to a relative lack of suppression since the presence of IgE-enhancing factors has also been convincingly described [13, 15].

Basically, regulation of IgE in the immune system seems to operate at three different levels:

1. A T/B cell network, which may involve complicated ramifications [16] and ultimately govern the induction of IgE-binding factors.
2. IgE-binding factors, which are produced by induced but not antigenically primed T cells, and which appear to influence IgE formation most directly since they act on IgE-bearing B cells.

3. Glycosylation-enhancing or -suppressing factors, which appear to determine whether the IgE-binding factors will ultimately have an enhancing or suppressive effect on IgE formation.

IgE Regulation and the T/B Cell Network

According to Katz et al. [16] IgE interacts with B cells to provoke the production of a factor termed EIR_B (IgE-induced regulant from B cells) which induces B cells to express Fc_ε receptors. These $Fc_\varepsilon R^+$ B cells themselves produce a factor influencing IgE secretion, termed SFA (suppressor factor of allergy). The production of SFA is considerably enhanced in the presence of Lyt-1^+ T cells. SFA can also be produced by Lyt-1^+ T cells and apparently counterbalances the effect of Lyt-1^+ T cells on the expression of Fc_ε receptors by B cells.

$Fc_\varepsilon R^+$ B cells also provide signals to Lyt-2^+ T cells to produce an EIR_T, which acts on Lyt-2^+ T cells to express Fc_ε receptors. The same Lyt-2^+ T cells produce an inhibitory factor, termed EIR_i, which inhibits the expression of Fc_ε receptors by B cells. Another inhibitory factor of Fc_ε receptor induction acts indirectly by blocking Lyt-1^+ T cells, which counterbalance the inhibitory effect of EIR_i. The ultimate effect is an enhancement of IgE production, hence the name “enhancing factor of allergy” (EFA) for that factor produced by a still undefined subset of T cells.

The existence of these various factors has been inferred from experiments performed with cell populations more or less depleted of the one or other subset and also with their supernatants; however, the molecular characterization of these factors has not yet been fully achieved. The relationship between the postulated SFA, EFA, EIR_T, EIR_B, and EIR_i and IgE-binding factors described by other groups has not yet been clarified, although it has been stated that EIRs have no IgE-binding properties.

IgE-Binding Factors

IgE-binding factors produced by T cells have now been described by several groups in mice [17], rats [14, 18], and man [4, 19–21]. In several experimental systems, the target of action of the IgE-binding factors appears to be the IgE-bearing B cell: the factors seem to influence the differentiation of IgE-bearing B cells into IgE-secreting cells.

While T cells from spleen or peripheral blood, when induced by lectins, or supernatants from activated lymphocytes containing interferon gamma, but possibly also other lymphokines, have been shown to produce IgE-binding factors, such factors have also been described in supernatants from T-T cell hybridomas [19, 20] and from B cells carrying Fc_ε receptors [22]. Several authors have claimed that the production of IgE-binding factors requires the presence of IgE [14] or, even more, of aggregated IgE [23]; however, in our hands this does not seem to be an absolute requirement [20].

The physicochemical properties of IgE-binding factors seem to bear similarities between various animal species: a pronounced molecular heterogeneity has been reported and IgE-binding moieties of 60000, 30000, and 15000 daltons seem to occur in the supernatants of activated T cells or T cell hybridomas [19, 20]. Although a rat IgE binding factor has recently been produced by genetic engineering [24], the inclusion in the product of some viral protein has left the precise structure of the IgE-binding protein somewhat unclear. Antibodies prepared against the Fc_ε receptor of B cell lines carrying large numbers of IgE receptors (e.g., WiI 2, RPMI 8886) cross-react with T cell Fc_ε receptors [25] and, according to some reports [22, 37], also bind to IgE-binding factors derived from T cells or from B cells. Accordingly, there is some suspicion that a structural relationship exists between IgE-binding proteins detectable in cell culture supernatants and Fc_ε receptors. However, the Fc_ε receptors isolated from B cell lines [26] appear to be larger molecules than the moieties found in culture supernatants, which are suspected of being fragments of the former.

The precise mode of action of IgE-binding factors on IgE-bearing B cells is not yet known. In many ways, there might be similarities in the isotypic regulation achieved by Fc receptors for other immunoglobulins, such as IgG [27] or IgA [28], and that observed for IgE. In all instances, the blocking effect of the corresponding Ig-binding factors is strictly isotype-specific and appears to act late in the differentiation of Ig-committed B cells to Ig-secreting cells. Still somewhat confusing is the observation that the increase in Fc_ε receptors on T

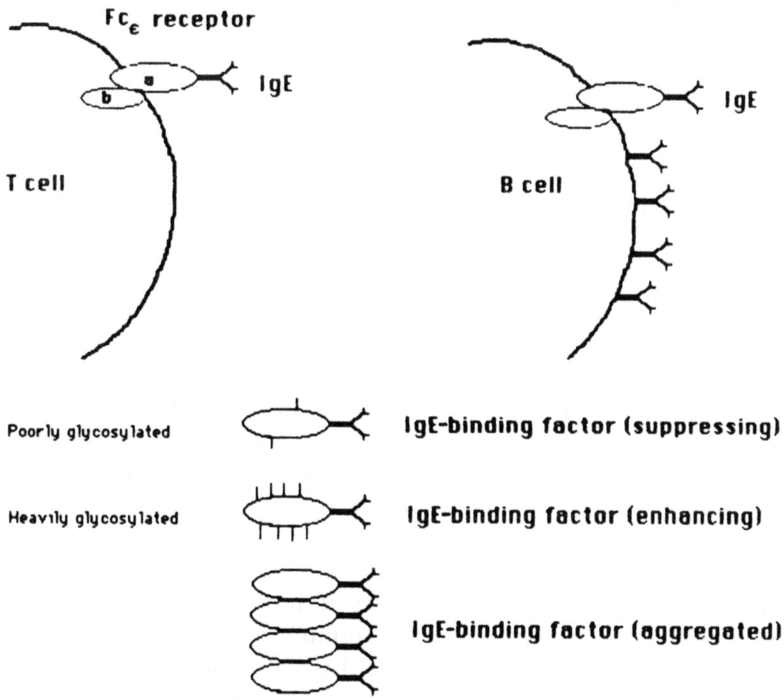

Fig. 1. Possible relationships between Fc_ε receptors and IgE-binding factors

Table 2. Main features of IgE-binding factors

T cell-derived IgE-suppressing factor(s)

- Binds to IgE
- Present in various molecular sizes of 60000, 30000, and 15000 daltons
- Binds to IgE-bearing B cells through surface IgE and IgE receptors ($Fc_\varepsilon R$)
- Reduces expression of Fc_ε receptors
- Suppresses intracytoplasmic synthesis of IgE by activated B cells
- Moderately glycosylated: binds to peanut agglutinin

T cell-derived IgE-enhancing factor (s)

- Binds to IgE
- Present in various molecular sizes of 60000, 30000, and 15000 daltons
- Binds to IgE-bearing B cells through surface IgE and IgE receptors ($Fc_\varepsilon R$)
- Probably derived from Fc_ε receptors on T cells
- Influences expression of $Fc_\varepsilon R$
- Heavily glycosylated, binds to concanavalin A
- Cell proliferation not required for production (produced in the G1 phase of the cell cycle, like most lymphokines)

Table 3. Detection of IgE-binding factors in cell culture supernatants by the nitrocellulose immunodot technique

Sample deposited as dot on nitrocellulose	Revealing antibody/antigen			
	$IgE^{I\,125}$	$IgE^{I\,125}$ + anti-$IgE^{I\,125}$	Anti-$IgE^{I\,125}$	Anti-$IgE^{I\,125}$ +IgE 5 μg
Blocking solution	126[a]	264	247	1011
Crude supernatant from T cell hybridoma	175	381	248	1689
Con A-Sepharose eluate from T cell hybridoma supernatant				
Concentrated 11 ×	2448	7526	288	17467
Dil. 1:5.5	295	450	279	10239
Dil. 1:11	208	390	290	2160

[a] cpm

cells observed after induction by IgE or aggregated IgE [29] may also be associated with the production of IgE-enhancing or IgE-suppressing factors. Present concepts on the relationships between Fc_ε receptors and IgE-binding factors with T and B cells are schematically represented in Fig. 1, and the main features described for IgE-binding factors are summarized in Table 2.

Thanks to a sensitive and specific binding assay (Table 3), we have recently been able to analyze various moieties of human IgE-binding factors which may be purified by a sequence of column chromatographic separations (Con A-sepharose, IgE-sepharose, and HPLC). Production of such factors in large amounts from human T cell hybridomas or B cell lines should permit new approaches and mass production by genetic engineering.

Glycosylation-Enhancing and -Suppressing Factors

Since different adjuvants, such as *Bordetella pertussis* or complete Freund's adjuvant, induce the formation of IgE-binding factors with opposite biological activities but do not directly induce IgE biosynthesis, it has been speculated that lymphoid cells may indeed modulate the expression and biological activity of IgE-binding factors. Since IgE-suppressing and -enhancing IgE-binding factors differ in their affinity for lentil lectins [14], it is probable that the lymphoid factors modulating the biological activity of IgE-binding factors act upon their glycosylation during biosynthesis [18]. Further studies by Ishizaka's group have revealed the existence of at least two factors produced by T cells that influence the glycosylation of IgE-binding factors:

1. A *glycosylation-inhibiting factor* (GIF) which inhibits the assembly of N-linked oligosaccharides on IgE-binding factors during their biosynthesis. In the mouse this factor is produced upon antigen stimulation by Lyt-2^+, I-J^+ T suppressor cells [30]. It has a molecular weight of 25000–30000 in the mouse, and of 15000 in the rat. It binds to anti-I-J alloantibodies and also to monoclonal antibodies against lipomodulin. GIF is therefore postulated to be a fragment of phosphorylated lipomodulin, a phospholipase-inhibiting protein [31]. In recent experiments in mice it has been reported that GIF also has affinity for antigen, which raises the matter of possible relationships between GIF and antigen-specific T cell-suppressive factor(s).

2. A *glycosylation-enhancing factor* (GEF) which enhances the assembly of N-linked oligosaccharides to IgE-binding factors and provides them with selective potentiating activity upon the IgE response. This factor is produced by helper T cells in response to some adjuvants such as *Bordetella pertussis* [34], aluminum hydroxide [33], or parasitic infestation with *Nippostrongylus brasiliensis* [32]. GEF appears to be a kallikrein-like enzyme of about 15000 daltons which induces the activation of phospholipase. GEF induces from T cells the release of both GIF and arachidonate. It also induces the release of histamine from mouse mast cells [35], apparently through similar biochemical mechanisms (phospolipid methylation, increase in intracellular cAMP and Ca uptake) to those observed upon bridging of IgE receptors. Similar effects, both on enhanced glycosylation of IgE-binding factors and on histamine release from mouse mast cells, may be achieved by bradykinin [35].

Relationships Between IgE-Binding Factors and IgE Receptors on T and B Cells

There are indications that IgE-binding factors are closely related in their functions, and possibly even in their structure, to Fc_ε receptors of T or B cells. Procedures or health states leading to the induction of IgE-binding factors also affect the percentage of lymphocytes demonstrating Fc_ε receptors [36]. However, there is no apparent agreement as yet on the effect of various IgE-modulating factors and the expression of Fc_ε receptors. While rat IgE-suppressing factor decreases but IgE-enhancing factor enhances the expression of Fc_ε receptors on rat lymphocytes [14], mouse suppressor and enhancing factors of allergy (SFA and EFA respectively) have both been reported to reduce the expression of Fc_ε receptors in mouse lymphoid cells.

Although the molecular sizes reported for IgE-binding factors isolated from lymphoid cell or T cell hybridoma culture supernatants (15000, 30000 and 60000 daltons) are markedly different from the reported molecular size of Fc_ε receptors extracted from lymphoid cell membranes, antibodies reacting with the Fc_ε receptors of IgE-bearing B cells have been reported to interact with IgE-binding factors isolated from B [25] or T [37] cell supernatants. Accordingly, some structural relationships are postulated. It may well turn out that IgE-binding factors isolated from culture supernatants are indeed fragments from Fc_ε receptors.

It is not yet known in which way and through which molecular mechanisms IgE-binding factors may regulate the function of IgE-bearing B cells. However, this mode of isotypic regulation is probably not unique for the IgE-producing system, since accumulating evidence suggests that similar mechanisms operate for IgG [27] and IgA [28] regulation.

Conclusion

Isotypic IgE regulation seems to depend upon complex interactions of various factors in the T/B cell network, of IgE-binding factors which may be part of T and/or B cell Fc_ε receptors, and of factors affecting the glycosylation of IgE binding factors.

The emerging understanding of isotypic IgE regulation and of its abnormalities in atopic states opens up new perspectives in the control and treatment of IgE-mediated allergic diseases.

References

1. Ishizaka K, Ishizaka T (1983) Immunology of IgE-mediated hypersensitivity. In: Middleton E, Reed C, Ellis E (eds) Allergy: principles and practice. 2nd edn. Mosby, St. Louis, pp 43–73
2. Katz DH, Bargatze RF, Bogowitz CA, Katz LR (1979) Regulation of IgE antibody production by serum molecules. IV. Complete Freund's adjuvant induces both enhancing and suppressive activities detectable in the serum of low and high responder mice. J Immunol 122:2184–2190
3. Buckley RH, Sampson HA (1981) The hyperimmunoglobulinemia E syndrome. In: Franklin EC (ed), Clinical immunology update. Elsevier/North Holland, New York, p 147
4. Geha RS (1984) Regulation of IgE synthesis in man. Curr Concepts Allergy Clin Immunol 15:1–4

5. Buckley RH, Becker WG (1978) Abnormalities in the regulation of human IgE synthesis. Immunol Rev 41:288
6. Tada T, Taniguchi M, Okumura K (1971) Regulation of homocytotropic antibody formation in the rat. II. Effect of X-irradiation. J Immunol 106:1012–1018
7. Tada T (1975) Regulation of reaginic antibody formation in animals. Prog Allergy 19:122
8. Katz DH (1978) The allergic phenotype: manifestation of "allergic breakthrough" and imbalance in normal "damping" of IgE antibody production. Immunol Rev 41:77–108
9. Vaz NM, deSouza CM, Maier LC (1974) Genetic control of immune responsiveness in mice to ovalbumin in (C57BLxDBA/2)F_1 mice. Int Arch Allergy Appl Immunol 46:275
10. Frick OL, German DF, Mills J (1979) Development of allergy in children. I. Association with virus infections. J Allergy Clin Immunol 63:228–241
11. Chiorazzi N, Fox DA, Katz DH (1976) Hapten-specific IgE antibody response in mice. VI. Selective enhancement of IgE antibody production by low doses of X-irradiation and cyclophosphamide. J Immunol 117:1629–1637
12. Chiorazzi N, Fox DA, Katz DH (1977) Hapten-specific IgE antibody response in mice. VII. Conversion of IgE "non-responder" strains to IgE "responders" by elimination of suppressor T cell activity. J Immunol 118:48–54
13. Björksten B, Ahlstedt S (1984) Relevance of animal models for studies of immune regulation of atopic allergy. Allergy 39:317–327
14. Ishizaka K (1984) Regulation of IgE synthesis. Ann Rev Immunol 2:159–182
15. Katz DH, Bargatze RF, Bogowitz CA, Katz LR (1979) Regulation of IgE antibody production by serum molecules. IV. Complete Freund's adjuvant induces both enhancing and suppressive activities detectable in the serum of low and high responder mice. J Immunol 122:2184–2190
16. Katz DH (1984) Regulation of the IgE system: experimental and clinical aspects. Allergy 39:81–106
17. Kishimoto T, Hirai Y, Suemura M, Nokanishi K, Yamamura Y (1978) Regulation of antibody response in different immunoglobulin classes. IV. Properties and functions of IgE-class specific suppressor factors released from DNP-mycobacterium-primed T cells. J Immunol 121:2106–2112
18. Ishizaka K, Yodoi J, Suemura M, Hirashima M (1983) Isotype-specific regulation of the IgE-binding factors. Immunol Today 4:192–196
19. Huff T, Ishizaka K (1984) Formation of IgE-binding factors by human T cell hybridomas. Proc Natl Acad Sci USA 81:1514–1518
20. Weck de AL, Stadler BM, Knutti-Müller J, Ruff P, Hofstetter H, Lüdin C, Heusser C (1985) Factors influencing human IgE synthesis in vitro and in vivo. Int Archs Allergy Appl Immunol 77:38–44
21. Kishimoto T, Deguchi H, Suemura M, Yamamura Y (1983) Regulation of human IgE response by IgE class-specific suppressor T cells or suppressor factor(s). Monogr Allergy 18:75–82
22. Sarfati M, Rector E, Wong K, Rubio-Trujillo M, Sehon AH, Delespesse G (1984c) In vitro synthesis of IgE by human lymphocytes. II. Enhancement of the spontaneous IgE synthesis by IgE-binding factors secreted by RPMI 8866 lymphoblastoid B cells. Immunology 53:197
23. Uede T, Sandberg K, Bloom BR, Ishizaka K (1983) IgE-binding factors from mouse T lymphocytes. I. Formation of IgE-binding factors by stimulation with homologous IgE and interferon. J Immunol 130:649–654
24. Martens CL, Huff TF, Jardieu P, Trounstine ML, Coffman RL, Ishizaka K, Moore KW (1985) cDNA clones encoding IgE-binding factors from a rat-mouse T-cell hybridoma. Proc Natl Acad Sci USA 82:2460–2464
25. Rector E, Nakajima T, Rocha C, Duncan D, Lestourgeon D, Mitchell RS, Fischer J, Sehon AH, Delespesse G (1985) Detection and characterization of monoclonal antibodies specific to IgE receptors on human lymphocytes by flow cytometry. Immunology 55:481–488
26. Meinke GC, Magro AM, Lawrence DA, Spiegelberg HL (1978) Characterization of an IgE receptor isolated from cultured B-type lymphoblastoid cells. J Immunol 121:1321
27. Vaquero C, Fridman WH, Moncuit J, Provost M-A, Falcoff E, Gelabert MJ, Neauport-Sautes C (1984) Isolation and partial characterization of messenger RNA, from murine T cell hybrids, coding for suppressive immunoglobulin G-binding factor. J Immunol 133:482–488

28. Adachi M, Yodoi J, Noro N, Masuda T, Uchino H (1984) Murine IgA binding factors produced by Fc alpha R(+) T cells: role of Fc gamma R(+) cells for the induction of Fc alpha R and formation of IgA binding factor in con A-activated cells. J Immunol 133:65–71
29. Ishizaka K (1985) Isotope-specific T cell factors for the IgE response. CRC Crit Rev Immunol 5:229–262
30. Iwata M, Huff TF, Ishizaka K (1984) Modulation of the biologic activities of IgE-binding factor. V. The role of glycosylation-enhancing factor and glycosylation-inhibiting factor in determining the nature of IgE-binding factors. J Immunol 132:1286–1293
31. Uede T, Hirata F, Hirashima M, Ishizaka K (1983) Modulation of the biologic activities of IgE-binding factors. I. Identification of glycosylation inhibiting factor as a fragment of lipomodulin. J Immunol 130:878–884
32. Suemura M, Yodoi J, Hirashima M, Ishizaka K (1980) Regulatory role of IgE-binding factors from rat T lymphocytes. I. Mechanisms of enhancement of IgE response by IgE-potentiating factor. J Immunol 125:148–154
33. Uede T, Huff TF, Ishizaka K (1982) Formation of IgE-binding factors by rat T lymphocytes. V. Effect of adjuvant for the priming immunization on the nature of IgE-binding factors formed by antigenic stimulation. J Immunol 129:1384–1390
34. Hirashima M, Yodoi J, Ishizaka K (1981) Regulatory role of IgE-binding factors from rat T lymphocytes. V. Formation of IgE-potentiating factors by T lymphocytes from rats treated with *Bordetella pertussis* vaccine. J Immunol 126:838–842
35. Ishizaka T, Iwata M, Ishizaka K (1985) Release of histamine and arachidonate from mouse mast cells induced by glycosylation-enhancing factor and bradykinin. J Immunol 134:1880–1887
36. Spiegelberg HL (1984) Structure and function of Fc receptors for IgE on lymphocytes, monocytes and macrophages. Adv Immunol 35:61
37. Huff TF, Yodoi J, Uede T, Ishizaka K (1984) Presence of an antigenic determinant common to rat IgE potentiating factor, IgE-suppressive factor, and Fc epsilon receptors on T and B lymphocytes. J Immunol 132:406–412

The IgE Receptor of Mast Cells and Basophils

A. Kulczycki

Washington University School of Medicine, 660 South Euclid Avenue, St. Louis, MO 63110, USA

Abstract

Mast cells and basophils express large numbers of surface receptors which bind homologous IgE with high affinity ($K_A > 10^{10}$ M^{-1}). The IgE-receptor is *not* as species-specific as previously suspected. Apposition of adjacent IgE receptors is the critical event initiating histamine release, although the mechanisms by which receptor bridging activates the cell are not clear. Each IgE receptor appears to be composed of one 50000 M_r α-chain, one 32000 M_r β-chain, and two 9000 M_r γ-chains. The heavily glycosylated α-component binds IgE, can be labeled by surface iodination, and is phosphorylated in response to antigenic cross-linking of receptors (Hempstead et al., PNAS 80: 3050 '83). Recent data (F.-T. Liu et al., PNAS 82:4100, 1985) show that a 31000 M_r protein resembling β-chain also binds to IgE and anti-receptor antibodies and has a proline-rich N-terminus.

Introduction

Mast cells and basophils (and neoplastic cells derived from them) express cell surface receptors which have extremely high affinity for IgE. Monomeric IgE molecules are bound to these receptors and displayed on the mast cell/basophil surface. Subsequently, multivalent antigen may bind to adjacent receptor-bound IgE molecules and initiate mediator release. The primary physiologic role of IgE receptors thus appears to be transducing antigen's cross-linking signal in order to generate and release mediators involved in allergic responses. The specificity of the IgE receptors (or Fc_ε receptors) on basophils for IgE was first shown in studies with human peripheral blood leukocytes [1, 2]. More detailed studies of the structure, function, and expression of the high-affinity Fc_ε receptors have been made possible by using the rat basophilic leukemia (RBL) cell line [3].

The Interaction of IgE and IgE Receptors

The binding of IgE to cell surface IgE receptors is a temperature-dependent and reversible reaction [3, 4]. The studies of this interaction are consistent with a simple biomolecular forward (binding) reaction and a first-order backward (dissociation) reaction:

$$[\text{IgE}] + [\text{receptor}] \underset{k_{-1}}{\overset{k_1}{\rightleftharpoons}} [\text{IgE-receptor complex}],$$

where the forward rate constant, k_1, is approximately 1×10^5 l/mol-s at 37° C [4]. The rather ordinary k_1 value together with the usually low concentrations of IgE explains why IgE binding requires very long "latent" periods in vivo in the passive cutaneous anaphylaxis (PCA) reaction. The backward rate constant, k_{-1}, of $< 10^{-5}$/s indicates an affinity constant, K_a ($= k_1/k_{-1}$), of the order of 10^{10} l/mol [4]. The affinity of human IgE for the human Fc_ε receptor appears to be of a similar order of magnitude [5].

Initially, the interaction of IgE with its receptor had been considered to be a species-specific or "homocytotropic" reaction. However, rat IgE and mouse IgE have been found to bind quite well to human IgE receptors [6, 7] and human IgE has been found to bind rat IgE receptors [8]. Thus, the term "homocytotropic" can no longer be used to describe IgE antibodies.

Studies on the rate of sequential digestion of IgE by trypsin in the presence and absence of IgE receptor suggest that the $C_\varepsilon 3$ (penultimate) domains of IgE are bound to receptor [9]. Resonance energy transfer studies indicate that the $C_\varepsilon 2$ domain of receptor-bound IgE is only 35–52 Å from the membrane surface, implying either (a) that the C-terminal domain of IgE is buried deeply in the membrane, (b) that the Fc region of IgE is held at an angle to the cell surface, or (c) (most probably) that IgE is bent near its receptor-binding site [10].

Structure of Mast Cell/Basophil IgE Receptors

The high affinity IgE receptor of mast cells and basophils now appears to comprise four subunits; one α-component, one β-component, and two γ-components [11]. The surface-exposed α-component was the first subunit recognized. It was purified from rat mast cells and rat basophilic leukemia cells that had been surface labeled by using ^{125}I and lactoperoxidase, the cells were solubilized, and the α-component was immunoprecipitated because of its affinity for IgE [12]. The ability of IgE to inhibit surface iodination of the α-component clearly demonstrated that IgE bound to the α-component [12, 13]. The α-component was characterized as an ~ 50000 M_r glycoprotein in SDS-polyacrylamide gels [13] and a similar ^{125}I-labeled α-component has been isolated from human basophils [6, 7]. The α-component appears as a broad band in SDS-polyacrylamide gels and in isoelectric focusing gels, and such microheterogeneity appears to be a result of N-linked carbohydrate moieties [14]. The rat α-component contains about 30% carbohydrate and only a modest proportion of hydrophobic amino acids [15]. It has been claimed that two independent enzymatic digestion fragments of the rat α-component, a 34000 M_r "α_1" and a more heavily glycosylated 30000 M_r "α_2", can be resolved [16].

The first evidence that the receptor consisted of multiple components was obtained when the IgE receptor was isolated from rat basophilic leukemia cells biosynthetically labeled with ^{3}H-labeled amino acids. A 33000 M_r molecule (now termed the β-component) was discovered which copurified with the α-component [17, 18] and these two subunits could be cross-linked by chemical reagents [18]. The 33000 M_r β-component is not a glycoprotein [14, 17] nor is it a fragment of the α-component [14]. The β-component comprises two distinct regions [19]; the larger appears to have a segment within the plasma membrane since it can be labeled with 5-iodonaphthyl-1-nitrene [19, 20].

Recent studies suggest that the β-component might also have some affinity for IgE. In these studies a 31000 M_r macromolecule derived from rat basophilic leukemia cell mRNA is recognized by rabbit antibodies to IgE receptor components and the 31000 M_r protein binds specifically to IgE, yet it is clearly not a fragment of the α-component [21]. The sequence of this 31000 M_r IgE-binding molecule (which may represent β-component) is unusual for its concentration of proline (five prolines within a span of 16 amino acid residues) near its N-terminus [21].

Attention to the detergent–lipid ratio is important in stabilizing interactions between components [22]. Maintenance of the detergent–lipid ratio within a narrow appropriate range has allowed an increased yield of β-component during purification [22]. It has also led to the discovery that two additional ~ 9000 M_r molecules (termed "γ-chains"), linked to each other by disulphide bonding, are associated noncovalently with each α- and β-component [23]. It now appears that the β-component and/or the γ-components serve to anchor the α-component to the cell membrane since the presence of β- and γ-components seems to correlate with the ability to incorporate purified IgE receptor into liposomes [24].

The Role of Mast Cell/Basophil IgE Receptors in Release of Mediators

Numerous studies have demonstrated that receptor-bound IgE molecules must be brought into apposition in order for mast cells and basophils to release mediators [reviewed in 25]. By using antibodies to the IgE receptor it was formally demonstrated that it is the apposition of the receptors which is the necessary and sufficient signal to initiate mediator release [26, 27]. IgE antibodies can thus be viewed as extensions of the receptors which impart antigen specificity to the degranulation process. Furthermore, when the apposition of IgE receptors is reversed the process of granule exocytosis stops [28].

There has been increasing interest in the possibility that IgE receptor's function might involve ion channel formation. Cross-linking of IgE receptors by multivalent antigen appears to cause a depolarization of the plasma membrane of the basophil [29]. The decrease in membrane potential occurs independently of mediator release and is rapidly reversed by monovalent antigen [29]. The depolarization data are consistent with a view that the apposition of IgE receptors opens ion channels which are partially selective for calcium [29]. It has been suggested that the calcium-selective ion channels might actually be the same molecules that bind cromolyn [30], since conductance perturbations of artificial membrane bilayers containing cross-linked cromolyn binding proteins are similar to bilayers containing cross-linked IgE receptors (which are presumably associated with cromolyn binding proteins) [30].

It is also of interest that the IgE receptor components can be phosphorylated [31, 32] and that increased phosphorylation of the receptor α-component can be induced by antigen [31]. Phosphorylation of the α-component (which alters the charge and probably the confirmation of the component) is attractive as a potential mechanism for regulating the mediator release process.

Expression of Mast Cell and Basophil IgE Receptors

Mast cells and analogous RBL cells express large numbers of IgE receptors on their surfaces. It is estimated that there are 300000 receptors per rat mast cell [33] and 300000 to 1400000 receptors per RBL cell [4]. Smaller-sized human basophils have approximately 40000 to 100000 receptors per cell [34]. With RBL cells it has been shown that the density of IgE receptors varies according to the cell cycle. Cell cultures in their "stationary" phase of growth (when most cells are in the G_1 phase of the cell cycle) synthesize and express the greatest number of receptors per cell [35]. Although nonglycosylated nascent α-components (extracted from cells grown in the presence of tunicamycin) are capable of binding both to IgE and to antireceptor antibodies, the α-component of the IgE receptor must be glycosylated before it can be expressed on the cell surface [14].

Membrane proteins can be classified in two groups [36]. "Migrant" proteins such as the LDL and transferrin receptors recycle from one membrane-containing organelle to another via "coated pits." "Resident" proteins such as histocompatibility and theta antigens do not recycle. Both unoccupied IgE receptors and occupied IgE receptors are diffusely distributed on the plasma membrane in studies with RBL cells [37, 38] and they appear to function as "resident" proteins in plasma membrane. The attachment of plasma cell-derived IgE to the Fc_ε receptor can be considered for practical purposes as irreversible so that IgE could be viewed as a "resident alien" protein on the basophil/mast cell surface.

Cross-linking of IgE receptors (under physiological conditions by antigen, under experimental conditions by antibodies to IgE or to receptor, or by IgE aggregates) is required for receptor redistribution [37] and for internalization of receptor [39]. When receptor-bound IgE molecules bind to a multivalent antigen they become indirectly cross-linked, they initiate histamine release from the cell (above), and the IgE molecules together with their receptors and their bound antigen are internalized. However, the IgE receptor is not recycled nor is it replaced by active synthesis of new receptor [39]. Therefore the IgE receptor still does not appear to fit the description of a "migrant" receptor.

The internalization of multivalent antigen bound to antigen-specific IgE molecules (bound, in turn to Fc_{ε} receptors) does serve to remove both antigen and IgE antibody from the cell surface. It may account, at least in part, for the "antigen-specific desensitization" phenomenon observed when low concentrations of a specific antigen render a mast cell or basophil unresponsive to further challenge with that antigen yet responsive to a different antigen.

Involvement of IgE Receptors in Allergic Diseases

To put the IgE receptor activation sequence in perspective, it may be useful to remind ourselves that in the etiology of a given individual's asthma or rhinitis, IgE receptors may have a known role, a potential role, or no role at all (Fig. 1). The classical pathway of extrinsic allergic disease, in which high affinity IgE receptors are clearly involved in pathogenesis of the disease, is emphasized in this figure (and the figure is not meant to be comprehensive). Allergens bind to receptor-bound IgE antibodies, which brings high-affinity IgE receptors into apposition and activates mast cells to produce a variety of mediators – some of which lead directly to asthma and/or rhinitis. Several surveys indicate that "extrinsic" allergens do play an important etiologic role in the majority of patients

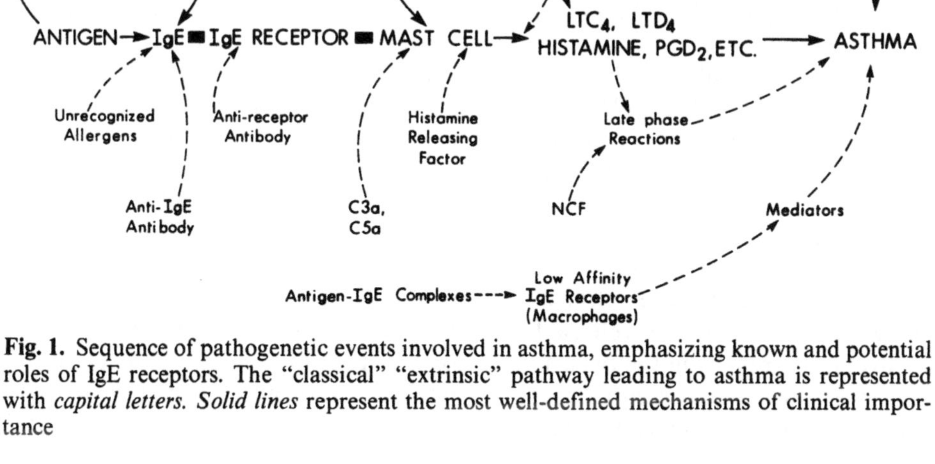

Fig. 1. Sequence of pathogenetic events involved in asthma, emphasizing known and potential roles of IgE receptors. The "classical" "extrinsic" pathway leading to asthma is represented with *capital letters. Solid lines* represent the most well-defined mechanisms of clinical importance

with asthma [25]. (Although numerous antigens are well-known causes of asthma, the antigen most commonly implicated is derived from the house dust mite *Dermatophagoides,* e.g., in one study 85% of unselected asthmatic children appeared to be allergic to *Dermatophagoides* [40].) Obviously, the lower affinity IgE receptors of lymphocytes (Fc_{ε} receptors) can play an important role in the etiology of asthma because they regulate the synthesis of IgE [41].

There are a variety of potential roles for IgE receptors in the pathogenesis of allergic diseases. First, it is very likely that additional antigens, presently unrecognized, will in the future be implicated in the etiology of immediate hypersensitivity reactions.

Second, it has been suggested that spontaneous autoantibodies against IgE or IgE receptors could conceivably be involved in idiopathic asthma [25] because several groups have found a high frequency of various autoantibodies in patients with idiopathic asthma and because antibodies deliberately produced against IgE or IgE receptors can induce mediator release. Recently, anti-IgE autoantibodies of the IgG class were found in 93% of atopic asthmatics and 72% of nonatopic asthmatics, compared with 7% (1 of 15) of normal individuals [42]. The anti-IgE antibody levels were correlated with the total IgE levels in the sera of 76 individuals studied. Gel filtration studies suggested that the anti-IgE autoantibodies were present in the immune complex form (bound to IgE) in asthmatic patients' sera. The autoantibodies appeared to mediate reversed-type immediate hypersensitivity reactions in the skin of normal individuals, which suggests that anti-IgE autoantibody might play a pathogenetic role in asthma [42].

Third, IgE immune complexes might also be involved in the pathogenesis of allergic diseases. It has been shown that allergic patient populations frequently have elevated levels of IgE-containing immune complexes [43]. It is known that aggregates containing IgE can induce mediator release in vitro from macrophages [44]; it is presumed that complexes bind to lower-affinity IgE receptors and that they might be involved in the pathogenesis of asthma. Another cell type potentially involved with IgE complexes and asthma pathogenesis is the sensitized T cell. Most dust-allergic patients (but not controls) have T-lymphocytes which are sensitized to the antigen P_1 of house dust [45]. The sensitized cells (apparently T helper cells) are probably involved in the production of antibody but may also be involved in the delayed manifestations of asthma.

Not all paths culminating in asthma involve IgE receptors (Fig. 1). Aspirin sensitivity occurs in 8%–14% of all asthmatics and does not involve IgE or IgE receptors. It is known that aspirin and nonsteroidal anti-inflammatory drugs inhibit the cyclooxygenase pathway of arachidonic acid metabolism, but their precise site(s) and mechanism(s) of producing asthma are not known. Certain other drugs are known to cause nonimmunologic release of mediators from mast cells in vitro (e.g., opiates, polymyxin, radiocontrast dyes, mannitol) and are sometimes important clinically. The anaphylatoxins, C3a and C5a, are known to cause mediator release from mast cells in vitro, and recently a 20000 M_r histamine-releasing factor has been isolated from human mononuclear cells. However, the clinical significance of these latter substances is not clear. It is known that mast cell-derived mediators and neutrophil chemotactic factor may produce late-phase allergic reactions (which may involve eosinophils, neutrophils, monocytes, and lymphocytes). Late phase reactions also seem to have a potentially important role in the pathogenesis of asthma.

References

1. Ishizaka K, Tomioka H, Ishizaka T (1970) Mechanisms of passive sensitization. I. Presence of IgE and IgG molecules of human leukocytes. J Immunol 105:1459
2. Sullivan AL, Grimley PM, Metzger H (1971) Electron microscopic localization of IgE on the surface membrane of human basophils. J Exp Med 124:1403
3. Kulczycki A, Isersky C, Metzger H (1974) The interaction of IgE with rat basophilic leukemia cells. I. Evidence for specific binding of IgE. J Exp Med 139:600
4. Kulczycki A, Metzger H (1974) The interaction of IgE with rat basophilic leukemia cells. II. Quantitative aspects of the binding reaction. J Exp Med 140:1976
5. Ishizaka T, Soto C, Ishizaka K (1973) Mechanisms of passive sensitization. III. Number of IgE molecules and its receptor sites on human basophil granulocytes. J Immunol 111:500
6. Hempstead BL, Parker CW, Kulczycki A Jr (1979) Characterization of the IgE receptor isolated from human basophils. J Immunol 123:2283
7. Conrad DH, Wingard JR, Ishizaka T (1983) The interaction of human and rodent IgE with the human basophil IgE receptor. J Immunol 130:327
8. Sterk AR, Barrett KE, Metcalfe DD, Ishizaka T (1985) Binding of human IgE to rodent mast cells and basophils. Fed Proc 44:585
9. Perez-Montfort R, Metzger H (1982) Proteolysis of soluble IgE receptor complexes: localization of sites on IgE which interact with the Fc receptor. Mol Immunol 19:1113
10. Holowka D, Baird B (1983) Structural studies on the membrane-bound IgE-receptor complex. 2. Mapping of distances between sites on IgE and the membrane surface. Biochemistry 22:3475
11. Metzger H, Rivnay B, Henkart M, Kanner B, Kinet J-P, Perez-Montfort R (1984) Analysis of the structure and function of the receptor for immunoglobulin E. Mol Immunol 21:1167
12. Conrad DH, Froese A (1976) Characterization of the target cell receptor for IgE. II. Polyacrylamide gel analysis of the surface IgE receptor from normal rat mast cells and from rat basophilic leukemia cells. J Immunol 116:319
13. Kulczycki A, McNearney TA, Parker CW (1976) The rat basophilic leukemia cell receptor for IgE. I. Characterization as a glycoprotein. J Immunol 117:661
14. Hempstead BL, Parker CW, Kulczycki A Jr (1981) The cell surface receptor for IgE. Effect of tunicamycin on molecular properties of receptor from rat basophilic leukemia cells. J Biol Chem 256:10717
15. Kanellopoulos JM, Liu TY, Poy G, Metzger H (1980) Composition and subunit structure of the cell receptor for IgE. J Biol Chem 255:9060
16. Goetze A, Kanellopoulos J, Rice D, Metzger H (1981) Enzymatic cleavage products of the α subunit of the receptor for IgE. Biochemistry 20:6341
17. Kulczycki A Jr, Parker CW (1979) The cell surface receptor for IgE. I. The use of repetitive affinity chromatography for the purification of a mammalian receptor. J Biol Chem 254:3187
18. Holowka D, Hartmann H, Kanellopoulos J, Metzger H (1980) Association of the receptor for IgE with an endogenous polypeptide on rat basophilic leukemia cells. J Recept Res 1:41
19. Holowka D, Metzger H (1982) Further characterization of the β component of the receptor for IgE. Mol Immunol 19:219
20. Holowka D, Gitler C, Bertovici T, Metzger H (1981) Reaction of 5-iodonaphthyl-1-nitrene with the IgE receptor on normal and tumor mast cells. Nature 289:806
21. Liu F-T, Albrandt K, Mendel E, Kulczycki A Jr, Orida NK (1985) Identification of an IgE-binding protein by molecular cloning. Proc Natl Acad Sci USA 82:4100

22. Rivnay B, Wank SA, Poy G, Metzger H (1982) Phospholipids stabilize the interaction between the α and β subunits of the solubilized receptor for IgE. Biochemistry 21:6922
23. Perez-Montfort R, Kinet JP, Metzger H (1983) A previously unrecognized subunit of the receptor for IgE. Biochemistry 22:5722
24. Rivnay B, Rossi G, Henkart M, Metzger H (1984) Reconstitution of the receptor for IgE into liposomes. Reincorporation of purified receptors. J Biol Chem 259:1212
25. Kulczycki A Jr (1981) Role of IgE and IgE receptors in bronchial asthma. J Allergy Clin Immunol 68:5
26. Ishizaka T, Ishizaka K, Conrad DH, Forese A (1978) A new concept of triggering mechanisms of the IgE-mediated histamine release. J Allergy Clin Immunol 61:320
27. Isersky C, Taurog JD, Poy G, Metzger H (1978) Triggering of cultured neoplastic mast cells by antibodies to the receptor for IgE. J Immunol 121:549
28. Kagey-Sobotka A, MacGlashan DW, Lichtenstein LM (1982) Role of receptor aggregation in triggering IgE-mediated reactions. Fed Proc Fed Am Soc Exp Biol 41:12
29. Kanner BI, Metzger H (1983) Crosslinking of the receptors for immunoglobulin E depolarizes the plasma membrane of rat basophilic leukemia cells. Proc Natl Acad Sci USA 80:5744
30. Mazurek N, Schindler H, Schurholz T, Pecht I (1984) The cromolyn binding protein constitutes the Ca^{2+} channel of basophils opening upon immunological stimulus. Proc Natl Acad Sci USA 81:6841
31. Hempstead BL, Parker CW, Kulczycki A Jr (1983) Selective phosphorylation of the IgE receptor in antigen-stimulated rat mast cells. Proc Natl Acad Sci USA 80:3050
32. Fewtrell C, Goetze A, Metzger H (1982) Phosphorylation of the receptor for IgE. Biochemistry 21:2004
33. Conrad DH, Bazin H, Sehon AH, Froese A (1975) Binding parameters of the interaction between rat IgE and rat mast cell receptors. J Immunol 114:1688
34. Ishizaka T, Soto C, Ishizaka K (1973) Mechanisms of passive sensitization. III. Number of IgE molecules and its receptor sites on human basophil granulocytes. J Immunol 111:500
35. Isersky C, Metzger H, Buell DN (1975) Cell cycle-associated changes in receptors for IgE during growth and differentiation of a rat basophilic leukemia cell line. J Exp Med 141:1147
36. Brown MS, Anderson RGW, Goldstein JL (1983) Recycling receptors: The round-trip itinerary of migrant membrane proteins. Cell 32:663
37. Carson DA, Metzger H (1974) Interaction of IgE with rat basophilic leukemia cells. IV. Antibody-induced redistribution of IgE receptors. J Immunol 113:1271
38. Isersky C, Rivera J, Mims S, Triche TJ (1979) The fat of IgE bound to rat basophilic leukemia cells. J Immunol 122:1926
39. Isersky C, Rivera J, Segal DM, Triche T (1983) The fat of IgE bound to rat basophilic leukemia cells. II. Endocytosis of IgE oligomers and effect on receptor turnover. J Immunol 131:388
40. Morrison Smith J, Disney ME, Williams JD, Goels ZA (1969) Clinical significance of skin reaction to mite extracts in children with asthma. Br Med J 2:723
41. Ishizaka K (1984) Regulation of IgE synthesis. In: Paul WE, Fathman CG, Metzger H (eds) Annual of review of immunology Vol 2. Annual Reviews Inc., Palo Alto, California, p 159
42. Nawata Y, Koike T, Yanagisawa T, Iwamoto I, Itaya T, Yoshida S, Tomioka H (1984) Anti-IgE autoantibody in patients with bronchial asthma. Clin Exp Immunol 58:348
43. Stevens WJ, Bridts CH (1984) IgG-containing and IgE-containing circulating immune complexes in patients with asthma and rhinitis. J Allergy Clin Immunol 73:276
44. Dessaint J-P, Waksman BH, Metzger H, Capron A (1980) Cytophilic binding of IgE to the macrophage. Cell Immunol 51:280
45. Rawle FC, Mitchell EB, Platts-Mills TAE (1984) T cell responses to the major allergen from the house dust mite *Dermatophagoides pteronyssinus,* antigen P: comparison of patients with asthma, atopic dermatitis, and perennial rhinitis. J Immunol 133:195

IgE Receptors on Lymphocytes

H. L. Spiegelberg

Research Institute of Scripps Clinic, 10666 North Torrey Pines Road, La Jolla, CA 92037, USA

Abstract

Peripheral blood lymphocytes (PBL), B and T cells from nonatopic donors, patients with allergic rhinitis and/or asthma ("mild atopic", 300 – 900 IU IgE/ml), severe atopic dermatitis (1000 – 40000 IU IgE/ml) and the hyper-IgE Syndrome (> 7000 IU IgE/ml) were examined for IgE and IgG Fc receptor positive cells ($Fc_\varepsilon R$, $Fc_\gamma R$). Nonatopic donors had 1.2 ± 1% $Fc_\varepsilon R^+$ PBL, > 95% being B cells with < 0.1% $Fc_\varepsilon R^+$ T cells. Patients with mild atopic disease in remission had 1.6 ± 1% $Fc_\varepsilon R^+$ PBL; however, they showed transient increases in both $Fc_\varepsilon R^+$ B cells (3 – 6%) and T cells (0.2 to 1.2%) lasting for several weeks. Patients with severe atopic dermatitis or the Hyper-IgE Syndrome had 7 ± 3% $Fc_\varepsilon R^+$ PBL, > 95% being B cells and always < 0.1% $Fc_\varepsilon R^+$ T cells; these patients also had significantly fewer $Fc_\gamma R^+$ T cells (3 ± 1%) than nonatopic (11 ± 4%) and mildly atopic (7 ± 4%) patients.

T cells and non-T cells were separated by rosetting with neuraminidase treated sheep erythrocytes and Ficoll-Hypaque centrifugation. The two cell fractions were then reacted with a panel of monoclonal mouse antibodies to lymphocyte surface antigens, followed by fluoresceinated $F(ab')_2$ goat anti-mouse Ig and then rosetted for detection of $Fc_\varepsilon R$ and $Fc_\gamma R$ on the immunofluorescence positive cells. Both $Fc_\varepsilon R^+$ and $Fc_\gamma R^+$ T cells reacted with the same set of monoclonal antibodies. They were Lyt3$^+$ and OKT11$^+$ positive (sheep erythrocyte receptor) OKT3 (T receptor associated protein) and OKT4 (helper T cells) negative. Approximately 20% reacted with antibody OKT8 (suppressor T cells) and 80% with OKM1 which reacts with monocytes, K and NK cells. The $Fc_\varepsilon R^+$ T cells were most likely large granular lymphocytes; it is unknown whether the cells belong to the T cell or monocyte cell series. E rosette depleted cells from patients with atopic dermatitis or the Hyper-IgE Syndrome had 56 ± 18% sIgM$^+$/IgD$^+$, 45 ± 9% $Fc_\varepsilon R^+$ and 47 ± 21% $Fc_\gamma R^+$ cells; 92 ± 2% of the $Fc_\varepsilon R^+$ and 9 ± 7% of the $Fc_\gamma R^+$ cells were IgM$^+$/IgD$^+$ and 3 ± 4% of the $Fc_\varepsilon R^+$ and 30 ± 22% of the $Fc_\gamma R^+$ cells were B73.1$^+$ (NK cell marker), indicating that most of the $Fc_\varepsilon R^+$ non-T cells of these patients were B cells. The data indicate that most of the B cells of severe atopic patients are $Fc_\varepsilon R^+$ and that these patients are deficient in $Fc_\varepsilon R^+$ and $Fc_\gamma R^+$ OKT8$^+$/OKM1$^+$, large granular lymphocytes which lack the T3 pan T cell marker but have the sheep erythrocyte receptor.

Rats infected with the parasite *Nippostrongylus brasiliensis* showed a large increase of $Fc_\varepsilon R^+$ cells and small percentages of $Fc_\varepsilon R^+$ T cells that were W3/25^- (helper T) and $OX8^+$ (suppressor T) which persisted long after the decline of the parasitically induced elevated serum IgE level.

Both the data obtained in man and in rats suggest that the $Fc_\varepsilon R^+$ lymphocytes are involved in IgE regulation; however, their precise function is as yet not established.

Introduction

IgE antibodies are mainly responsible for acute allergic (atopic) diseases. They bind to high affinity IgE Fc receptors ($Fc_\varepsilon R$) on mast cells and basophilic granulocytes. Reaction of the cell-bound IgE with allergens causes cross-linking of $Fc_\varepsilon R$ which induces the release of histamine and other vasoactive substances [1]. In relation to all other Ig classes, IgE is present in the serum at the lowest concentration. Most healthy subjects have less than 200 ng IgE/ml. Even patients with severe allergic disease seldom have more than 10 µg IgE/ml.

Because certain parasites induce formation of large quantities of IgE, the major role of IgE may be defense against parasites [2]. In geographical areas free of parasitic infestation, it appears that IgE antibodies are not essential for the host's defense system. In such areas, IgE may even be harmful by causing allergic diseases. Therefore, it appears feasible to search for natural or synthetic compounds that down-regulate or even eliminate IgE antibody formation.

IgE Receptors on Lymphocytes

IgE formation is most likely regulated by T cells [1]. However, the precise mechanism of the T cell mediated IgE suppression is unknown. Several years ago, we discovered that subpopulations of lymphocytes bear $Fc_\varepsilon R$ [3]. The $Fc_\varepsilon R$ on lymphocytes differ from those on mast cells in two ways: first, they bind IgE with a lower affinity than mast cells, and second, the cells expressing the $Fc_\varepsilon R$ increase as a result of IgE formation [4]. Rats [5, 6] and mice [7] infected with the parasite *Nippostrongylus brasiliensis*, as well as patients with severe atopic dermatitis [8], have much higher percentages of $Fc_\varepsilon R^+$ lymphocytes than normal rats and mice and healthy humans. This observation suggests that $Fc_\varepsilon R^+$ lymphocytes may be involved in the regulation of IgE antibody formation.

Lymphocytes expressing $Fc_\varepsilon R$ were identified in our laboratory with a rosette assay [3]. Aldehyde-fixed ox erythrocytes were coated with monomeric or bis-diazotized benzidine-aggregated IgE and the rosette forming cells enumerated. The percentage of $Fc_\varepsilon R^+$ peripheral blood lymphocytes (PBLs) was approximately 1% in healthy nonatopic humans and in patients with mild atopic disease (< 1000 IU IgE/ml) in remission. Most of the $Fc_\varepsilon R^+$ lymphocytes in these subjects were B cells. Pure T cell preparations contained < 0.1% $Fc_\varepsilon R^+$ cells. Tonsil and spleen lymphocytes, which contain higher percentages of B cells than PBLs, have 5% – 10% of $Fc_\varepsilon R^+$ cells, also mainly B cells [9]. However,

Table 1. Effect of systemic corticosteroid treatment of $Fc_{\varepsilon}R$ expression on lymphocytes and monocytes in patients with atopic dermatitis

	% $Fc_{\varepsilon}R^+$ cells	
	Lymphocytes	Monocytes
Nonatopic [10]	1.2±0.6	18± 8
Atopic dermatitis [6]	7.2±2.6	68±22
Atopic dermatitis in remission [4]	2.5±1.2	25±12
Atopic dermatitis + corticosteroids [5]	0.2±0.2	3± 3

the percent and absolute numbers of $Fc_{\varepsilon}R^+$ lymphocytes increases transiently in nonatopic apparently healthy subjects and in patients suffering from seasonal allergic rhinitis [10]. The increase involves both $Fc_{\varepsilon}R^+$ B and T cells and lasts several weeks [11]. In contrast, patients with atopic dermatitis [8] or the hyper-IgE syndrome [12] having > 1000 IU IgE/ml always show a significantly elevated percentage of $Fc_{\varepsilon}R^+$ lymphocytes (7% ± 2%). The increase of $Fc_{\varepsilon}R^+$ lymphocytes in the patients with extremely high IgE serum levels is the result of an increase of $Fc_{\varepsilon}R^+$ B cells, since < 0.1% $Fc_{\varepsilon}R^+$ T cells and only few NK cells have been detected in these patients [11, 12].

As shown in Table 1, the expression of $Fc_{\varepsilon}R$ on lymphocytes and monocytes is affected by systemic corticosteroid treatment. Such treated patients had a lower percentage of $Fc_{\varepsilon}R^+$ PBLs than the normal control donors. The reduction in the percentage of $Fc_{\varepsilon}R^+$ PBLs in atopic patients after systemic corticosteroid treatment occurred in a relatively short time. Patients having 6%–8% $Fc_{\varepsilon}R^+$ lymphocytes had < 1% 1 week after corticosteroid treatment. The percentage of monocytes expressing the same type of $Fc_{\varepsilon}R$ as lymphocytes [4] was also found to diminish after corticosteroid treatment. Whether the disappearance of $Fc_{\varepsilon}R^+$ lymphocytes from the circulation has a down-regulatory role on IgE formation in man is not established. Yodoi et al. [13] reported that rats treated with dexamethasone form suppressor rather than enhancing IgE binding factors in vitro.

To examine the nature of the $Fc_{\varepsilon}R^+$ T cells, they were stained with monoclonal antibodies to T cell subsets followed by IgE rosette formation. This allowed direct identification of the phenotype of the IgE rosetting T cells [11]. The $Fc_{\varepsilon}R^+$ T cells reacted with monoclonal antibodies to the T cell's sheep erythrocyte receptor (Lyt3, OKT11) but not with antibody OKT3, which detects a T cell receptor associated antigen present on most peripheral blood T cells. Approximately 20% of the $Fc_{\varepsilon}R^+$ T cells reacted with antibody OKT8 (suppressor T cells), whereas no OKT4+ (helper T cells) IgE rosetting T cells were detected. Approximately 80% of the $Fc_{\varepsilon}R^+$ T cells reacted with the monoclonal antibody OKM1 which was prepared against monocytes and also reacts weakly with large granular lymphocytes, suggesting that $Fc_{\varepsilon}R^+$ T cells are large granular lymphocytes. T cells having IgG Fc receptors ($Fc_{\gamma}R$) reacted with the same monoclonal antibodies to T cell markers as $Fc_{\varepsilon}R^+$ T cells, suggesting that both $Fc_{\varepsilon}R^+$ T cells belong to the same T cell subset. Rat IgE rosetting T cells reacted with the monoclonal antibody OX8, which detects suppressor T cells, whereas no $Fc_{\varepsilon}R^+$ T cells reacting with antibody W3/25$^+$ (helper T cells) were detected, suggesting that rat $Fc_{\varepsilon}R^+$ T cells belong to the same T cell subsets as human $Fc_{\varepsilon}R^+$ T cells. The numbers of $Fc_{\varepsilon}R^+$ T cells were very small both in humans and rats, usually less than 1%.

Despite the fact that the above described findings of $Fc_{\varepsilon}R^+$ lymphocytes have been known for some time, three major issues with regard to the function of these cells remain to be resolved: a) the exact mechanism of induction of $Fc_{\varepsilon}R^+$ lymphocytes, (b) the function of $Fc_{\varepsilon}R^+$ T cells, and (c) the role of $Fc_{\varepsilon}R$ on B cells.

The expression of $Fc_{\varepsilon}R$ on lymphocytes is most likely induced as a result of IgE formation. Yodoi et al. [14] first suspected that IgE induces the $Fc_{\varepsilon}R$ and showed that normal rat mesenteric lymph node cells become $Fc_{\varepsilon}R^+$ after overnight incubation with IgE. The same observation was made by Chen et al. [15] in mice and we showed that injection of native but not heat denatured IgE induces $Fc_{\varepsilon}R^+$ lymphocytes in rats [6]. In contrast, culturing of human cells with IgE or injection of IgE into rhesus monkeys did not induce $Fc_{\varepsilon}R^+$ lymphocytes [8]. This suggests that factors other than or in addition to IgE are involved in $Fc_{\varepsilon}R$ induction. We repeatedly observed significant increases of $Fc_{\varepsilon}R^+$ lymphocytes in healthy donors having very low and constant serum IgE levels [10]. Rats [4–6] and mice [7] have much higher percentages of $Fc_{\varepsilon}R^+$ lymphocytes than humans and monkeys. Perhaps the rodents' cells are "preactivated" by some as yet unknown factors to respond with $Fc_{\varepsilon}R$ formation. Activators could be products of parasites as well as bacterial and viral antigens. Perhaps such substances induce $Fc_{\varepsilon}R$ to enhance IgE antibody production. This hypothesis should be testable by measuring the percentage of $Fc_{\varepsilon}R^+$ lymphocytes in rats and mice injected with antigens which might induce IgE formation.

The $Fc_{\varepsilon}R^+$ T cells reacted with monoclonal antibodies to the T cell subset typical for suppressor and $Fc_{\gamma}R^+$ T cells. $Fc_{\gamma}R^+$ T cells have been shown to suppress pokeweed mitogen induced IgG formation in vitro [16]. Therefore, both $Fc_{\varepsilon}R^+$ and $Fc_{\gamma}R^+$ T cells may have an isotype down-regulatory function. However, in vivo functional studies similar to those described by Hoover and Lynch [17] for the down-regulatory effect of $Fc_{\alpha}R^+$ lymphocytes will be necessary to elucidate the function of $Fc_{\varepsilon}R^+$ T cells. Fc receptor positive T cells may regulate the Ig isotype through Ig binding factors. Fridman et al. [18] first described an IgG binding factor which presumably represents fragments of $Fc_{\gamma}R$ shed from T cells that down-regulates IgG formation in vitro. Ishizaka and his colleagues [19] described analogous IgE binding factors that are produced by rat or mouse $Fc_{\varepsilon}R^+$ T cells which either up- or down-regulate IgE formation in vitro. Although these factors have been known for over 5 years, it has not yet been shown whether they have an effect on IgG or on IgE formation in vivo. It appears not too surprising that these factors bind to membrane bound IgG or IgE on B cells and affect Ig synthesis of these cells in vitro. However, whether the binding factors produced by T cells will reach B cells in vivo is less clear. Because of the high Ig serum concentrations, one would expect them to be absorbed onto circulating Ig before they can reach B cells. It is also possible that the $Fc_{\varepsilon}R$ on the T cells allow the T cells to recognize B cells having membrane bound IgE and that the $Fc_\varepsilon R^+$ T cells down-regulate IgE synthesis of these B cells by direct cell contact [4].

As described above, the great majority of $Fc_\varepsilon R^+$ lymphocytes are B cells. In patients with severe atopic diseases, 50%–90% of the peripheral blood B-lymphocytes are $Fc_\varepsilon R^+$ [8, 11, 12]. The function of the $Fc_\varepsilon R$ on B cells is not understood. Because incubation of lymphocytes with IgG immune complexes results in inhibition of B cell proliferation in vitro, it has been postulated that Fc receptors on B cells may have a down-regulatory role on antibody formation [20]. However, this hypothesis is difficult to adapt for $Fc_\varepsilon R$. If $Fc_\varepsilon R$ on B cells have a down-regulatory role on IgE formation, one would expect patients with such disorders as atopic dermatitis or hyper-IgE syndrome to have low IgE levels because an average of 70% of their B cells are $Fc_\varepsilon R^+$. Therefore, it is possible that $Fc_\varepsilon R$ on B cells may have an up-regulatory role. Addition of Fc fragments of all classes induces B cell proliferation [21], a finding which is in agreement with this hypothesis.

In summary, the following hypothesis for IgE regulation is proposed based on findings of $Fc_\varepsilon R^+$ lymphocytes in man and rats. Certain antigens, particularly parasite antigens and allergens, induce $Fc_\varepsilon R$ on B cells, and this process is enhanced by newly formed IgE in the environment of the B cells. These receptors play an up-regulatory role on IgE antibody formation. Subsequently, $Fc_\varepsilon R$ are induced on a subset of T cells, presumably by the increasing IgE concentration. The $Fc_\varepsilon R^+$ T cells react with the membrane IgE of B cells and suppress their IgE formation. The numerical deficiency of $Fc_\varepsilon R^+$ T cells in patients with atopic dermatitis or the hyper-IgE syndrome may explain their high IgE serum levels. In vivo functional studies in suitable animal models will be necessary to examine the validity of this hypothesis.

Acknowledgments. This is publication no. 4008 IMM from the Research Institute of Scripps Clinic and Research Foundation, La Jolla, California 92037, USA. This work was supported by grants from the United States Public Health Service AI 10734. The author thanks Kathleen Canning for editorial assistance and Margaret Stone for preparing the manuscript.

References

1. Ishizaka K, Ishizaka T (1978) Mechanisms of reaginic hypersensitivity and IgE antibody response. Immunol Rev 41:109
2. Jarrett EE (1978) Stimuli for the production of control of IgE in rats. Immunol Rev 41:52
3. Gonzalez-Molina A, Spiegelberg HL (1977) A subpopulation of normal human peripheral B lymphocytes that bind IgE. J Clin Invest 59:616
4. Spiegelberg HL (1984) Structure and function of Fc receptors for IgE on lymphocytes, monocytes and macrophages. Adv Immunol 35:61
5. Yodoi J, Ishizaka K (1979) Lymphocytes bearing Fc receptors for IgE. I. Presence of human and rat T lymphocytes with Fc_ε receptors. J Immunol 122:2577
6. Spiegelberg HL (1981) Lymphocytes bearing Fc receptors for IgE. Immunol Rev 56:199
7. Katona IM, Urban JF, Scher I, Kanellopoulos-Langevin C, Finkelman FD (1983) Induction of an IgE response in mice by *Nippostrongylus brasiliensis:* characterization of lymphoid cells with intracytoplasmic or surface IgE. J Immunol 130:350

8. Spiegelberg HL, O'Connor RD, Simon RA, Mathison DA (1979) Lymphocytes with IgE Fc receptors in patients with atopic disorders. J Clin Invest 64:714
9. Hellstrom UB, Spiegelberg HL (1979) Characterization of human lymphocytes bearing Fc receptors for IgE isolated from blood and lymphoid organs. Scand J Immunol 9:75
10. Spiegelberg HL, Simon RA (1981) Increase of lymphocytes with Fc receptors for IgE in patients with allergic rhinitis during the grass pollen season. J Clin Invest 68:845
11. Thompson LF, Mellon MH, Zeiger RS, Spiegelberg HL (1983) Characterization of T lymphocytes bearing Fc receptors for IgE (T_ε) and IgG (T_γ) with monoclonal antibodies. J Immunol 131:2772
12. Thompson LF, Spiegelberg HL, Buckley RH (1985) IgE Fc receptor positive T and B lymphocytes in patients with the hyper-IgE syndrome. Clin Exp Immunol 59:77
13. Yodoi J, Hirashima M, Ishizaka K (1981) Lymphocytes bearing Fc receptors for IgE. VI. Suppressive effect of glucocorticoids on the expression of Fc_ε-receptors and glycosylation of IgE binding factors. J Immunol 127:471
14. Yodoi J, Ishizaka T, Ishizaka K (1979) Lymphocytes bearing Fc receptors for IgE. II. Induction of Fc_ε receptor bearing rat lymphocytes by IgE. J Immunol 123:455
15. Chen SS, Bohn JW, Liu FT, Katz DH (1981) Murine lymphocytes expressing Fc receptors for IgE ($Fc_\varepsilon R$). I. Conditions for inducing $Fc_\varepsilon R^+$ lymphocytes and inhibition of the inductive events by suppressive factor of allergy (SFA). J Immunol 127:166
16. Moretta L, Webb SR, Grossi CE, Lydyard PM, Cooper MD (1977) Functional analysis of two human subpopulations: help and suppression of B cell responses by T cells bearing receptors for IgM (T_μ) or IgG (T_γ). J Exp Med 146:184
17. Hoover RG, Lynch RG (1983) Isotype-specific suppression of IgA: suppression of IgA responses in Balb/C mice by T_α cells. J Immunol 130:521
18. Fridman WH, Rabourdin-Combe C, Neaport-Sautes C, Gisler RH (1981) Characterization and function of T cell Fc_γ receptor. Immunol Rev 56:51
19. Ishizaka K (1985) Twenty years with IgE: from the identification of IgE to regulatory factors for the IgE response. J Immunol 135:1
20. Sidman CL, Unanue ER (1976) Control of B-lymphocyte function. I. Inactivation of mitogenesis by interaction with surface immunoglobulin and Fc-receptor molecules. J Exp Med 144:882
21. Berman MA, Spiegelberg HL, Weigle WO (1979) Lymphocyte stimulation with Fc fragments. I. Class, subclass and domain of active fragments. J Immunol 122:89

IgE and Allergic Diseases

S. G. O. Johansson
Department of Clinical Immunology, Karolinska Hospital, 10401 Stockholm, Sweden

Immediate-type hypersensitivity reactions seem to be mediated more or less exclusively by IgE antibodies [4–6]. Although other homocytotropic antibodies have been described, their role in diseases is still obscure. IgE must have a beneficial role in the immune defense system, though little is known about this function. Thus, measures of IgE sensitization, such as increased IgE levels and the presence of IgE antibodies in serum [11], are indications of allergy.

IgE-mediated, atopic allergy is common and seems to be increasing. In Sweden about 15% of all children have been reported to suffer from one of the atopic diseases (allergic rhinitis, allergic bronchial asthma, and atopic eczema) [7].

There is evidence from reviews in medical history as well as from comparative studies performed in the early 1950s that the incidence of allergic diseases in civilized countries is increasing [2, 8]. Similar data are available from the developing countries, where allergies were regarded as rare disorders some 30 years ago but are now increasingly common, especially in urban areas [2].

The cause of this increase in allergic diseases is not known. It may be speculated that pollution in the air is an indirect factor in increased IgE production. The most important pollutant has been found to be cigarette smoke. Both in studies in rats and in clinical studies, it has been observed that exposure to cigarette smoke stimulates IgE production [1, 12, 13]. One may speculate that other air pollutants, e.g., sulfur dioxide and other agents inducing chemical or mechanical irritation of the mucosal surfaces, have a similar influence.

Equally important seem to be microbial infections. During the course of some viral infections IgE levels increase quickly and steeply [6]. During the development of graft-versus-host reactions, increases in IgE production are common [9].

The question of IgE reactions against bacterial antigens has been discussed for many years. Regarding the response to *Staphylococcus aureus,* two binding sites of protein A on immunoglobulins have to be distinguished, namely the classical binding activity located on the Fc portion of immunoglobulin molecules and the "alternative protein A binding site" on the Fab part of IgG and IgE molecules [3].

Care of allergic patients in the form of prediction, prevention, diagnosis, and treatment is nowadays a concern not limited to specialists in allergology but rather extending to pediatricians, general practitioners, and others [8]. Immunological tests for IgE antibodies are useful adjuncts to conventional skin and provocation tests in diagnosis and follow-up of treatment.

Several hundred different allergens are known. However, only very few (in Europe probably less than ten) account for more than 95% of all allergies observed. New allergens are usually discovered in certain occupational settings. Thus, occupational allergy is becoming an increasingly important field. Allergy to storage mites among farmers is such an example. In a study of farmers in Sweden [10], we found that the prevalence of allergy to storage mites (*Acarus siro, Lepidoglyphus destructor, Tyrophagus putrescentiae,* and *Glycyphagus domesticus*) among all farmers in the area of Gotland was 6.2%. The corresponding prevalence among farmers with respiratory symptoms was as high as 15.4% and among those with atopic constitution 37.8%. The overall incidence of any form of immediate-type hypersensitivity was 40.0% (asthma 3.5%, asthma + rhinoconjuctivitis 10.6%, rhinoconjunctivitis 25.9%). The incidence of suspected allergic alveolitis was only 0.2%. Among these farmers allergies to common inhalant allergens such as pollens and house dust mites were much less common.

References

1. Bahna SL, Heiner DC, Myhre BA (1983) Immunoglobulin E pattern in cigarette smokers. Allergy 38:57
2. Foucard T (1985) The epidemiology of allergic disease in childhood. In: "Proceedings of the European Academy of allergology." Stockholm, pp 105–107
3. Inganäs M, Johansson SGO (1981) Influence of the alternative protein A interaction on the precipitation between human monoclonal immunoglobulins and protein A from *Staphylococcus aureus.* Int Arch Allergy Appl Immunol 65:91–101
4. Ishizaka K, Ishizaka T, Hornbrook MM (1966) Physicochemical properties of reaginic antibody. IV. Presence of a unique immunoglobulins as carrier of reaginic activity. J Immunol 97:75
5. Johansson SGO (1967) Raised levels of a new immunoglobulin (IgND) in asthma. Lancet 2:951
6. Johansson SGO (1981) The clinical significance of IgE. In: Franklin EC (ed) Clinical immunology update, New York, pp 123–145
7. Kjellman NIM (1983) Serum IgE and the predictive value of IgE determination. In: Buscino L (ed) Advances in pediatric allergy, vol 69. Excerpta Medica, Amsterdam
8. Middleton E, Ellis R, Reed CE (eds) (1984) Principles and practice of allergy. Mosby, St. Louis
9. Ringden O, Persson U, Johansson SGO (1983) Are increased levels a signal of an acute graft-versus-host reaction? Immunol Rev 71:57
10. van Hage-Hamsten M, Johansson SGO, Höglund S, Tüll P, Wirén A, Zetterström O (1985) Storage mite allergy is common in a farming population. Clin Allergy 15:555–564
11. Wide L, Bennich H, Johannsson SGO (1967) Diagnosis of allergy by an in-vitro test for allergen antibodies. Lancet 2:1105
12. Zetterström O, Osterman K, Machado L, Johansson SGO (1981) Another smoking hazard: raised serum IgE concentration and increased risk of occupational allergy. Br Med J 283:1215
13. Zetterström O, Nordvall SL, Björkstén B, Ahlstedt S, Stelander M (1985) Increased IgE antibody responses in rats exposed to tobacco smoke. J Allergy Clin Immunol 75:594–598

Mediators

Histamine and Allergic Diseases

J. Ring[1], F. Sedlmeier[1], D. von der Helm[1], T. Mayr[1], U. Walz[1], H. Ibel[1], H. Riepel[1], B. Przybilla[1], H.-J. Reimann[2], and W. Dorsch[3]

[1] Dermatologische Klinik und Poliklinik der Ludwig-Maximilians-Universität München, 8000 Munich, Federal Republic of Germany
[2] II. Medizinische Klinik der Technischen Universität München, 8000 Munich, Federal Republic of Germany
[3] Kinderpoliklinik der Ludwig-Maximilians-Universität München, 8000 Munich, Federal Republic of Germany

Abstract

Although known for almost 80 years, histamine (H) (β-imidazolylethylamine) still remains a fascinating substance for many researchers. In spite of great progress in knowledge of pharmacology and release mechanisms as well as the discovery of other potent mediators, the definition of the physiological role of histamine in health and disease remains incomplete. The role of H – among others – as mediator of immediate-type hypersensitivity diseases (both allergic and pseudo-allergic in origin) is rather well established. This *proinflammatory* effect involves predominantly H_1 receptors on mucosal cells, smooth muscle and vascular endothelium. Similarly well-defined is the H_2-mediated role of H in gastric acid secretion. Less well defined is the clinical relevance of cardiac H_1 and H_2 receptors (atrial H_1 receptors mediating negative dromotropic effects, while ventricular tachycardia is mediated by H_2 receptors) as well as the role of H as neurotransmitter in the human brain.

Recent interest has focussed on *antiinflammatory* effects of H as modulator of immune reactions acting predominantly on H_2 receptors on the surface of leukocytes (suppression of immediate and delayed type immune reactions).

H is produced and stored in mast cells and basophils; it can be released by a spectrum of immunologic and non-immunologic mechanisms involving active secretory processes. Differences regarding species and origin of cell population (connective tissue mast cells, bone marrow mast cells, mucosal mast cells or basophils) have to be considered.

A variety of factors have been found to influence the *"releasability"* of H secreting cells:

- *Age* (increases with age).
- *Sex* (higher values in females; inhibitory influence of androgens?).
- *Autonomic nervous system transmitters* (β-adrenergic, cholinergic) and
- *Cyclic nucleotides* (cAMP/cGMP).
- *Arachidonic acid metabolites* (cyclooxygenase inhibitors enhance, lipoxygenase inhibitors inhibit H release).
- *Negative feedback* by e.g. H itself (H_2 receptors).
- *Diseases:* in certain (mostly atopic) diseases altered in vitro H releasability characteristics have been described, their clinical relevance being supported by in vivo studies.

The term "Releasability" has to be defined very specifically regarding different cells, stimuli, modulating agents and disease states. E.g. while indomethacin enhances H release by anti-IgE or Ca-Ionophore, it significantly inhibits C5a-induced release reactions. Our findings argue against a general reduction of membrane "stability" for explanation of increased H releasability. It can be speculated that on the basis of certain releasability patterns, a characterization of subgroups of allergic diseases might be achieved.

H is one of the best studied mediators. In the treatment of H dependent reactions the following approaches are used or under investigation:

- H synthesis inhibitors
- H release blockers
- H_1 antagonists
  (new drugs with less sedating side-effects)
- H_1 antagonists + release blockers
- Combined H_1 and H_2 antagonists.

Introduction

Although known for almost 80 years, histamine (β-imidazolyl-ethylamine) (Fig. 1 a) still remains a fascinating substance for many researchers. It was first synthesized by Windaus und Vogt [199], and its organic origin was first shown in 1910 by Ackermann, who found it in ergot [1]; in the same year Dale and Laidlaw [30] reported that in vivo effects of this substance resembled the symptoms of anaphylaxis. Two years later, Führer [51] created the name "histamine" meaning "amine of the tissues." The major steps in the development of our knowledge of histamine are shown in Table 1 [1, 2, 11, 13, 18, 51, 65, 80, 89, 90, 94, 106, 132, 154, 163, 165, 168, 186, 195, 202]; the most important have been the development of antihistamines [18, 65, 93] and the introduction of the H_1- and H_2-receptor concept [2, 13].

Table 1. Major landmarks in the history of histamine

1907	Chemical synthesis	Windaus, Vogt
1910	Organic origin	Ackermann
1910	Effects resemble anaphylaxis	Dale, Laidlaw
1912	name (= "tissue amine")	Führer
1927	Natural occurrence in fresh tissues	Best et al.
1927	"Triple response"	Lewis
1937	Antihistamine (experimental)	Bovet, Staub
1940	In vitro histamine release	G. Katz
1942	Antihistamine ("Antergan")	B. Halpern
1953	Histamine in mast cells	Riley, West
1959	Fluorometric assay	Shore, Burkhalter
1964	In vitro H release from leukocytes	Lichtenstein, Osler
1966	H_1 receptor concept	Ash, Schild
1966	Enzymatic isotopic assay	Snyder et al.
1970	Mediator of pseudo-allergic reactions	Meßmer, Lorenz et al.
1972	H_2 antagonist (burimamide)	Black et al.

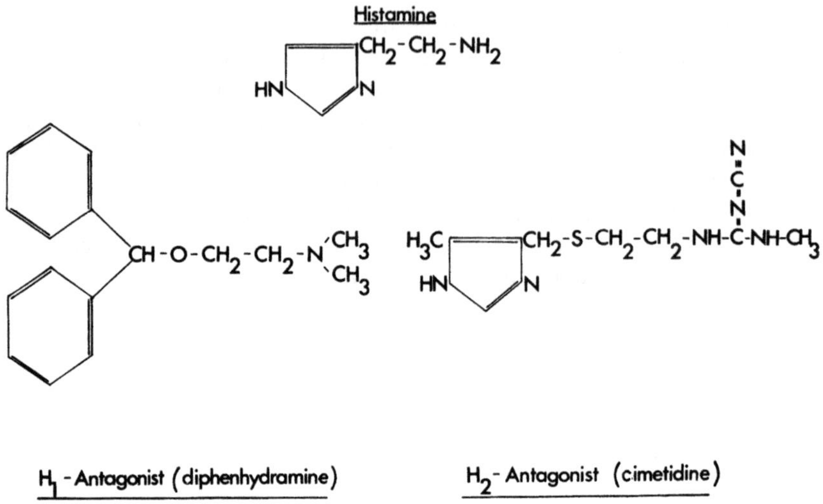

a

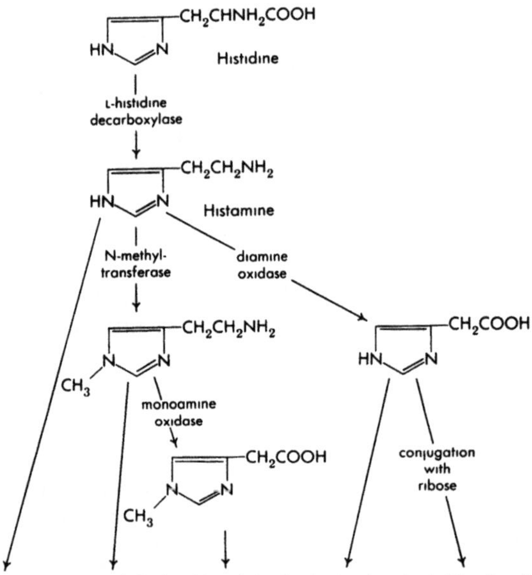

Histamine	N-Methyl-histamine	N-Methyl Imidazole Acetic Acid	Imidazole Acetic Acid	Imidazole Acetic Acid Riboside
2-3%	4-8%	42-47%	9-11%	16-23%

b

Fig. 1. **a** Chemical structure of histamine and H_1 and H_2 antagonists. **b** Histamine metabolism [from 38, 155]

Methods of Histamine Determination

There are various techniques to detect histamine in biological fluids (Table 2). For decades the bioassay, mostly performed on the guinea-pig ileum, was the standard method [2, 30, 195]. Today, the most commonly used method is a fluorometric assay which is used in several modifications [94, 165], including the automated histamine analyzer developed by Siraganian [168]. This technique is especially useful for in vitro histamine release studies from cell suspensions.

In protein-rich samples, e.g., plasma, many authors prefer the isotopic enzymatic assay, originally developed by Snyder [174] and modified by Beaven and co-workers [9, 10, 71]. Of course, histamine and especially its metabolites can be measured by high performance liquid chromatography (HPLC) [76, 174]. Perhaps in the future radioimmunoassays or enzyme immunoassays for histamine will become available [66].

Table 2. Histamine assays

Bioassay (guinea pig ileum)
Fluorometric assay
Isotopic-enzymatic assay
High performance liquid chromatography (HPLC)
Radioimmunoassay?

Histamine Distribution and Metabolism

Histamine occurs almost ubiquitously in living nature. It is contained in many plants (Table 3), bacteria, and animals [38, 62, 172, 173, 194]. The dangerous so-called scombroid fish poisoning, not infrequent in Japan, is caused by histamine intoxication due to histamine synthesizing bacteria (e.g., *E. aerogenes* or *K. pneumoniae*) in various fish [173].

Table 3. Histamine content of various plants [172, 197]

Family	Genus and species	Histamine content (μg/g)
Urticaceae	*Urtica dioica*	40–140
Chenopodiaceae	*Spinacia oleracea,*	14–290
	Ch. bonus Henricus	40
Papaveraceae	*Chelidonium maius*	10–107
Rutaceae	*Citrus vulgaris*	17
Gramineae	*Lolium perenne*	7
Leguminosae	*Trifolium repens*	13

Table 4. Human tissue histamine in different organs [127]

Organ	Histamine (μg/g)
Lung ($n = 20$)	
Trachea	9.2±2.3
Bronchi	16.7±5.3
Tissue	21.3±7.1
Stomach ($n = 40$)	
Fundus	39.6±5.4
Corpus	24.8±6.3
Antrum	17.3±3.1
Gut ($n = 10$)	
Duodenum	13.4±4.0
Jejunum	22.6±4.7
Ileum	19.2±6.4
Colon	9.9±2.7
Rectum	8.4±2.3

Of special interest in this context are reports that certain plants tend to produce increased amounts of amines under stress conditions like hyperosmolarity or SO_2 [171]. This reminds us of the human situation, where we can measure increased amounts of histamine in stress [128, 163].

In the human organism histamine is found in different concentrations in various tissues. Especially high concentrations are found in the stomach, lung tissue, and ureter [129] (see Table 4).

Histamine is metabolized via two pathways, namely a diaminooxidase pathway leading to imidazole acetic acid and a methyltransferase pathway leading to N-methylhistamine and N-methylimidazoleacetic acid (Fig. 1 b) [38, 155].

Effects of Histamine

The definition of the physiological role of histamine in health and disease remains incomplete. We know that histamine exerts powerful effects mainly by two receptors (Table 5) [13, 38, 52]. For each receptor specific antagonists are available (Table 6). The stimulatory or inhibitory effects of histamine on various organs or cells are summarized in Table 7.

The role of histamine as a mediator of immediate-type hypersensitivity diseases (both allergic and pseudo-allergic in origin) is quite well established. The "triple response" according to Lewis [89] involves initial redness, axon reflex, and wheal formation – the typical "wheal and flare" reaction (Fig. 2). This proinflammatory effect predominantly involves H_1 receptors on mucosal cells, on the smooth muscle of gut and bronchi, and on the vascular endothelium [5, 30, 38, 97, 139, 202, 205] but also H_2 receptors on skin vessels [100].

Table 5. Physiological and pathophysiological histamine effects

Proinflammatory	$H_1 + H_2$
Antiinflammatory	H_2
Gastric secretion	H_2
Cardial conduction	$H_1 + H_2$
Central neurotransmitter?	H_3 ?

Table 6. Histamine H_1 and H_2 agonists and antagonists

	H_1		H_2
Agonists	2-Methyl-histamine		4-Methyl-histamine
	2-2-Pyridylethylamine		Impromidine
	2-2-Thiazolylethylamine		Dimaprit
Antagonists	Classical antihistamines		Burimamide
	– Ethanolamines	(e.g., Diphenhydramine)	Metiamide
	– Alkylamines	(e.g., Dimetindene)	Cimetidine
	– Ethylenediamines	(e.g., Bamipine)	Ranitidine
	– Phenothiazines	(e.g., Promethazine)	
	– Others	(Clemastine)	
	Newer nonsedating drugs		
	– Terfenadine		
	– Astemizole		

Table 7. Histamine effects in human organs

Organ	Stimulatory	Inhibitory	None/negligible
Vessels			
Large veins (> 80 μm)	+	–	–
Arterioles, venules (20–30 μm)	–	+	–
Permeability of "capillaries" (postcapillary venules)	+	–	–
Extravascular smooth muscle			
Bronchi, gut	+	–	–
Uterus, bladder, gallbladder, iris	–	–	+
Stomach (secretion)	+	–	–
Salivary glands	+	–	–
Heart			
Rate, force, output	+	–	–
AV conduction	–	+	–
Ventricular arrhythmia	+	–	–
Nervous system			
Sensory fibers	+	–	–
Central effects	(+) ?	–	–
Endocrine system			
(adrenal medulla)	–	–	+
Leukocytes	–	+	–

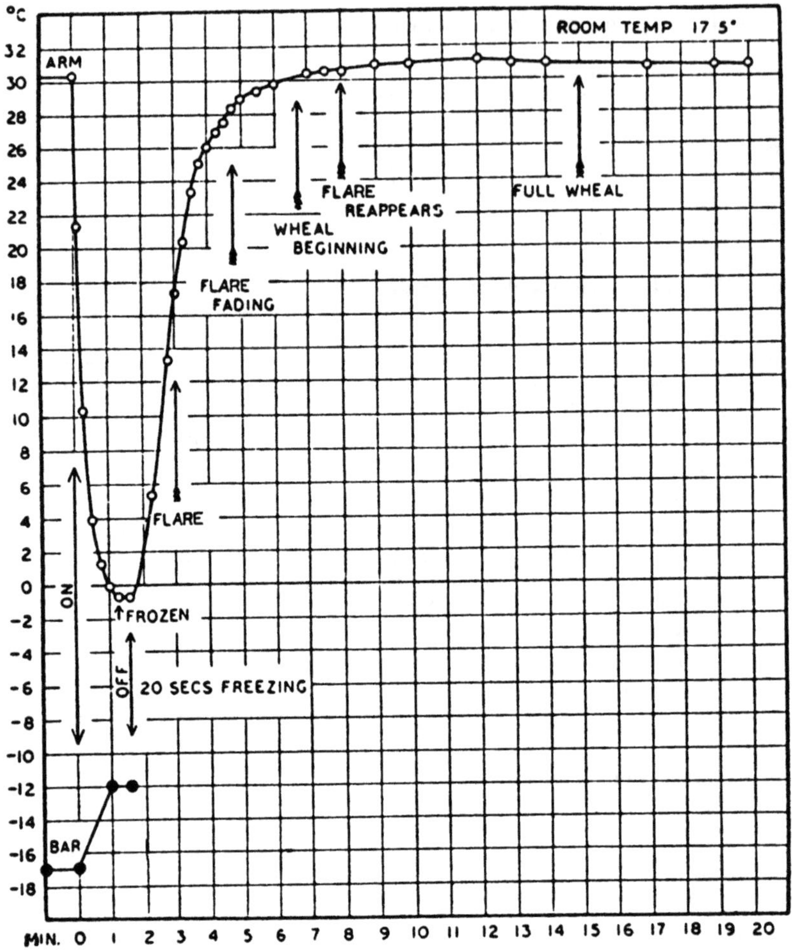

Fig. 2. Diagram from the original work of Lewis on the wheal and flare response after application of freezing temperature to the skin [89]

Similarly well defined is the H_2-mediated role of histamine in the induction of gastric acid secretion [13, 38]. Less well defined is the clinical relevance of histamine receptors on the heart. Here atrial H_1 receptors seem to mediate negative dromotropic effects, while H_2 agonists have positive inotropic effects but at the same time can induce ventricular arrhythmia [88, 115] or be involved in myocardial ischemia [8].

Histamine exerts powerful effects on peripheral nerves, namely sensory fibers inducing itch sensations [31, 63, 64, 176]. Its role in the central nervous system as a possible neurotransmitter substance has been shown in many animals: it influences behavior and arousal reactions, not all of which can be blocked by classical H_1 or H_2 antagonists [112, 181]. This has led to the postulation of a possible new class of "H_3" receptors [53, 161]. Little is known about

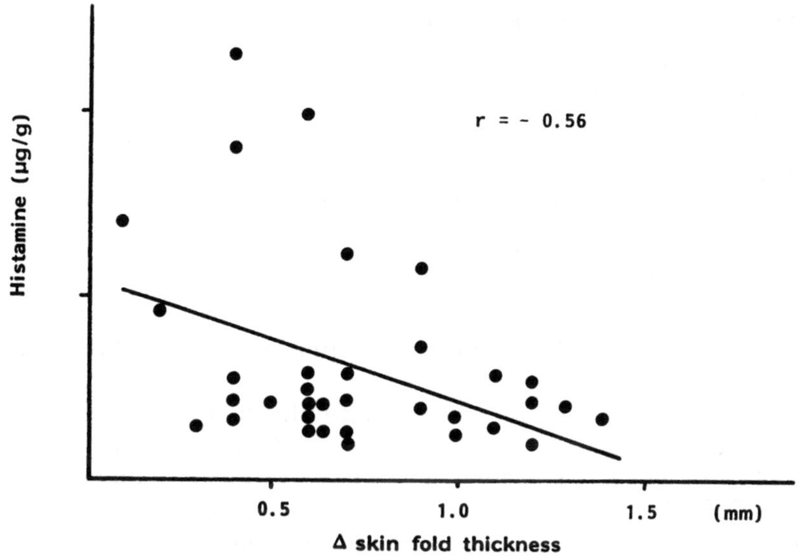

Fig. 3. Correlation between intensity of allergic contact dermatitis (guinea pigs sensitized to dinitrochlorobenzene, measured as increase in skin fold thickness after 48 h) and skin histamine content

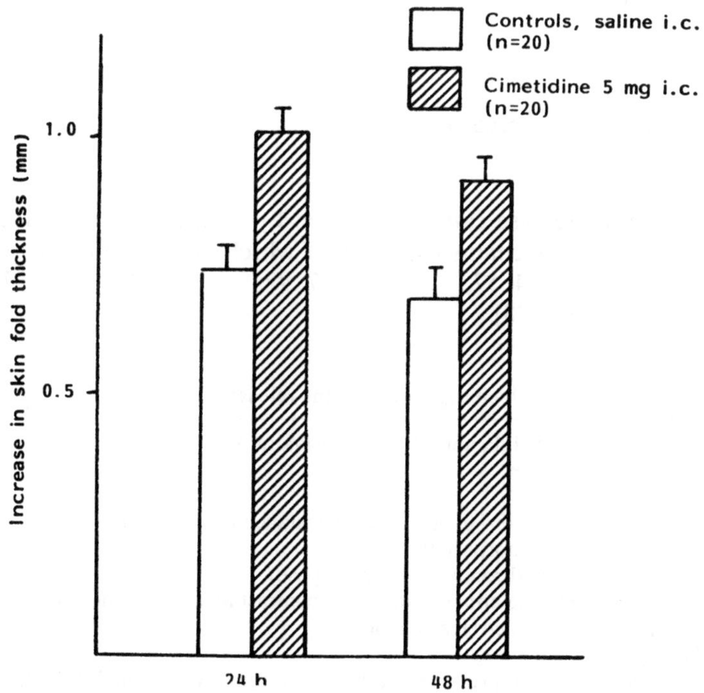

Fig. 4. Influence of intradermal pretreatment with the H_2 antagonist cimetidine upon intensity of allergic contact dermatitis (DNCB) in guinea pigs

Table 8. Immune reactions inhibited by histamine

Mast cells and basophils (mediator release)
Neutrophil function (chemotaxis, phagocytosis, enzyme release)
Eosinophils
Macrophages (complement production)
Lymphocyte proliferation and lymphokine production
Lymphocyte cytotoxicity
Concanavalin A-induced suppressor cell activity

possible histamine effects in wound healing and epidermal proliferation [38, 99, 151].

Recent interest has focused on anti-inflammatory effects of histamine as a modulator of immune reactions acting predominantly on H_2 receptors on the surface of leukocytes, thereby inhibiting a variety of immune reactions (Table 8) [17, 21, 91, 120–122, 148, 150, 160]. These are not only in vitro data. Like other groups [3, 148], we too were able to inhibit the induction of contact allergic reactions in guinea pigs by histamine [104]. There was an indirect correlation between skin histamine content and the intensity of contact dermatitis reactions (Fig. 3). At the same time, after pretreatment with an H_2 antagonist (cimetidine), the skin fold thickness as a parameter of contact dermatitis was significantly increased (Fig. 4). The negative effect of histamine upon mast cell mediator release will be discussed later.

Histamine Release

Histamine release can be triggered by a variety of substances (Table 9) acting by different mechanisms, many of which are by no means yet established [5, 6, 23, 33, 46, 48, 54, 57, 73, 84, 86, 87, 92, 96, 110, 119, 123, 127, 134, 135, 149, 157, 169, 183, 192, 198].

Table 9. Stimuli which trigger histamine release

IgE (allergen, anti-IgE, anti-εR, Concanavalin A)
Calcium-Ionophore
Complement
Basic compounds (48/80, polylysine, substance P, synacthen)
Opiates (codeine, morphine)
Enzymes (trypsin, thrombin, phospholipase)
Drugs (relaxants, gelatin, radiographic contrast media, i.v. anesthetics)
Cytokines (histamine-releasing factor)
Detergents
Physical (cold, heat, pressure, mechanical trauma, vibration, UV light)
Chemical (hyperosmolar, acid, and alkaline solutions)
Hypoxia

Table 10. Differences between mast cells and basophils regarding mediator release (data from Lichtenstein et al., Bienenstock et al., Pearce et al.)

	Connective tissue mast cells	Mucosal mast cells	Basophils
Releasers			
48/80	+	–	–
Anti-IgE	+	+	+
Ionophores	+	+	+
C5a	+	(±)	+
Codeine	+	–	–
Kinin	+	–	–
Substance P	+	–	–
Trypsin	+	±	+
Inhibitors			
Glucocorticoids	–	+	+
Cromolyn	+	±	–
Ketotifen	+	?	+
Doxantrazole	+	+	?
ETYA	+	?	+
Histamine	±	?	+
Quercetin	+	+	+

When we talk about histamine release and the effects of different triggers or inhibitors we have to differentiate clearly between different species and different types of histamine-containing cells [40]. Differentiation between "connective tissue mast cells" = "heparin-containing mast cells" (corresponding to rat peritoneal mast cells) and "mucosal mast cells" = "chondroitin sulfate-containing mast cells" (similar to bone marrow-derived mast cells in the mouse) seems especially important. Table 10 shows a simplified review of the differences between various histamine-containing cells with regard to different releasers and inhibitors; most of the relevant work has been performed by the groups of Lichtenstein [92], Bienenstock [12], and Pearce [41, 117].

Factors Influencing Histamine Releasability

Apart from the above-mentioned differences regarding species and the origin of cell populations, there are interindividual differences in the amount of histamine released in response to the same stimulus. This characteristic has been called "*releasability*" [26, 27] and is defined as the *capacity of mediator-secreting cells to release preformed or newly synthesized mediators* [27, 137, 143]. Histamine is one of the best studied substances. The best established mechanism is the IgE-mediated reaction. There are, however, other stimuli and other mediators of possible clinical importance.

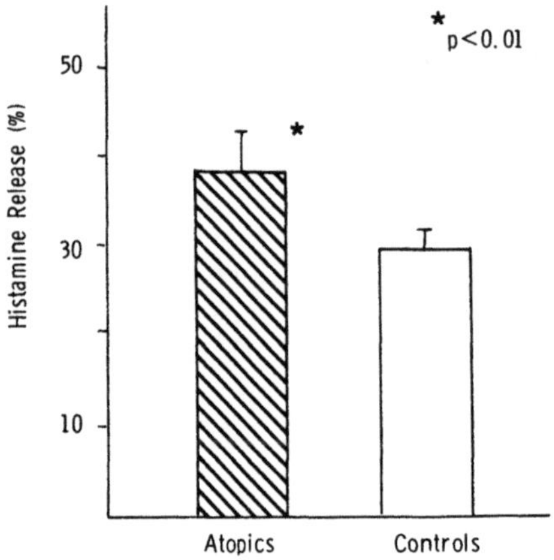

Fig. 5. Speed of histamine release: comparison of histamine release occurring within the first 5 min after anti-IgE-stimulation from basophils of atopics and normal individuals [192]

Table 11. Factors influencing histamine releasability

Nerval influence (autonomic, endorphins, neuropeptides)
Cyclic nucleotide system (cAMP/cGMP)
Arachidonic acid metabolites
Negative feedback
Age
Sex
Microbial infection
Disease

The most important clinically relevant aspects of mediator release are *quantity* (the total amount of mediators) and *quality* (the nature of different mediators or the combination of mediators released). The *speed* of the release reaction might also be a critical factor. In a recent study we found a significantly increased speed of histamine release during the first 5 min after stimulation with anti-IgE in atopics compared with nonatopic controls (Fig. 5) [192]. The duration of the *refractory phase* might prove to be a critical factor for clinical effects of mediator release [48, 81, 145, 205]. The *sensitivity of certain end-organs or cells* to histamine or other mediators influences the outcome of the clinical reaction too; this parameter has been found to be changed in some allergic conditions [29, 114, 176, 195, 207]. Melanin pigmentation might equally influence histamine reactions in the skin [189].

The origin and nature of increased releasability is not known. A variety of factors have been found to influence "releasability" of histamine-secreting cells (Table 11). In the following the most important aspects of this question will be briefly discussed.

Cyclic Nucleotide System

Leukocytes of atopic individuals show a decreased response of cyclic adenosine monophosphate (cAMP) to *β*-adrenergic stimuli [21, 22, 67, 116, 131, 138]. This impaired β-adrenergic reactivity might be explained by the findings of Hanifin, who described elevated levels of the cAMP-inactivating enzyme phosphodiesterase in leukocytes of patients with atopic eczema [67], this marker already being present in neonates [70].

Autonomic Nervous System

Since the first description of the β-adrenergic blockade as a possible explanation for the atopic abnormality in bronchial asthma by Szentivanyi [180], many authors have put forward the concept of a dysregulation of the autonomic nervous system in patients with atopic eczema [7, 15, 19, 67, 85, 116, 124, 139, 143, 203]. Together with a decreased cAMP response to adrenergic stimuli we observed an increased response of cGMP to cholinergic stimulation [138].

There are controversial data regarding the effect of cholinergic stimulation upon histamine release from mast cells and basophils in different species [14, 22, 43, 76, 77, 157, 177]. We found significant augmentation of anti-IgE-induced histamine release from basophils after incubation in vitro with carbamylcholine [141], especially when the suspensions were preincubated for 10 min with carbamylcholine. This increase was more pronounced in atopics than normals (Fig. 6). When the pretreatment with carbamylcholine was combined with the muscarinic antagonist atropine the cholinergic enhancement was abolished (Fig. 7), suggesting a specific effect of carbamylcholine on muscarinic receptors of basophil leukocytes in these patients. These in vitro observations of autonomic mediator dysregulation are supported by in vivo studies showing increased responses of pupillary constriction or blood pressure to α-adrenergic and cholinergic stimulation in atopic individuals [69].

The above findings might be important with regard to the well-known clinical influence of psychosomatic interactions in atopic diseases [15, 146, 197].

Negative Feedback Mechanism

Histamine is able to inhibit its own release (Fig. 8) when added to an anti-IgE-stimulated basophil suspension [91]. This effect seems to be an H_2-mediated reaction; it can be induced by the specific H_2 agonist impromidine (Fig. 9) and blocked by cimetidine, leading to increased histamine release [182]. The concentrations necessary to block release reactions are rather high; however, in the direct environment of the mast cell, this effect might play a physiological role under in vivo conditions.

Arachidonic Acid Metabolites

Arachidonic acid metabolites obviously play a regulating role in mediator release [54, 59, 84, 101, 118, 143, 144, 177, 190]. The precise role of single products

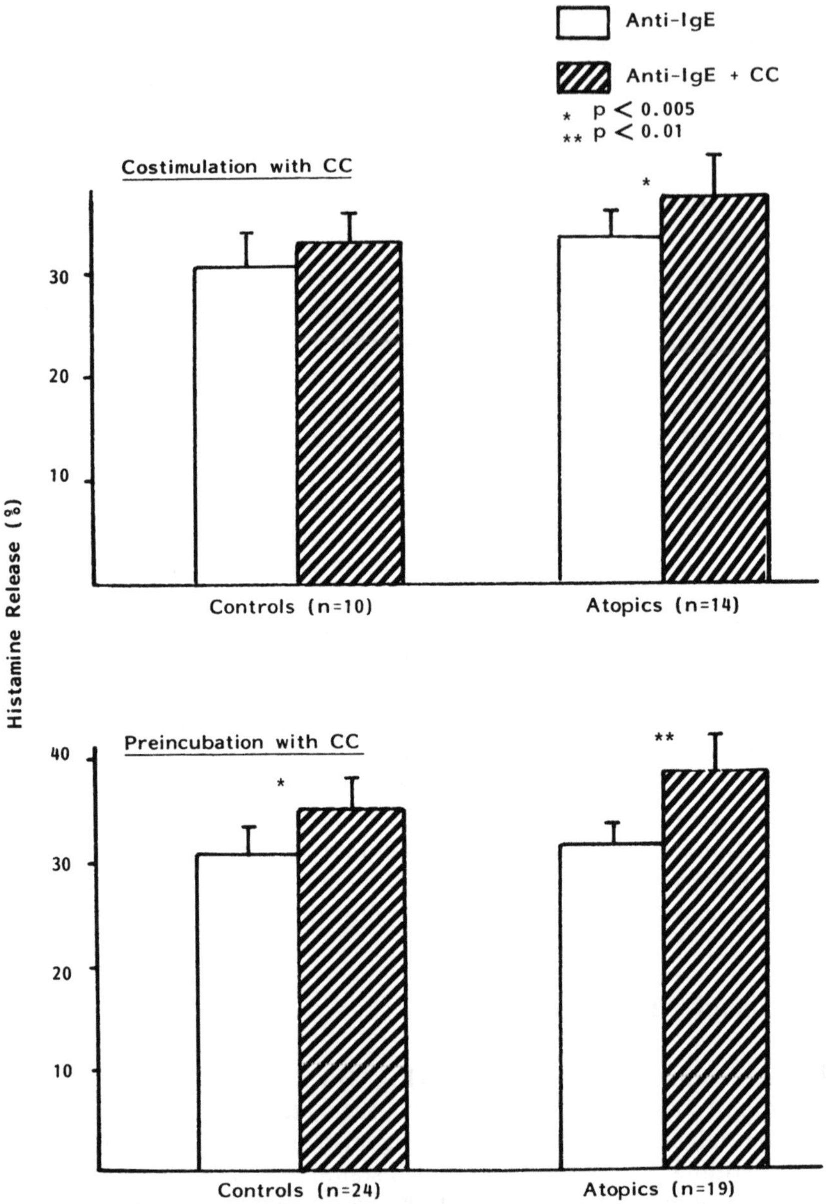

Fig. 6. Influence of cholinergic stimulation using carbamylcholine (*CC*) in vitro upon anti-IgE-induced histamine release from basophils of atopics and normals. There is a significant increase after preincubation of the cell suspensions with carbamylcholine

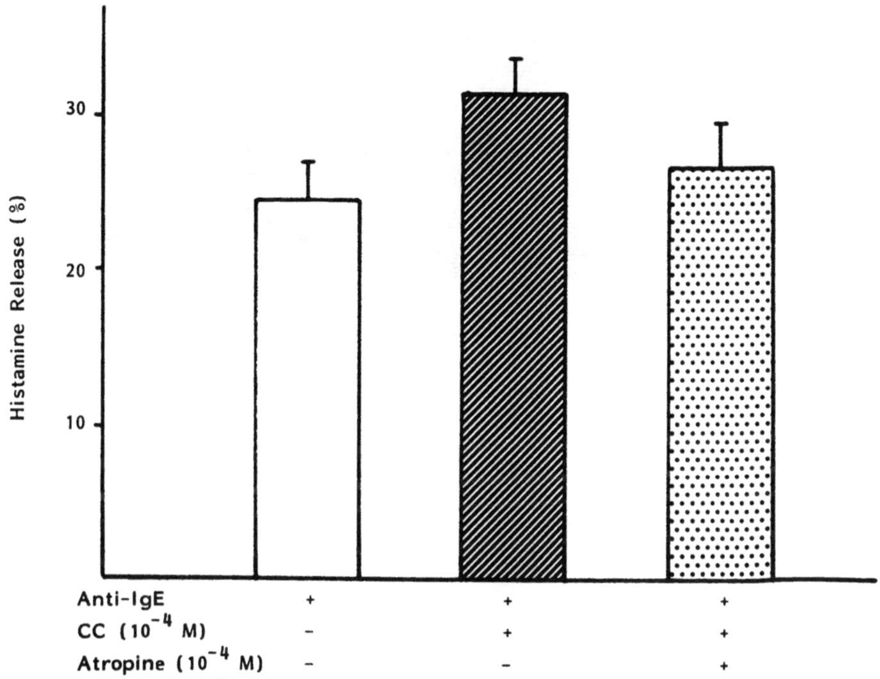

Fig. 7. The addition of atropine is able to abolish the enhancing effect of carbamylcholine (*CC*) upon anti-IgE-induced histamine release in vitro ($n = 15$)

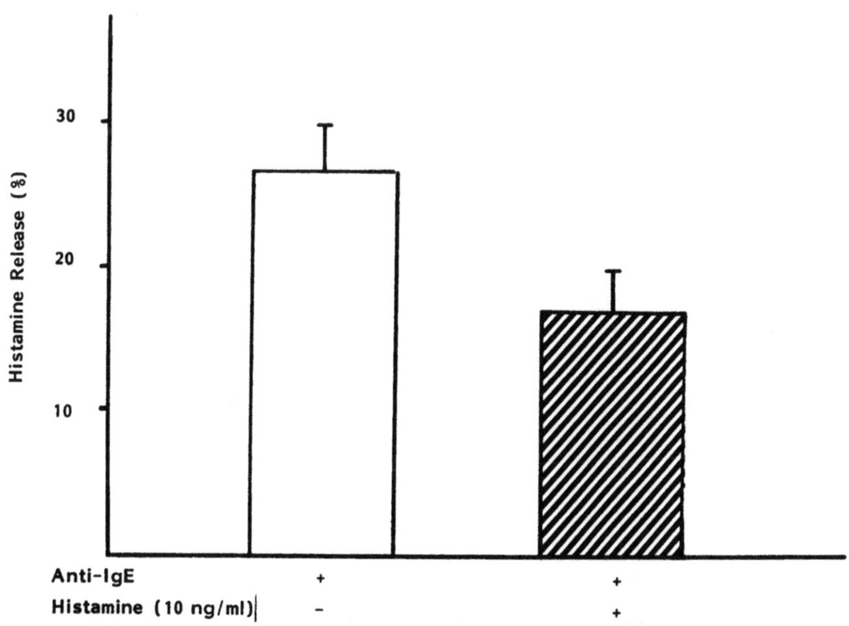

Fig. 8. Histamine is able to inhibit its own release: after preincubation with histamine there is significantly reduced histamine release from basophil leukocytes in vitro ($n = 15$)

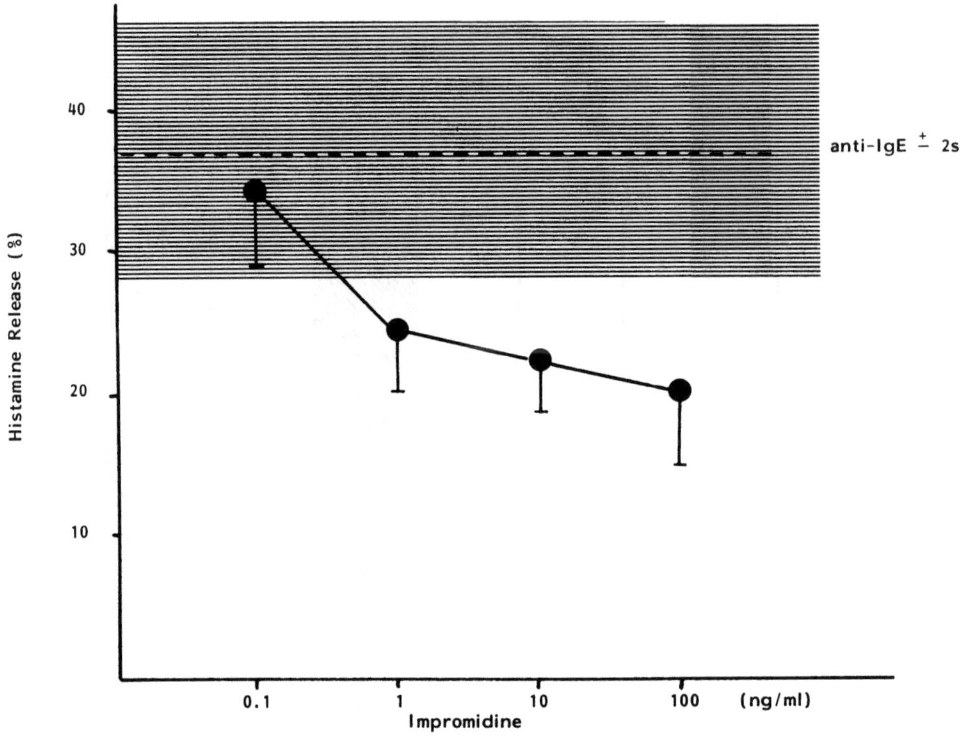

Fig. 9. Dose-dependent inhibition of histamine release from human leukocytes by the H_2 agonist impromidine

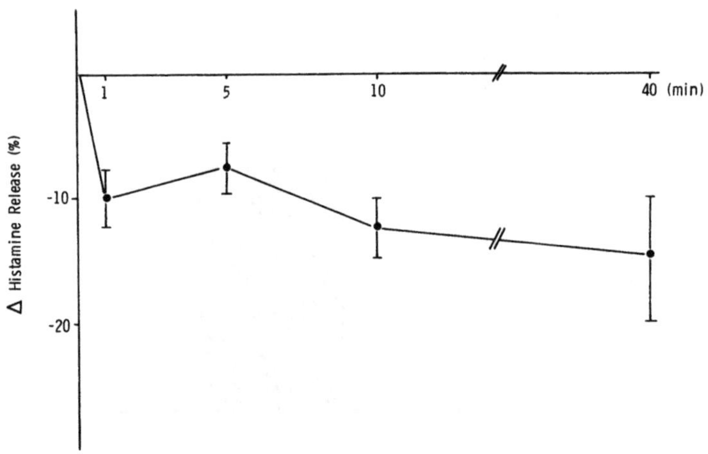

Fig. 10. Inhibition of anti-IgE-induced histamine release from human basophils in vitro by exogenous addition of PGE 2 [192]

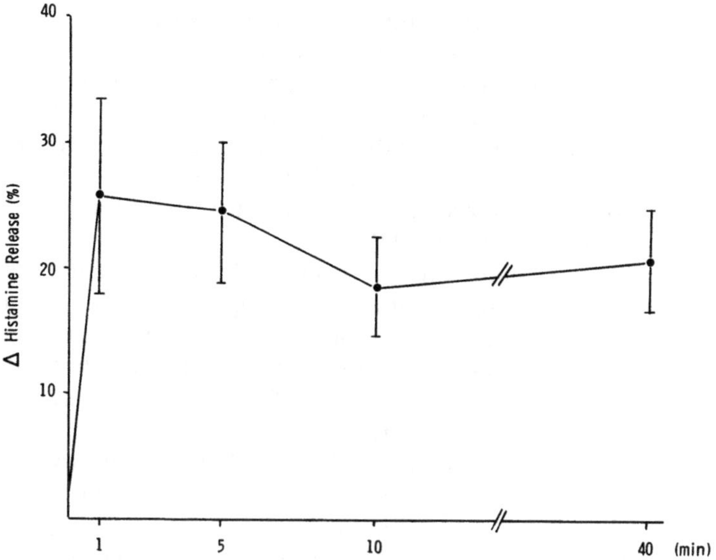

Fig. 11. Enhancement of anti-IgE-induced histamine release from basophil leukocytes in vitro by preincubation with the cyclooxygenase inhibitor indomethacin [192]

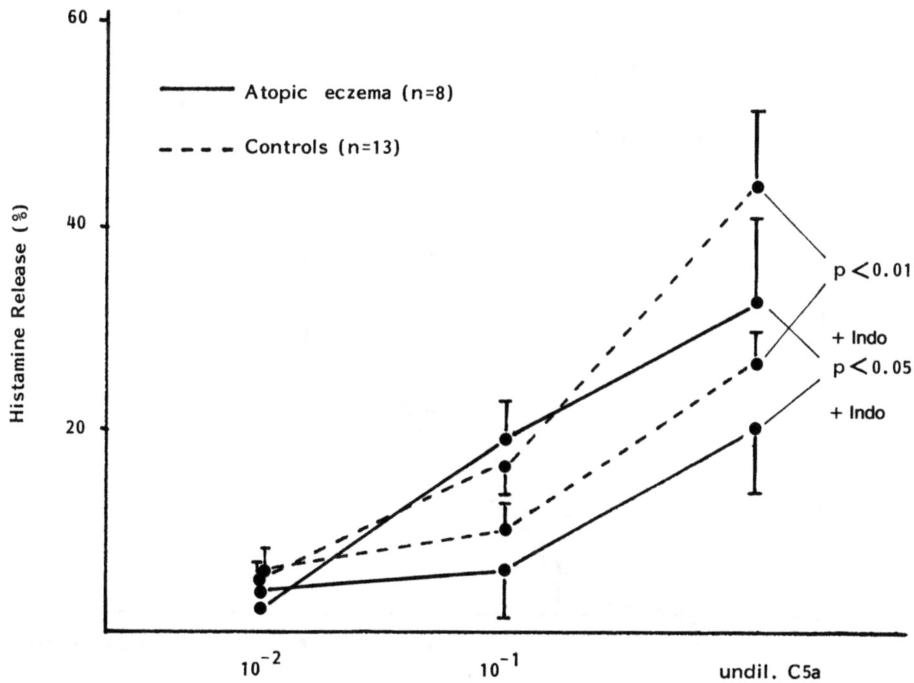

Fig. 12. While indomethacin (Indo) increases anti-IgE-induced histamine release, it significantly inhibits release reactions induced by activated complement (C5a) both in atopics and normals [144]

of the cyclooxygenase or lipoxygenase pathway in different pathological conditions, however, has not yet been established.

Among prostaglandins, PGE_2 inhibits histamine release induced by various stimulators in atopics and normals after exogenous addition (Fig. 10). Concomitantly with anti-IgE induced histamine release we observed a slight increase in PGE_2 production by the leukocyte suspension. This endogenous PGE_2 production was increased after preincubation with reduced glutathione, a coenzyme of PGE_2 isomerase [192].

On the other hand, cyclooxygenase inhibitors enhance histamine release, especially after anti-IgE stimulation (Fig. 11). While indomethacin enhances histamine release to a variety of stimuli it is surprising to note that it clearly inhibits complement-induced histamine reactions in both atopics and normals [45, 144] (Fig. 12). This might be of therapeutic interest in complement-dependent diseases, e.g., urticarial vasculitis.

It becomes clear from these findings that releasability is not a single parameter and not only a "leakage of mast cells," but rather has to be evaluated differently for each specific stimulus.

Lipoxygenase inhibitors like eicosatetraenoic acid inhibit histamine release in a dose-dependent fashion [92] in atopics and normals (Fig. 13). The endogenous lipoxygenase inhibitor 15-HETE, however, showed no inhibitory effect

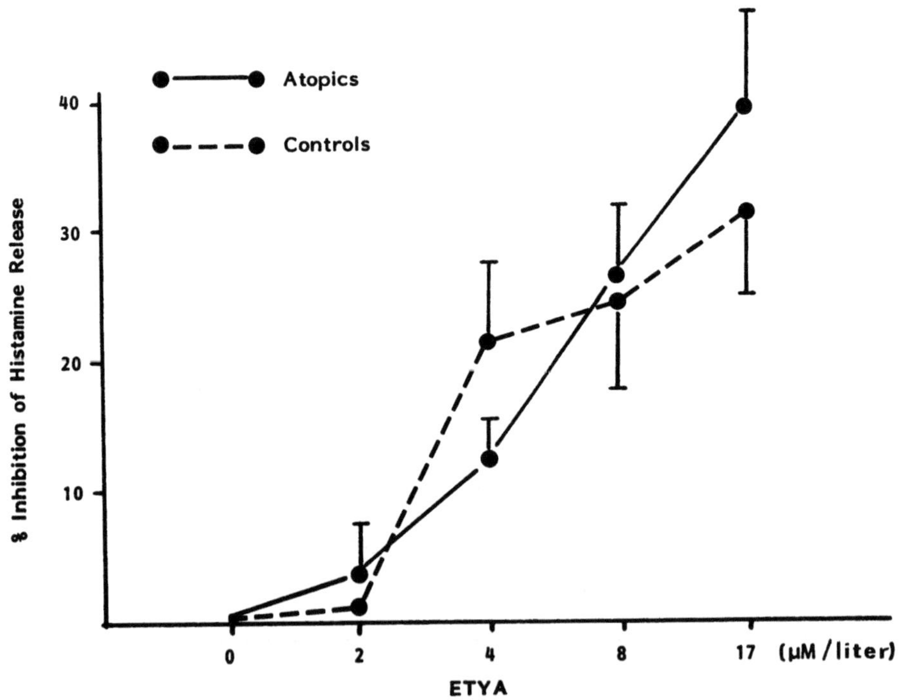

Fig. 13. Dose-dependent inhibition of anti-IgE-induced histamine release from human leukocytes by exogenous addition of the lipoxygenase inhibitor eicosatetrayonic acid (*ETYA*) ($n = 8$) [37]

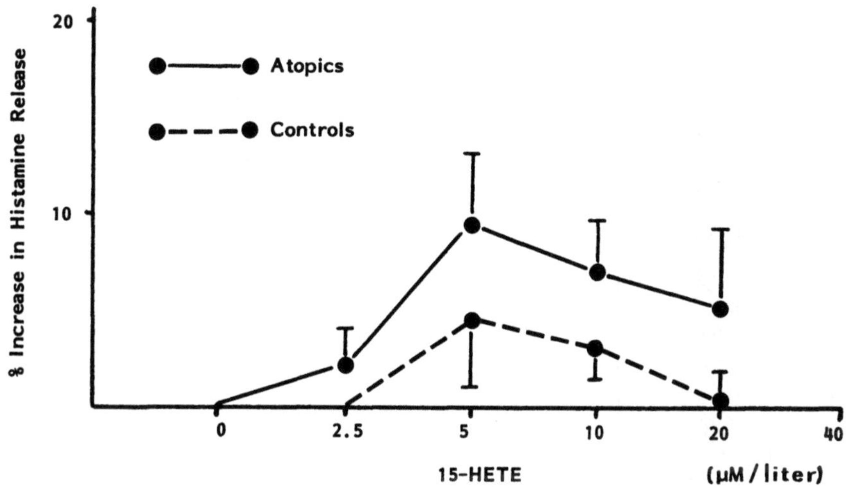

Fig. 14. Slightly enhancing effect of preincubation with the endogenous lipoxygenase inhibitor 15-hydroxyeicosatetraenoic acid (*15-HETE*) on anti-IgE-induced histamine release from peripheral leukocytes of atopics ($n = 13$) and normals ($n = 5$)

upon histamine release; on the contrary, there was a slight enhancing effect which was more pronounced in the atopic population (Fig. 14). 15-HETE was also able to partially reverse the inhibitory effect of the lipoxygenase inhibitor nordihydroguaretic acid upon histamine release (Fig. 15).

Conditions with Altered Histamine Releasability

It has been shown by many groups that under certain conditions and especially in atopic diseases patients show altered releasability patterns (Table 12) [4, 22,

Table 12. Histamine releasability of peripheral basophils: clinical studies using anti-IgE as stimulus

Disease	Releasability	Authors
Urticaria	Decreased	Kern and Lichtenstein [82]
Intrinsic asthma	Decreased	Virchow and Strassburg [191]
Intrinsic asthma	Normal	Findlay and Lichtenstein [47]
Intrinsic asthma	Increased	Assem and Attallah [4]
"Atopy"	No correlation to serum IgE	Conroy et al. [26]
Extrinsic asthma	Decreased	Ring et al. [136]
Allergic rhinitis	Increased	Assem and Attallah [4]
Atopic eczema	Increased	Ring [138]
Atopic eczema	Increased	Venencie et al. [190]
Atopic eczema	Increased	Butler et al. [22]
Atopic eczema	Increased	Marone et al. [102]
Atopic eczema	Increased	Ring and Walz [144]

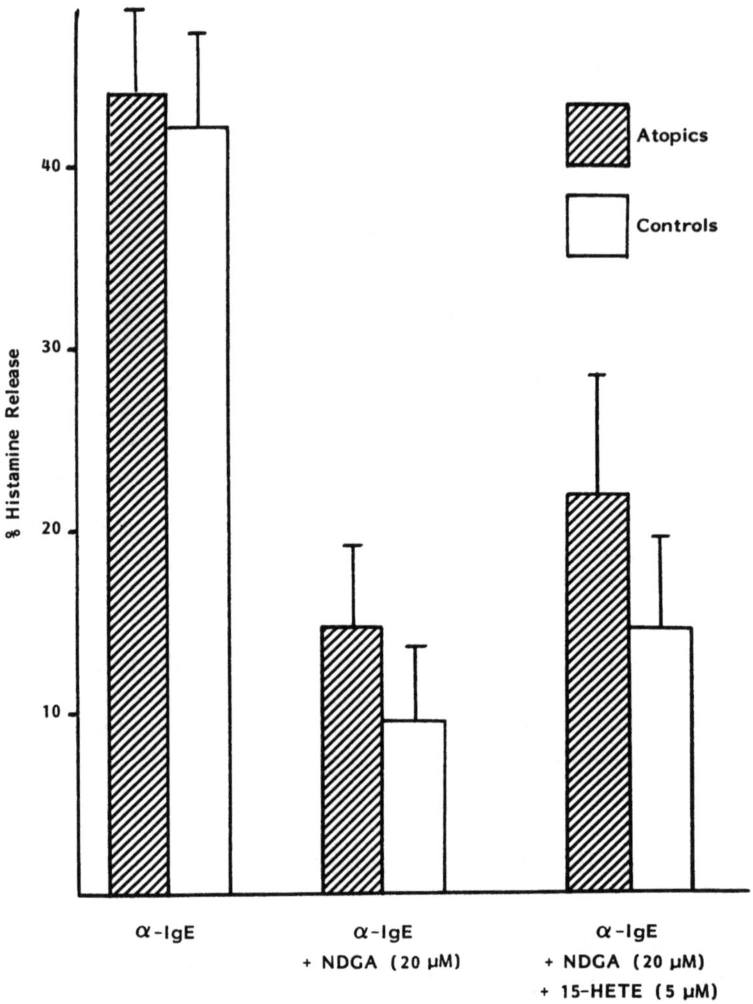

Fig. 15. Partial reversal by preincubation with 15-HETE of the inhibitory effect of nordihydroguaretic acid (*NDGA*) upon anti-IgE-induced histamine release (atopics: $n = 8$; normals: $n = 5$)

26, 47, 82, 102, 136, 137, 144, 188, 189]. In most studies basophils of atopic individuals released increased amounts of histamine after stimulation with anti-IgE and other stimuli.

Conditions with a known histamine influence or elevated histamine levels in the blood or tissues are listed in Table 13 [10, 34, 36, 39, 49, 56, 58, 71, 74, 75, 79, 83, 108, 110, 111, 119, 130, 133, 140, 162, 166, 179, 185, 201].

It might be of interest that stress alone is sufficient to induce histamine release [129], as can be seen from the example of a patient who developed a striking increase in plasma histamine at a dental surgery when pain occurred during the treatment (Fig. 16).

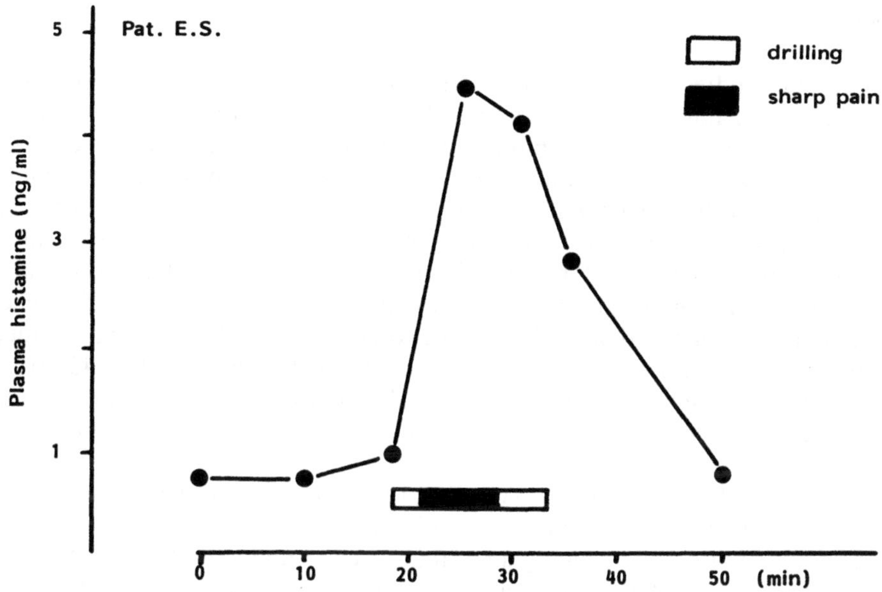

Fig. 16. Increase in plasma histamine concentration in a patient undergoing dental treatment without further medication [145]

Table 13. Conditions with known histamine influence or histamine elevation

Urticaria
Anaphylactoid reactions (allergic, pseudo-allergic)
Itch
Bronchial asthma
Atopic eczema
Gastric ulcer
Mastocytosis
Chronic myeloid leukemia
Ulcerative colitis
Wound healing?
Keloid formation?

Microbial Infection

Several bacterial and viral infections are connected with increased histamine releasability patterns in vitro and in animal experiments [21, 72, 103].

Age

Among the factors influencing histamine releasability, age has to be considered. Marone et al. have found that histamine releasability tends to increase with age [101]. Therefore studies comparing histamine releasability have to be performed with carefully age-matched controls.

Sex

In several studies we found significantly increased histamine release from the leukocytes of female donors compared with males of the same control or patient group (Fig. 17). In preliminary studies we observed that androgen, namely dihydrotestosterone can inhibit anti-IgE-induced histamine release from human basophils [60]. This led us to speculate about possible influences of androgenic hormones in allergic diseases, especially with regard to the clinical finding that atopic eczema often clears during puberty and that there is a clear predominance of females among adult patients while there is no sex difference in the frequency of the disease in childhood [19, 124, 203]. Hormonal influences upon allergic or immune reactions merit further investigation [16, 42, 61, 170]. Histamine is likely to be involved in prolactin secretion [164]. The antiandrogenic effect of cimetidine seems to be independent of its H_2 antagonist action [200].

It is well known that dry skin is a prerequisite and crucial factor in the pathogenesis of atopic eczema [19, 124]. Patients with atopic eczema have significantly smaller sebaceous glands than the normal population [55]. So one might speculate that a relative androgen deficiency could be a pathogenic factor in atopic eczema.

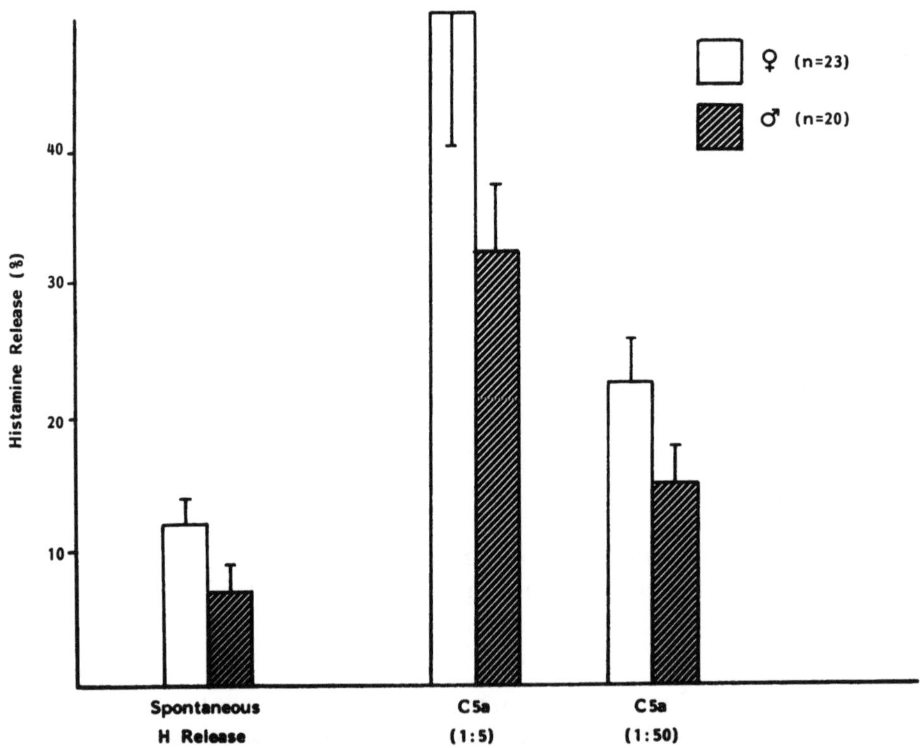

Fig. 17. Comparison of C5a-induced histamine release from leukocytes of male and female donors. There are significantly higher values in females

Therapeutic Approaches

Therapeutic approaches to histamine-mediated diseases can act at three levels, namely histamine synthesis inhibition, histamine release blockade, and histamine antagonism at the end-organ (Table 14).

Histamine synthesis inhibitors include drugs inhibiting the enzyme histidine decarboxylase. There are so far no convincing clinical studies with these drugs. In a study of short-term treatment with the HDC-blocker (+)-catechin in patients with food allergy [126], we found a significant decrease in gastric mast cell histamine content (Fig. 18). However, long-term clinical studies should be performed before this treatment can be recommended for allergic conditions.

Mast cell blockers play a central role in the prophylaxis of allergic reactions. The cromoglycate receptor seems to be involved in calcium binding [105]. Newer derivatives of cromolyn acting on different mast cell subpopulations are undergoing clinical trials and seem promising, e.g., nedocromil sodium. Many drugs acting by different mechanisms also have potent mast cell blocking effects, like glucocorticosteroids (on mucosal mast cells and basophils) [156] or drugs acting at the cAMP level (e.g., β_2 agonists).

Interesting drugs for clinical research include flavonoids [107], calcium antagonists [25], lipoxygenase inhibitors, and immunomodulators such as inosiplex, which was recently shown by Schmutzler et al. [158] to inhibit histamine release.

Histamine antagonists have been in clinical use since 1942. They represent powerful drugs in the treatment of acute urticaria and mild anaphylactoid re-

Table 14. Therapeutic approaches in histamine-mediated diseases (clinical and experimental)

Histamine synthesis inhibitors
- Tritoqualine (?)
- (+)-Catechin

Histamine release blockers
- DNCG
- Corticosteroids
- cAMP-active drugs (β_2 agonists, theophylline, PGE_2)
- ATPase inhibitors (ouabain)
- Flavonoids
- Ca antagonists
- Inosiplex
- Lipoxygenase inhibitors (ETYA)

Histamine antagonists
- H_1 antagonists
- H_1 antagonists without central effects
- H_1 antagonists + H release blockers
- H_2 antagonists
- H_1 + H_2 antagonists

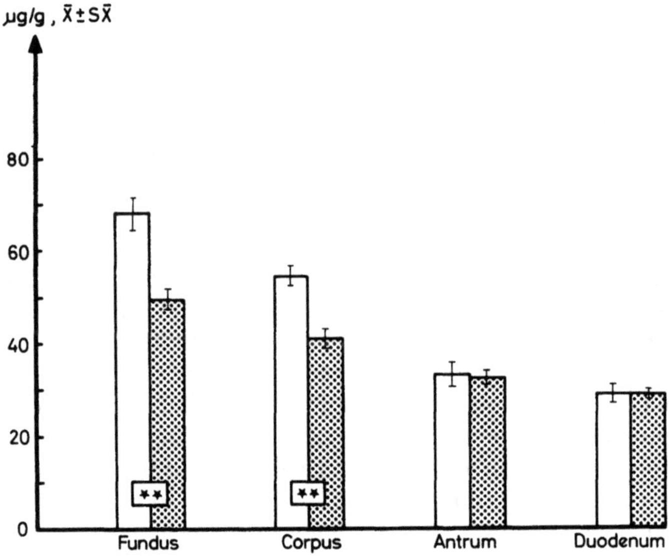

Fig. 18. During 8 days treatment of volunteers with the histidine decarboxylase inhibitor (+)-catechin there is a significant decrease in total histamine content of gastric mucosa [126]

actions. Their major drawback is the relatively pronounced sedative side-effect [38].

Many other drugs, e.g., dopamine [24] or psychopharmacological agents [159], are able to suppress histamine-induced skin reactions. This is of eminent practical importance with regard to skin test procedures [139, 159].

In recent years new H_1 antagonists have been synthesized (e.g., terfenadine or astemizole) which act specifically with the H_1 receptor and have almost no sedative side-effects in that they do not cross the blood-brain barrier. Drugs simultaneously showing histamine antagonistic effects and mast cell blocking properties are another new development; here ketotifen and oxatomide have to be mentioned.

The role of histamine H_2 antagonists in allergic diseases is still controversial. There are several reports of beneficial effects of H_2 antagonists (mostly combined with H_1 antagonists) in urticaria and anaphylactoid reactions [20, 35, 44, 95, 98, 109, 147]. Many controlled studies have led to divergent results: in some placebo-controlled studies there was a significant improvement in the H_1-H_2 combination group compared with H_1 antagonists alone [109], whereas in other studies a significant difference was not observed [28, 32, 50].

Our group was involved in a multicenter trial in Germany. In this study selected patients with chronic urticaria were treated in a cross-over protocol for 4 weeks each, with either placebo, the H_1 antagonist chlorpheniramine, or the combined H_1-H_2 regimen chlorpheniramine plus cimetidine. The efficacy was evaluated using a scoring system counting wheals and assessing subjective irritation by the disease. During the 4-week cross-over protocol there was no significant difference between the combined group and the group receiving H_1 antagonist alone, results in both groups being significantly superior to the placebo group. However, in the parameters "body surface involved" and "irritation by wheals" there was a trend toward greater efficacy of the combined H_1-H_2 regimen.

Following the period of three 4 week cross-over protocols, the patients were treated for another 3 months with one regimen of their own choice. None of the patients selected placebo treatment. Approximately half requested H_1 antagonists, the other half the combined treatment. When these groups were compared during another 3 months of follow-up, there was a markedly more pronounced improvement in the combined treatment group; however, these results were not statistically significant. Nevertheless, one can safely state that among patients with chronic urticaria there is a subgroup who clearly benefit from combined H_1-H_2 antagonist treatment. In certain cases H_2 antagonists alone have been effective [44].

Anaphylactoid reactions to a variety of drugs have been shown to be mediated by histamine [33, 34, 96, 106, 110, 119, 134]. In gelatine-induced anaphylactoid reactions in man [95], as after intravenous narcotics [119], it was found that anaphylactoid reactions were reduced significantly when pretreatment was given with combined H_1-H_2 antagonists. This led us to perform a similar study involving H_1-H_2 antagonists as a pretreatment regimen for

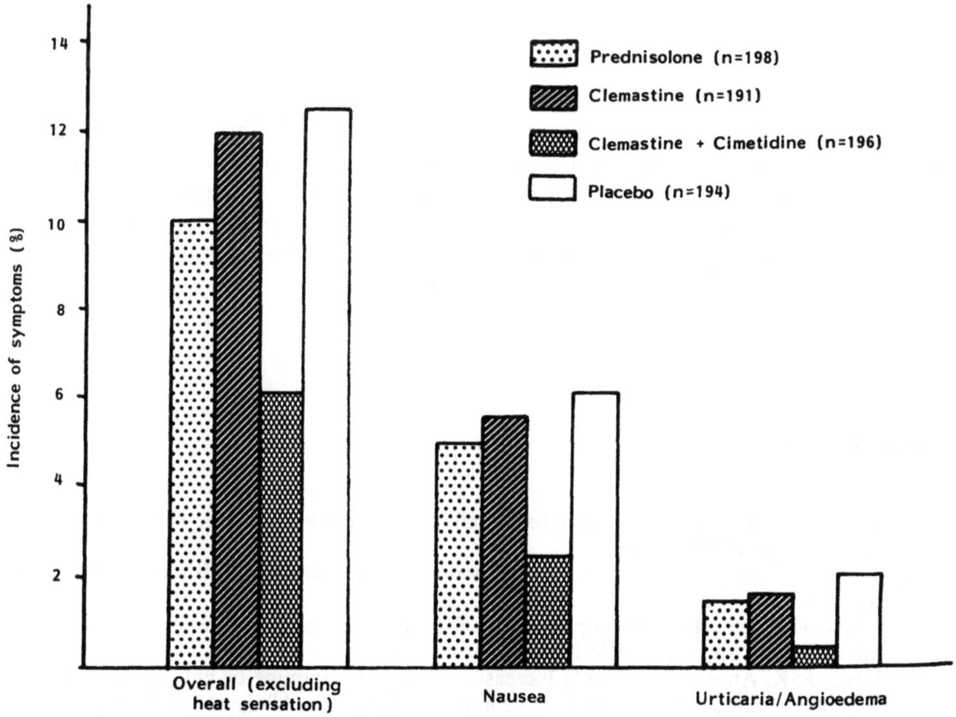

Fig. 19. Effect of intravenous prophylaxis with different regimens upon the incidence of subjective and objective side-reactions to radiographic contrast media infusion [together with Rothenberger and Clauß, 142]

Table 15. Prophylactic intravenous pretreatment in four groups of patients prior to infusion of 100 ml 60% meglumine diatrizoate (Urovist)

	I (n = 198)	II (n = 191)	III (n = 196)	IV (n = 194)
Pretreatment	Prednisolone	Clemastine	Clemastine + cimetidine	Saline
Trade name	Solu-Decortin	Tavegil	Tavegil + Tagamet	–
Dose	250 mg	0.03 mg/kg	0.03 mg/kg + 5 mg/kg[a]	5 ml 0.9%

[a] In patients with impaired creatinine clearance dose was reduced to 2 mg/kg

prophylaxis of radiographic contrast media (RCM)-induced anaphylactoid reactions. In this study four regimens were compared (Table 15). Five minutes after intravenous pretreatment, 100 ml of RCM (meglumine diatrizoate) (Urovist) were administered and the patients were examined for possible subjective and objective side-effects. In this prospective placebo-controlled trial in 800 patients undergoing urography we found a significant reduction in side-reactions in the H_1-H_2-pretreated group as compared with the placebo group. Figure 21 shows the results for the overall symptoms (excluding "heat sensation"), nausea, and urticaria/angioedema [142].

Conclusions

Although histamine is only one of many possible and detrimental mediator substances of allergy, its effects are well known and specific antagonists are available. This has led to considerable therapeutic improvements in a variety of allergic diseases. Let us hope that in the near future similar progress can be achieved in the development of specific antagonists of other potent mediator substances.

References

1. Ackermann B (1910) Über den bakteriellen Abbau des Histidins. Hoppe-Seyler's Z Physiol Chem 65:504–510
2. Ash ASF, Schild HO (1966) Receptors mediating some actions of histamine. Br J Pharmacol 27:427–439
3. Askenase PW (1980) Immunopathology of parasitic diseases: involvement of basophils and mast cells. Springer Semin Immunopathol 2:417
4. Assem ESK, Attallah NA (1981) Increased release of histamine by anti-IgE from leukocytes of asthmatic patients and possible heterogenicity. Clin Allergy 11: 367–375
5. Austen KF (1971) Histamine and other mediators of allergic reactions. In: Samter M (ed) Immunologic diseases, 2nd edn. Little, Brown, Boston, pp. 332–355
6. Bach MK (1982) Mediators of anaphylaxis and inflammation. Annu Rev Microbiol 36:371–413

7. Bandmann HJ (1962) Ekzeme und ekzematoide Dermatitiden im frühen Kindesalter. In: Miescher G, Storck H (eds) Entzündliche Dermatosen I. Springer, Berlin Göttingen Heidelberg, pp 320–368 (Handbuch der Haut- und Geschlechtskrankheiten, vol 2, part 1)
8. Baumann G, Permanetter B, Wirtzfeld A (1984) Possible value of H_2-receptor agonists for treatment of catecholamine-insensitive congestive heart failure. Pharamacol Ther 24:165–177
9. Beaven MA, Jacobsen ST, Horakova Z (1972) Modification of enzymatic isotopic assay of histamine and its application to measurement of histamine in tissues, serum and urine. Clin Chim Acta 37:91–103
10. Beaven MA, Robinson-White A, Roderick NB, Kauffman GL (1982) The demonstration of histamine release in clinical conditions: a review of past and present assay procedures. Klin Wochenschr 60:873–881
11. Best CH, Dale HH, Dudley HW, Thorpe WV (1927) The nature of the vasodilator constituents of certain tissue extracts. J Physiol (Lond) 62:397–417
12. Bienenstock J, Befus AD (1980) Mucosal immunology. Immunology 41:249–270
13. Black JW, Duncan WAM, Durant CJ, Ganellin CR, Parsons EM (1972) Definition and antagonism of histamine H_2-receptors. Nature 236:385–390
14. Blandina P, Barattini M, Fantozzi R, Masini E, Mannaioni PF (1983) Histamine release by vagal stimulation. Agents Actions 13:179–182
15. Borelli S (1967) Psyche und Haut. In: Grotton HA (ed) Grundlagen und Grenzgebiete der Dermatologie. Springer, Berlin Heidelberg New York, pp 264–568 (Handbuch der Haut- und Geschlechtskrankheiten, vol 8)
16. Bosse K, Ladebeck H (1972) Die kutane Histaminquaddel in Korrelation zum Zyklus der Frau. Z Hautkr 47:365–370
17. Bourne HR, Lichtenstein LM, Melmon KL, Henney CS, Weinstein Y, Shearer GM (1974) Modulation of inflammation and immunity by cyclic AMP. Science 184:19–28
18. Bovet D, Staub AM (1937) Action protectrice des éthers-phénoliques au cours de l'intoxication histaminique. C R Soc Biol (Paris) 124:547–549
19. Braun-Falco O, Ring J (1984) Zur Therapie des atopischen Ekzems. Hautarzt 35: 447–454
20. Breathnach SM, Allen R, Ward AM, Greaves MW (1983) Symptomatic dermographism: natural history, clinical features, laboratory investigations and response to therapy. Clin Exp Dermatol 8:463–476
21. Busse WW (1979) Histamine: mediator and modulator in inflammation. In "Chemical messengers of the inflammatory process" (JC Houck, ed.) Elsevier, Amsterdam New York Oxford, pp 1–47
22. Butler JM, Ebertz M, Chan SC, Stevens SR, Sobieszozuk D, Hanifin JM (1985) Basophil histamine release in atopic dermatitis and its relationship to disordered cyclic nucleotide metabolism. Acta Derm Venereol [Suppl] (Stockh) 114:55–60
23. Casale TB, Bowman S, Kaliner M (1984) Induction of human cutaneous mast cell degranulation by opiates and endogenous opioid peptides: evidence for opiate and nonopiate receptor participation. J Allergy Clin Immunol 73:775–781
24. Casale TB, Shelhamer JH, Parrillo JE, Kaliner M (1984) Dopamine inhibition of histamine-mediated cutaneous responses. J Allergy Clin Immunol 73:837–841
25. Cerrina J, Denjean A, Alexandre G, Lockhart A, Duroux P (1981) Inhibition of exercise-induced asthma by a calcium antagonist, nifedipine. Am Rev Respir Dis 123:156–160
26. Conroy MC, Adkinson NF, Lichtenstein LM (1977) Measurement of IgE on human basophils; relation to serum IgE and anti-IgE-induced histamine release. J Immunol 118:1317–1324
27. Conroy MC (1981) Releasability – a new dimension in basophil and mast cell reactivity. In: Ring J, Burg G (eds) New trends in allergy. Springer, Berlin Heidelberg New York, pp 40–45
28. Cook J, Shuster S (1979) Lack of effect of H_2 blockade in chronic urticaria. Br J Dermatol 101:21–22
29. Czarnetzki B (1983) Increased monocyte chemotaxis towards leukotriene B_4 and platelet activating factor in patients with inflammatory dermatoses. Clin Exp Immunol 54:486–492

30. Dale HH, Laidlaw PP (1910) The physiological action of β-imidazolylethylamine. J Physiol. (Lond) 41:318–344
31. Davies MG, Greaves MW (1980) Sensory responses of human skin to synthetic histamine analogues and histamine. Br J Clin Pharmacol 9:461–465
32. Diller G, Orfanos CE (1983) Behandlung der idiopathischen Urticaria mit H_1- und H_2-Antagonisten. Ergebnisse einer Crossover-Doppelblind-Langzeitstudie. Z Hautkr 58:785–793
33. Doenicke A, Lorenz W (1982) Histamine release in anesthesia and surgery. Premedication with H_1- and H_2-receptor antagonists: indications, benefits and possible problems. Klin Wochenschr 60:1039–1045
34. Doenicke A, Lorenz W (eds) (1985) Histamin und Histamin-Rezeptor-Antagonisten. Springer, Berlin Heidelberg New York Tokyo
35. Dorsch W, Reimann HJ, Neuhauser J (1982) Histamine$_1$-histamine$_2$ antagonism: effect of combined clemastine and cimetidine pretreatment on allergen and histamine-induced reactions of the guinea pig lung in vivo and in vitro. Agents Actions 12:113–118
36. Dorsch W, Ring H, Reimann HJ, Geiger R (1982) Mediator studies in skin blister fluid from patients with dual skin reactions. J Allergy Clin Immunol 70:236–244
37. Dorsch W, Ring J, Riepel H (1984) Effect of 15-hydroxyeicosatetraenoic acid (15-HETE) on anti-immunoglobulin E- and calcium ionophore-induced histamine release from human leukocytes. Int Arch Allergy Appl Immunol 73:274–279
38. Douglas WW (1984) Autacoids. In: Gilman AG et al. (eds) The pharmacological basis of therapeutics, 6th edn. Mac Millan, New York, pp 608–646
39. Drake-Lee AB, Bickerton R, McLanglan P (1984) Free histamine in nasal polyp fluid. Rhinology 22:133
40. Dvorak AM, Galli SJ, Schulan ES, Lichtenstein LM, Dvorak HF (1983) Basophil and mast cell degranulation: ultrastructural analysis of mechanisms of mediator release. Fed Proc 42:2510–2515
41. Ennis M, Truneh A, White JR, Pearce FL (1981) Inhibition of histamine secretion from mast cells. Nature 289:186–187
42. Fabry H (1976) Immunsuppressive Wirkung des Gelbkörperhormons? Z Hautkr 51 [Suppl 2]:137–143
43. Fantozzi R, Moroni F, Masini E, Blandina P, Mannaioni PF (1978) Modulation of the spontaneous histamine release by adrenergic and cholinergic drugs. Agents Actions 8:347–351
44. Farnam J, Grant JA, Guernsey BG, Jorizzo JL, Petrusa ER (1984) Successful treatment of chronic idiopathic urticaria and angioedema with cimetidine alone. J Allergy Clin Immunol 73:842–845
45. Farnam J, Grant JA, Lett-Brown MA, Hunt C, Thueson DO, Giclas C (1984) Complement- and IgE-mediated release of histamine from basophils in vitro. J Immunol 134:541–547
46. Findlay SR, Dvorak AM, Kagey-Sobotka A, Lichtenstein LM (1981) Hyperosmolar triggering of histamine release from human basophils. J Clin Invest 67:1604
47. Findlay SR, Lichtenstein LM (1980) Basophil "releasability" in patients with asthma. Am Rev Respir Dis 122:53–59
48. Foreman JC, Garland LG, Mongar JL (1976) The role of calcium in secretory processes: model studies in mast cells. Symp Soc Exp Biol 139:193–218
49. Frewin DB, Jonsson JR, Head RJ, Russell WJ, Beal RW (1984) Histamine levels in stored human blood. Transfusion 24:502–504
50. Frosch PJ, Schwanitz HJ, Macher E (1984) A double blind trial of H_1 and H_2 receptor antagonists in the treatment of atopic dermatitis. Arch Dermatol Res 276:36–40
51. Fühner H (1912) Das Pituitrin und seine wirksamen Bestandteile. Münch med Wochenschr 59:852–853
52. Ganellin R (1981) Medical chemistry and dynamic structure-activity analysis in the discovery of drugs acting at histamine H_2 receptors. Med Chem 24:913–920
53. Garbarg M, Arrang JM, Quach TT, Trung-Tuong E, Yeramian E, Schwartz JC (1985) Betahistine and cerebral histamine receptor. European Histamine Research Society, 14th meeting, Aachen abstract 7.4

54. Gillespie E, Valentine MD, Lichtenstein LM (1972) Cyclic cAMP metabolism in asthma; studies with leukocytes and lymphocytes. J Allergy Clin Immunol 53:27–33
55. Gloor M, Wirth H, Swoboda U (1980) Is sebosuppression by cimetidine an antiandrogenic effect? Acta Derm Venereol (Stockholm) 61:262–264
56. Granerus G, Weinfeld A, Westin J (1983) Histamine symptoms and histamine metabolism in chronic granulocytic leukaemia. Agents Actions 13:251–255
57. Grant JA, Dupree E, Goldman AS, Schultz DR, Jackson AL (1975) Complement-mediated release of histamine from human leukocytes. J Immunol 114:1101–1107
58. Greaves MW, McDonald, Gibson W (1973) Effect of nonsteroid anti-inflammatory and antipyretic drugs on prostaglandin biosynthesis by human skin. J Invest Dermatol 61:127–129
59. Greaves MW, Marks R, Robertson I (1977) Receptors for histamine in human skin blood vessels. Br J Dermatol 97:225
60. Grevers-Colorian J, Przybilla B, Ring J (1985) Hemmung der Anti-IgE induzierten Histaminfreisetzung (HF) durch 5-α-Dihydrotestosteron (DHT). Arch Dermatol Res (in press)
61. Guillet G, Jeune R (1983) Urticarial vasculitis with shock, leukopenia and thrombocytopenia, possibly due to anaphylatoxin release. Br J Dermatol 108:605–608
62. Guggenheim M (1958) Die biogenen Amine in der Pflanzenwelt. In: Ruhland W (ed) Handbuch der Pflanzenphysiologie, vol 8. Springer, Berlin Göttingen Heidelberg, pp 889–989
63. Hägermark Ö, Strandberg K, Grönneberg R (1979) Effects of histamine receptor antagonists on histamine-induced responses in human skin. Acta Derm Venereol (Stockholm) 59:297–300
64. Hägermark Ö (1983) Pruritus: pathogenesis and therapeutic trials. In: Kukita A, Seiji M (eds) Proceedings of the 16th international congress on dermatology. University of Tokyo Press, Tokyo pp 61–68
65. Halpern BN (1942) Etude expérimentale des antihistaminiques de synthèse. Essais de chimiothérapie des états allergiques. Arch Int Pharmacodyn Ther 68:339
66. Hammar E, Berglund A, Hedin A, Norrman A, Rustas K, Ytterström U, Akerblom E (1985) An enzyme immunoassay for histamine based on monoclonal antibodies. European Academy of Allergology, Stockholm, Abstract vol 162
67. Hanifin JM (1983) Clinical and basic aspects of atopic dermatitis. Semin Dermatol 2:5–19
68. Harries MG, Burge PS, O'Brien I, Cromwell O, Pepys J (1979) Blood histamine levels after exercise testing. Clin Allergy 9:437–441
69. Henderson WR, Smith L, Kaliner M (1978) Alpha-adrenergic response in asthma. Clin Res 26:447A
70. Heskel N, Chan SC, Stevens SR, Hanifin JM (1983) Leukocyte cAMP-phosphodiesterase as a marker for atopy in neonates. Clin Res 31:101A
71. Horakova Z, Keiser HR, Beaven MA (1977) Blood and urine histamine levels in normal and pathological states as measured by a radiochemical assay. Clin Chim Acta 79:447–456
72. Ida S, Hooks JJ, Siraganian RP, Notkins AL (1977) Enhancement of IgE-mediated histamine release from human basophils by viruses: role of interferon. J exp Med 145:892–906
73. Ishizaka T, Hirata F, Ishizaka K, Axelrod J (1980) Stimulation of phospholipid methylation, Ca^{++} influx and histamine release by bridging of IgE receptors on rat mast cells. Proc Natl Acad Sci USA 77:1901–1908
74. Johnson HH, De Oreo GA, Lascheid WP, Mitchell F (1960) Skin histamine levels in chronic atopic dermatitis. J Invest Dermatol 34:237–243
75. Juhlin L (1967) Localization and content of histamine in normal and diseased skin. Acta Derm Venereol (Stockh) 42:218–226
76. Kaliner M (1977) Human lung tissue and anaphylaxis. Evidence that cyclic nucleotides modulate the immunologic release of mediators through effects on microtubular assembly. J Clin Invest 60:951–957
77. Kaliner M (1984) Hypotheses on the contribution of late-phase allergic responses to the understanding and treatment of allergic diseases. J Allergy Clin Immunol 73:311–315

78. Kallos P, Kallos M (1980) Histamine and some other mediators of pseudo-allergic reactions. In: Dukor et al. (eds) Pseudo-allergic reactions: involvement of drugs and chemicals. Karger, Basel, pp 28–51
79. Kaplan AP, Beaven MA (1976) In vivo studies of the pathogenesis of cold urticaria, cholinergic urticaria and vibration induced swelling. J Invest Dermatol 67:327–332
80. Katz G (1940) Histamine release from blood cells in anaphylaxis in vitro. Science 91:221
81. Kazimierczak W, Meier HL, MacGlashan DW, Lichtenstein LM (1984) An antigen-activated DFP-inhibitable enzyme controls basophil desensitization. J Immunol 132:399–405
82. Kern F, Lichtenstein LM (1976) Defective histamine release in chronic urticaria. J Clin Invest 57:1369–1375
83. König W (1978) Die immunbiologische Rolle des Histamins und seine Bedeutung für die Allergiediagnostik. Immunität Infektion 1:38–46
84. König W, Bohn A (1981) Membrane biochemical events in mast cell and basophil activation and secretion. Behring-Inst Mitt 68:30–50
85. Korting GW (1954) Zur Pathogenese des endogenen Ekzems. Thieme, Stuttgart
86. Kownatzki E (1984) Entzündungsmediatoren. Allergologie 7:195–203
87. Laxenaire MD, Moneret-Vautrin DA, Boileau S, Moeller R (1982) Adverse reactions to intravenous agents in anaesthesia in France. Klin Wochenschr 60:1006–1009
88. Levi R, Capurro N, Lee CH (1975) Pharmacological characterization of cardiac histamine receptors: sensitivity to H_1 and H_2 receptor agonists and antagonists. Eur J Pharmacol 30:328–335
89. Lewis T (1927) The blood vessels of the human skin and their responses. Shaw, London
90. Lichtenstein LM, Osler AG (1964) Studies on the mechanisms of hypersensitivity phenomena. IX. Histamine release from human leukocytes by ragweed pollen antigen. J Exp Med 120:507–530
91. Lichtenstein LM, Gillespie E (1973) Inhibition of histamine release by histamine is controlled by an H_2 receptor. Nature 244:287
92. Lichtenstein LM, Schleimer RP, Kagey-Sobotka A, Adkinson NF, Adam GK, Schulman ES, MacGlashan DW (1983) Studies with purified human basophils and mast cells. Monogr Allergy 18:259–264
93. Loew ER, MacMillan R, Katser ME (1946) The antihistamine properties of Benadryl, β-dimethylaminoethyl benzhydryl ether hydrochloride. J Pharmacol Exp Ther 86:229–238
94. Lorenz W, Reimann HJ, Barth H, Kusche J, Meyer R, Doenicke A, Hutzel M (1972) A sensitive and specific method for the determination of histamine in human whole blood and plasma. Hoppe-Seyler's Z Physiol Chem 353:911–920
95. Lorenz W, Doenicke A, Dittmann I, Hug O, Schwarz B (1977) Anaphylaktoide Reaktionen nach Applikation von Blutersatzmitteln beim Menschen. Verhinderung dieser Nebenwirkung von Haemoccel durch Praemedikation mit H_1- und H_2-Rezeptorantagonisten. Anaesthesist 26:644–648
96. Lorenz W, Doenicke A (1978) Histamine release in clinical conditions. Mount Sinai J Med 45:357–386
97. Majno G, Shea SM, Leventhal M (1969) Endothelial contraction induced by histamine-type mediators. An electron microscopic study. J Cell Biol 42:647–672
98. Mansfield LE, Smith JA, Nelson HS (1983) Greater inhibition of dermographia with a combination of H_1 and H_2 antagonists. Ann Allergy 50:264–270
99. Marks R, Dykes PJ, Tan CY (1982) Histamine and epidermal proliferation. Br J Dermatol 107:15–20
100. Marks R, Greaves MW (1977) Vascular reactions to histamine and compound 48/80 in human skin: suppression by a histamine H_2-receptor blocking agent. Br J Clin Pharmacol 4:367
101. Marone G, Poto S, Columbo M, Quattrin S, Condorelli M (1983) Histamine release from human basophils in vitro: Effects of age of cell donor. Monogr Allergy 18:139–143
102. Marone G, Poto S, Giugliano R, Bonini S (1985) Studies on human basophil releasability. Int Arch Allergy Appl Immunol 77:103–106
103. Matsumura Y, Tan EM, Vaughan JH (1976) Histamine hypersensitivity in mice induced

by *Bordetella pertussis* or pharmacologic beta adrenergic blockade. J Allergy Clin Immunol 58:395–404
104. Mayr T (1984) Untersuchungen über den Einfluß von zirkadianen Rhythmen und Histamin H_2 Antagonisten auf Auslösung und Verlauf der allergischen Kontaktdermatitis beim Meerschweinchen. Thesis, University of Munich
105. Mazurek N, Schindler H, Schürholz T, Pecht I (1984) The cromolyn binding protein constitutes the Ca^{2+} channel of basophils opening upon immunological stimulus. Proc Natl Acad Sci USA 81:6841–6845
106. Messmer K, Lorenz W, Sunder-Plassmann L, Kloevekorn WP, Hutzel M (1970) Histamine release as cause of hypotension following rapid colloid infusion. Arch Pathol Pharm 267:433
107. Middleton E, Drzewiecki G, Krishnarao D (1981) Quercetin: an inhibitor of antigen-induced human basophil histamine release. J Immunol 127:546–550
108. Monchy de JGR, Keyzere JJ (1985) Urinary histamine and histamine metabolite excretion following insect sting anaphylaxis. European Histamine Research Society, 14th meeting, Abstract 11.10, Aachen
109. Monroe EW, Cohen SH, Kalbfleisch H, Schulz C (1981) Combined H_1 and H_2 antihistamine therapy in chronic urticaria. Arch Dermatol 117:404–407
110. Moss J, Philbin DM, Rosow CE, Basta SJ, Gelb C, Savarese J (1982) Histamine release by neuromuscular blocking agents in man. Klin Wochenschr 60:891–895
111. Neijens HJ, Raatgeep HC, Degenhart HJ, Kerrebijn KF (1982) Release of histamine from leucocytes and its determinants in vitro in relation to bronchial responsiveness to inhaled histamine and exercise in vivo. Clin Allergy 12:577–586
112. Nisticò G, Rotiroti D, De Sarro A, Naccari F, Stephenson JD (1980) Central effects of histamine and H_1 and H_2 receptor agonists and antagonists after intraventricular infusion in fowls. Res Comm Chem Pathol Pharmacol 27:431–450
113. Okazaki T, Ilea V, Okazaki A, Wicher K, Reisman R, Arbesman CE (1976) Inhibition of antigen-induced histamine release by ouabain. J Allergy Clin Immunol 57:454–462
114. Okuda M, Ohtsuka H, Sakaguchi K, Watase T (1983) Nasal histamine sensitivity in allergic rhinitis. Ann Allergy 51:51–55
115. Owen DAA, Parsons EM (1974) Histamine receptors in the cardiovascular system of the cat. Br J Pharmacol 51:123–124
116. Parker CW, Kennedy S, Eisen AZ (1977) Leukocyte and lymphocyte cyclic AMP response in atopic eczema. J Invest Dermatol 68:302–306
117. Pearce FL, Befus AD, Bienenstock J (1984) Mucosal mast cells. J Allergy Clin Immunol 73:819–823
118. Peters SP, Siegel MI, Kagey-Sobotka A, Lichtenstein LM (1981) Lipoxygenase products modulate histamine release in human basophils. Nature 292:455
119. Philbin DM, Moss J, Akins CW, Rosow CE, Katsuakira K, Schneider RC, VerLee TR, Savarese JJ (1981) The use of H_1 and H_2 histamine antagonists with morphine anesthesia: a double-blind study. Anesthesiology 55:292–296
120. Plaut M, Lichtenstein LM (1983) Cellular and chemical basis of the allergic inflammatory response. In: Middleton E, Reed CE, Ellis EF (eds) Allergy: principles and practice, vol 1, 2nd ed. Mosby St. Louis, pp 119–146
121. Polak L (1980) Immunological aspects of contact sensitivity. An experimental study. Monogr Allergy 15. Karger, Basel
122. Polmar SH (1985) Pharmacological modulation of immunoregulatory lymphocyte functions. Allergologie 8:309
123. Przybilla B, Ring J, Schwab U, Dorn M (1986) Nichtsteroidale Antirheumatika mit photosensibilisierender Wirkung. Allergologie 9:8–15
124. Rajka G (1975) Atopic dermatitis. Saunders, London, pp 1–169
125. Reimann HJ, Ring J, Wendt P, Lorenz R, Ultsch B, Swoboda K, Blümel G (1981) Der Histaminstoffwechsel des Magens bei Patienten mit Nahrungsmittelallergie. Verh Dtsch Ges Inn Med 87:823–826
126. Reimann HJ, Swoboda K, Wendt O, Blümel G, Schmidt U, Rakette S, Ultsch B (1980) Die Wirkung des HDC-Blockers (+)-Catechin auf die menschliche Magenschleimhaut bei akuten und chronischen Erkrankungen. Verh Dtsch Ges Inn Med 86:859–863

127. Reimann HJ, Emslander HP, Schlehe H, Goerg R, Wendt P (1982) Auswirkung der Hypoxie auf den Histaminstoffwechsel der Lunge. Verh Dtsch Ges Inn Med 88:407–409
128. Reimann HJ, Meyer HJ, Wendt P (1981) Stress and histamine. In: Ring J, Burg G (eds) New trends in allergy. Springer, Berlin Heidelberg New York, pp 50–56
129. Reimann HJ, Ring J, Schmidt U, Ultsch B, Lewin J, Wendt P, von Sanden H (1984) Der Einfluß von H_1- und H_2-Rezeptorantagonisten, Histidindecarboxylaseblockern und Mastzellmembranstabilisatoren auf den Histamingehalt des Magens bei Patienten mit Nahrungsmittelunverträglichkeit. Verh Dtsch Ges Inn Med 90:540–543
130. Reimann HJ, Ring J, Ultsch B, Wendt P (1985) Intragastral provocation under endoscopic control (IPEC) in food allergy: mast cell and histamine changes in gastric mucosa. Clin Allergy 15:195–202
131. Reinhardt D, Wagner J, Schumann HF (1974) Differentiation of H_1 and H_2 receptors mediating positive chrono- and inotropic response to histamine on atrial preparations of the guinea pig. Agents Actions 4:217–221
132. Riley JF, West GB (1952) Histamine in tissue mast cells. J Physiol (Lond) 117:72–73
133. Ring J (1978) Anaphylaktoide Reaktionen nach Infusion natürlicher und künstlicher Kolloide. Springer, Berlin Heidelberg New York
134. Ring J, Simon A, Arroyave CM (1978) Increased in vitro histamine release by radiographic contrast media in patients with history of incompatibility. Clin Exp Immunol 34:302–309
135. Ring J, O'Connor R (1979) In vitro histmaine and serotonin release studies in atopic dermatitis. Int Arch Allergy Appl Immunol 58:322–326
136. Ring J, Allen DH, Mathison DA, Spiegelberg HL (1980) In vitro releasability of histamine and serotonin: studies of atopic patients. J Clin Lab Immunol 3:85–91
137. Ring J, Mathison DA, O'Connor R (1981) In vitro cyclic nucleotide responsitivity of peripheral leucocytes and platelets in patients suffering from atopic dermatitis. Int Arch Allergy Appl Immunol 65:1–7
138. Ring J (1981) Increased vasoactive mediator releasability: a possible pathogenic factor of atopic dermatitits. Int Arch Allergy Appl Immunol 66 [Suppl 1]:156–158
139. Ring J (1982) Angewandte Allergologie. MMW-Verlag, München, pp 1–156
140. Ring J (1983) Plasma histamine concentration in atopic eczema. Clin Allergy 13:545–552
141. Ring J (1984) Reaktionsbereitschaft ("Releasability"): Veränderte Reaktionsmuster in der Freisetzung vasoaktiver Mediatoren. Untersuchungen am Beispiel der Histamin-Freisetzung aus menschlichen basophilen Leukozyten. Allergologie 7:41–48
142. Ring J, Rothenberger KH, Clauß W (1984) Combined histamine H_1-H_2-receptor antagonist pretreatment for prophylaxis of anaphylactoid reactions due to radiographic contrast media (RCM). J Allergy Clin Immunol 73:165
143. Ring J, Dorsch W (1985) Altered releasability of vasoactive mediator secreting cells in atopic eczema. Acta Derm Venereol [Suppl] (Stockh) 114:9–23
144. Ring J, Walz U (1985) Indomethacin enhances in vitro histamine release induced by anti-IgE and Ca-Ionophore but inhibits C5a-induced release reactions from basophils of atopics and normals. Int Archs Allergy Appl Immunol 77:225–227
145. Ring J (1985) Mediatoren bei allergischen Hautkrankheiten. Allergologie 8:69–78
146. Ring J, Palos E, Zimmermann F (1985) Psychosomatische Aspekte der Eltern-Kind-Beziehung bei atopischem Ekzem: Psychodiagnostische Testverfahren bei Eltern und Kindern und Vergleich mit somatischen Befunden. Hautarzt (in press)
147. Roberts LJ, Marney SR, Oates JA (1979) Blockade of the flush associated with metastatic gastric carcinoid by combined histamine H_1 and H_2 receptor antagonists. N Engl J Med 300:236–238
148. Rocklin RE (1976) Modulation of cellular immune response in vivo and in vitro by histamine receptor-bearing lymphocytes. J Clin Invest 57:1051–1058
149. Rossi SS, Miller RJ (1982) Regulation of mast cell histamine release by neurotensin. Life Sci 31:509–516
150. Roszkowski W, Plaut M, Lichtenstein LM (1977) Selective display of histamine receptors on lymphocytes. Science 195:683–685
151. Russell JD, Russell SB, Trupin KM (1977) The effect of histamine on the growth of cultured fibroblasts isolated from normal and keloid tissue. J Cell Physiol 93:389–394

152. Ruzicka T, Glück S (1983) Cutaneous levels and histamine releasability from the skin in atopic dermatitis and hyper-IgE-syndrome. Arch Dermatol Res 275:41–44
153. Ruzicka T, Simmet T, Peskar B A, Braun-Falco O (1984) Leukotrienes in skin of atopic dermatitis. Lancet 1:222–223
154. Schadewaldt H (1980) Geschichte der Allergie. Dustri, Deisenhofen
155. Schayer RW, Cooper AD (1956) Metabolism of C^{14} histamine in man. J Appl Physiol 9:481–483
156. Schleimer RP, Lichtenstein LM, Gillespie E (1981) Inhibition of basophil histamine release by anti-inflammatory steroids. Nature 292:454
157. Schmutzler W, Poblete-Freundt G, Rauch K, Schoenfeld W (1979) Response to immunological or cholinergic stimulation of isolated mast cells from man, guinea pig and rat. Monogr Allergy 14:288–291
158. Schmutzler W, Delmich K, Eichelberg D, Glück S, Greven T, Jürgensen H, Riesener KP, Risse G, Pult P (1985) The human adenoidal mast cell. Susceptibility to different secretagogues and secretion inhibitors. Int Archs Allergy Appl Immunol 77:177–178
159. Schöpf E (1981) Drug influences upon skin test reactivity. In: Ring J, Burg G (eds) New trends in allergy. Springer, Berlin Heidelberg New York, p 108
160. Schwartz A, Sutton SL, Askenase PW, Gershon RK (1981) Histamine inhibition of concanavalin A-induced suppressor T-cell activation. Cell Immunol 60:425–439
161. Schwartz A, Barbin G, Duchemin AM, Garbarg M, Palacios JM, Quach TT, Rose C (1980) Histamine receptors in the brain: characterization by binding studies and biochemical effects. In: Pepcu G, Kuhar MJ, Enna SJ (eds) Receptors for Neurotransmitters and Peptides. Raven, New York, pp 169–182
162. Sebahoun G, Verloet D, Charpin J, Carcassonne Y (1978) Histamine release reaction of basophils in chronic granulocyte leukaemia. Clin Pathol 31:749–752
163. Selye H (1965) The mast cells. Butterworth, Washington
164. Sharpe PC, Melvin MA, Mills JG, Groom GV, Burland WL (1980) Prolactin responses to histamine H_2 antagonists. Br J Pharmacol 68:A 0289
165. Shore PA, Burkhalter A, Cohn VH (1959) A method for the fluorometric assay of histamine in tissue. J Pharmacol Exp Ther 127:182–191
166. Simon RA, Stevenson DD, Arroyave CM, Tan EM (1977) The relationship of plasma histamine to the activity of bronchial asthma. J Allergy Clin Immunol 60:312–316
167. Simon EJ, Hiller JM (1978) The opiate receptors. Ann Rev Pharmacol Toxicol 18:371
168. Siraganian RP (1975) Refinements in the automated fluorometric histamine analysis system. J Immunol Methods 7:283–290
169. Siraganian RP, Hook WA (1977) Mechanisms of histamine release by formyl methionine-containing peptides. J Immunol 119:2078–2083
170. Slater JE, Kaliner MA (1985) Effect of sex steroids on basophil histamine release. J Allergy Clin Immunol 75:176
171. Slocum RD, Kaur-Sawhney R, Galston AW (1984) The physiology and biochemistry of polyamines in plants. Arch Biochem Biophys 235:283–303
172. Smith TA (1980) Enzyklopädie der Pflanzenphysiologie. Neue Serie 8:433–460
173. Smith AM, Hayden MA, McCay SG, Zapatka FA, Hamdy MK (1982) Detection and confirmation of histamine-producing bacteria. Bull Environ Contam Toxicol 29:618–623
174. Snyder SH, Baldessarini RJ, Axelrod J (1966) A sensitive and specific enzymatic isotopic assay for tissue histamine. J Pharmacol Exp Ther 153:544
175. Sondergard I (1982) Quantitative determination of 1,4-methylimidazoleacetic acid in urine by high performance liquid chromatography. Allergy 27:581–586
176. Stuckey MS, Witt CS, Schmitt LH, Warlow R, Lattimore M, Dawkins RL (1985) Histamine sensitivity influences reactivity to allergens. J Allergy Clin Immunol 75:373–376
177. Stüttgen G (1983) Pruritus, Pathophysiologie und therapeutische Konsequenzen. In: Braun-Falco O, Burg G (eds) Fortschritte der praktischen Dermatologie und Venerologie, vol 10. Springer, Berlin Heidelberg New York Tokyo, pp 1–12
178. Summerfield J (1980) Naloxone modulated the perception of itch in man. Br J Clin Pharmacol 10:180–183
179. Suschitzky JL, Sheard P (1984) The search for anti-allergic drugs for the treatment of asthma – problems in finding a successor to sodium cromaglycate. Prog Med Chem 21:1–61

180. Szentivanyi A (1968) The beta adrenergic theory of the atopic abnormality in asthma. J Allergy 42:203–221
181. Talbot S, Atkins P, Zweiman B (1984) Prolonged histamine release in cutaneous allergic reactions. J Allergy Clin Immunol 73, 147
182. Tauber R, Reimann HJ, Schmiedt E (1981) Hat das Histamin eine pathophysiologische Bedeutung bei Nierentumoren? In: Ziegler M (eds) Urologisch-nephrologische Probleme. 20. Tagung der Südwestdeutschen Gesellschaft für Urologie, Schnetztor, Konstanz, p 176
183. Taylor JE, Richelson E (1982) High affinity binding of (3H)doxepin to histamine H_1-receptors in rat brain; possible identification of a subclass of histamine H_1-receptors. Eur J Pharmacol 78:279–285
184. Tung R, Kagey-Sobotka A, Plaut M, Lichtenstein LM (1982) H_2 antihistamines augment antigen-induced histamine release from human basophils in vitro J Immunol 129:2113–2115
185. Thueson D, Speck L, Lett-Brown M, Grant A (1979) Histamine-releasing activity (HRA): II. Interaction with basophils and physiochemical characterization. J Immunol 123:633–639
186. Uehara M (1985) Clinical and histological features of dry skin in atopic dermatitis. Acta Derm Venerol [Suppl] (Stockh) 114:82–86
187. Ulmer WT, Zimmermann I, Bugalha de Almeida AA, Park HS (1982) Effects of exogenous and endogenous histamine on the respiratory system. Klin Wochenschr 60:991–996
188. Uvnäs B (1976) Modes of action of antigen-antibody reaction and compound 48/80 in histamine release. In: Johansson SGO, Strandberg K, Uvnäs B (eds) Molecular and biological aspects of the acute allergic reaction. Plenum, New York, pp 217–232
189. Van Niekerk CH, Prinsloo AEM (1985) Effect of skin pigmentation on the response to intradermal histamine. Int Arch Allergy Appl Immunol 76:73–75
190. Venencie PY, Lebel B, Saurat HJ (1981) Histamine release in atopic dermatitis of childhood. In: Ring J, Burg G (eds) New trends in allergy. Springer, Berlin Heidelberg New York, pp 224–230
191. Virchow C, Strassburg J (1978) Histamin-Freisetzung aus Leukozyten. Vergleich zwischen allergischem Asthma, Intrinsic Asthma und Normalpersonen. Prax Klin Pneumol 32:14–28
192. von der Helm D, Ring J, Dorsch W (1983) Prostaglandin influence on basophil releasability from atopic and normal individuals. J Allergy Clin Immunol 71:105
193. Wahn U (1985) Histamin als Mediator der allergischen Reaktion. Allergologie 8:47–50
194. Warren K, Dyer J, Merlin S, Kaliner M (1983) Measurement of urinary histamine: comparison of fluorometric and radioisotopic-enzymatic assay prodecures. J Allergy Clin Immunol 71:206–211
195. Wegner F, Hockamp R, Rutschke A, Becker B, Reinhardt D (1983) Superiority of the histamine release test above case history, prick test, and radio-allergosorbent test in predicting bronchial reagibility to the house dust mite in asthmatic children. Klin Wochenschr 61:43–47
196. Werle E (1940) Zur Kenntnis der Histidindecarboxylase und der Histaminase. Biochem Z 304:201
197. Werle E, Raub A (1944) Über Vorkommen, Bildung und Abbau biogener Amine bei Pflanzen unter besonderer Berücksichtigung des Histamins. Biochem Z 318:538–553
198. West GB (1961) The action of dextran in rats. Biochem Pharmacol 8:153–155
199. Whitlock FA (1976) Psychophysiological aspects of skin disease. Holt-Saunders, London
200. Wolff HH, Maciejewski W, Scherer R, Braun-Falco O (1978) Immunoelectromicroscopic examination of early lesions in histamine induced immune complex vasculitis in man. Br J Dermatol 99:13–24
201. Wilhelm OH, Kreusser W, Ritz E (1981) Parathyroid hormone elicits histamine release from mast cells. Miner Electrolyte Methods 6:29
202. Windaus A, Vogt W (1907) Synthese des Imidazolyläthylamins. Ber Dtsch Chem Ges 40:369
203. Winters SJ, Banks JL, Loriaux DL (1979) Cimetidine is an antiandrogen in the rat. Gastroenterology 76:504–508

204. Wirth H, Gloor M, Stoika D (1981) Sebaceous glands in uninvolved skin of patients suffering from atopic dermatitis. Arch Dermatol Res 270:167–169
205. Wolstenholme GEW, O'Connor CM (eds) (1956) Histamine. Little, Brown, Boston
206. Wüthrich B (1975) Zur Immunopathologie der Neurodermitis constitutionalis. Huber, Bern
207. Zimmermann I, Bugalho de Almeida AA, Ulmer WT (1980a) Allergen-induzierte Atemwegsobstruktion und Histaminkonzentration im arteriellen wie venösen Plasma. Res Exp Med 177:91–100
208. Zweifach BW (1973) Microcirculation. Ann Rev Physiol 35:117–150

Lipid Mediators and Inflammation

C. W. Parker

Howard Hughes Medical Institute Laboratory; Department of Internal Medicine, Division of Allergy and Immunology, Washington University School of Medicine, St. Louis, MO 63110, USA

Abstract

The role of arachidonic metabolites in the control of immunity in inflammation is reviewed with particular emphasis on the most recent observations and possible interactions between these products and other mediators. Continuing studies on the nature of the lipoxygenase involved in leukotriene synthesis will be discussed as will the nature of the enzymatic activity involved in the transfer of sulphur in leukotriene C, D and E.

The most important known lipid mediators of inflammation are either metabolites of long chain fatty acids, particularly arachidonic acid, or 1-alkyl-2-acetyl derivatives of phosphatidylcholine (platelet activating factor, PAF). This chapter will review the mediators derived from arachidonic acid with emphasis on the most recent findings, particularly in regard to the lipoxygenase products, which is a very active area. [1–6].

Arachidonic Acid Metabolites

Arachidonic acid (eicosatetraenoic acid, AA) is a C20 fatty acid with double bonds at the 5–6, 8–9, 11–12, and 14–15 positions. The multiplicity of double bonds provides a variety of potential mechanisms by which new products may be formed and helps explain the flexibility of AA as a precursor of bioreactive lipids. Since AA itself and most of its initial metabolites have 20 carbons, its metabolites have been termed eicosanoids. If esterification in neutral lipids and phospholipids is excluded, the two major routes of AA metabolism in mammalian cells are the lipoxygenase (LO) and cyclooxygenase (CO) pathways (Fig. 1).

Lipoxygenases differ in the location of the double bond on the AA molecule where enzymatic attack is initiated [7, 8]. They include the 12-LO (*top left*) in platelets (and other cell types), the 5-LO (*top right*) in a variety of leukocytes and mast cells, and a 15-LO (also found in leukocytes and other cell types, not shown). LOs produce monohydroperoxy fatty acids (HPETES) as their initial product, which in turn are converted to monohydroxy fatty acids (HETES), and various dihydroxy and trihydroxy fatty acids (diHETES and triHETEs, respectively). The term leukotriene has been applied to LO derivatives with at least three conjugated double bonds, which include leukotriene B and the sulfidoleukotrienes (leukotrienes C, D, and E). The CO pathway (*lower part* of Fig. 1) gives the endoperoxides PGG and PGH, which in turn are converted to prostacyclin, the various prostaglandins (PGs), or thromboxane A_2 (TxA_2), the precise pattern depending on the cell. The COs are associated with microsomes and show marked structural and enzymatic similarities in different cells and tissues. The LOs are primarily soluble enzymes which not only differ from one another in the site on the AA molecule where oxidation is initiated but presumably have more marked structural and mechanistic differences from one another than the COs. Frequently an eicosanoid may exist in several structural forms depending on the number, location, and configuration of the double bonds. The number of double bonds is indicated by a subscript (for example, when AA is converted to PGs two of the original four double bonds are lost so the usual PGE metabolite is PGE_2). With the leukotrienes, double bond rearrangement occurs but the original number of double bonds is typically maintained. C20 fatty acids with three (eicosatrienoic acid) or five (eicosapentaenoic acid) double bonds may also serve as eicosanoid precursors [provided the particular double bond(s) critical for LO or CO action is present]. Their corresponding metabolites, of course, either lack the missing double bond or have an extra one. As discussed below, although C20 fatty acids with three or five double bonds are normally much less prevalent in mammalian tissues than AA, dietary manipulations can be used to increase their levels in cells, affecting the relative amount, biologic activity, or catabolism of the various metabolites. However, since AA is normally by far the predominant eicosanoid precursor, in the ensuing discussion the emphasis will be on AA itself and its metabolites.

The AA in mammalian cells is primarily derived either from shorter chain essential fatty acid or AA itself in the diet and is carried to cells through the blood or lymphatic fluid. Almost all of the AA present in tissues is esterified in phospholipids and triglycerides. The rate-limiting step in AA metabolism is thought to be the availabiltiy of free AA which is released enzymatically by phospholipases or lipases at the time cells are activated by antigens and other

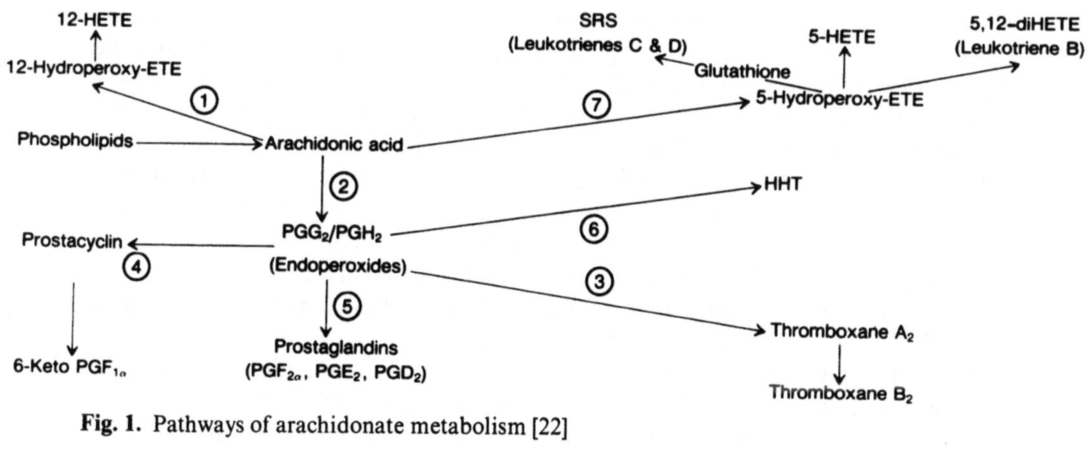

Fig. 1. Pathways of arachidonate metabolism [22]

stimuli. Ordinarily an activated cell is thought of as supplying its own unesterified AA, although it should be kept in mind that phospholipids, triglycerides, and unesterified fatty acids are present in the blood, bound in chylomicrons or reversibly to the lipoproteins and albumin, and may conceivably serve as another source of rapidly available AA. Moreover in areas of inflammation where high leukocyte densities are present, a cell may utilize AA derived from nearby cells as well as draw on its own intracellular pool.

Because of its apparent importance in inflammation and allergy the 5-LO pathway will now be considered in more detail. The products of the 5-LO pathway include the 5-hydroperoxide (5-hydroperoxy,6,8,11,14eicosatetraeonic acid, 5-HPETE); its epoxide rearrangement product (5,6epoxy7,9,11,14eicosatetraeonic acid, LTA_4); the sulfidoleukotrienes, which are thioethers with glutathione (LTC_4), cysteinyl glycine (LTD_4), or cysteine side chains (LTE_4) adjacent to the 5-OH group, 5 (S), 12 (R)-6 (*cis*), 8 (*trans*), 10 (*trans*), 14 (*cis*) eicosatetraenoic acid (LTB_4); and 5-HETE (5-hydroxy6,8,11,14eicosatetraenoic acid). While LTA_4, LTB_4, LTC_4, and R-HETE all can be produced nonenzymatically, under the usual conditions of cellular metabolism most of their formation is thought to be enzymatically mediated. LTA_4 is probably the major precursor of both LTB_4 and LTC_4. Peroxidation at CS requires double bonds at the 5 and 8 positions [9]. 5-HETE is formed from 5-HPETE or LTA_4 by the action of glutathione or other peroxidases, which are widely distributed enzymes capable of reducing the peroxy groups in a wide range of substrates, including long chain fatty acids. The available evidence would indicate that selenium and nonselenium glutathione peroxidases are both present in leukocytes [10]. 5-HETE is the predominant 5-LO product, usually accounting for more than 80% of the radiolabeled AA converted through this pathway. Small amounts of 5-HETE are incorporated covalently in ester linkage into phospholipids and triglycerides when the 5-LO enzyme is stimulated or 5-HETE is made available in the extracellular medium [11]. Similar incorporation occurs with 12-HETE although less readily than with 5-HETE. While confirmatory evidence is not yet available, the presence of hydroxylated fatty acids would be expected to affect the polarity of phospholipids in the membrane bilayer and might selectively alter membrane transport or enzyme activity. The formation of LTC_4 from LTA_4 is probably mediated by S-transfcrase enzymes. S-transferases are a heterogeneous group of enzymes which promote the reaction of reduced glutathione (by far the predominant intracellular thiol) and other thiols with a wide variety of epoxides, producing thioethers. S-transferases have been studied extensively in regard to their important role in drug detoxification. They are especially prominent in liver, where the major part of their activity is in the cytosol. The S-transferase involved in LTC_4 production (LTC_4 synthetase) is probably a different enzyme present primarily in the membranous fraction with considerable selectivity for LTA_4 [12–14], although further studies are needed. A requirement for this enzyme could help explain why cells that contain 5-LOs differ markedly in the amount of LTC_4 they produce.

Once formed, the thioether (sulfide) linkage shows considerable stability, although oxidation to a sulfoxide or sulfone has been demonstrated in polymorphonuclear leukocytes and almost certainly occurs in other tissues. One probable mechanism for oxidation of the sulfur in sulfidoleukotrienes is through reactive O_2 metabolites which have been shown to oxidize the methionyl sulfide group in F-Met-Leu-Phe [15]. The peptide side chain of LTC_4 is rapidly metabolized by intracellular and extracellular enzymes, producing LTD_4 and LTE_4 [16, 17]. The conversion to LTD_4 apparently involves conventional γ-glutamyl transferases. These enzymes are widely distributed in tissue and blood. They are inhibited by serine-borate complexes, which also prevent LTD_4 formation from LTC_4. Conversion of LTD_4 to LTE_4 has been described with aminopeptidases, and it seems likely that selected esterases and carboxypeptidases, including cathepsin H [18], can produce LTE_4 as well. The conversion of LTC_4 to LTD_4 is largely completed within 10–15 min in most tissues, including lung. LTE_4 formation from LTD_4 (or its sulfoxide or sulfone) is also rapid. Once formed, LTE_4 is relatively stable, although its sulfide group can be oxidized (see above) and enzymatic attack is also possible at C20 and other positions in the fatty acid chain. In mice and guinea pigs the predominant metabolite identified in urine and feces of mice after intravenous injection of LTD_3 has been LTE_3 [19]. Virtually nothing is presently known about the major metabolites of the sulfidoleukotrienes in man.

The production of LTB_4 from LTA_4 is thought to involve a specific enzyme (LTB_4 synthetase or LTA_4 hydrolase) which catalyzes the introduction of a hydroxy group from water or OH– at the 12 position. In addition to LTB_4 other diHETEs are formed from LTA_4 including 5S, 12S 6 (*trans*), 8 (*trans*), 10 (*trans*), 14 (*cis*) diHETE (6-*trans* LTB_4) and 5S, 12R dihydroxy6,8,10 (all *trans*), 14 (*cis*) diHETE as well as 2 isomeric 5,6dihydroxy7,9,11,14eicosatetraenoic acids [20]. Leukotrienes are also produced from the 15-hydroperoxide 15 (s) hydroperoxy5,8,11 *cis*-13-*trans*-eicosatetraenoic acid (15-HPETE). These isomers are always present to a limited extent when LTB_4 is generated biosynthetically, although they are almost certainly derived in part from spontaneous (nonenzymatic) rearrangement of LTB_4 during incubation, purification, or storage. Hemoproteins promote nonenzymatic conversions of the hydroperoxides which lead to leukotriene transformations. LTB_4 is metabolized successively to 20-hydroxy and 20-carboxy LTB_4 by enzymes present in leukocytes. The introduction of a third hydroxyl group elsewhere in the molecule is also possible. Two novel trihydroxy trienes, termed lipoxins, produced by 15-LOs in leukocytes [2] have also been described. Since they also appear to be highly active biologically, they are currently under intensive study. Keto, hydroxy-epoxy, or vinyl groups may also be introduced into AA during oxidation by LOs, particularly in vitro, when little or no O_2 is available. Vinyl derivatives can be cleaved to produce short hydrocarbon fragments which are volatile, although this has thus far been studied almost exclusively in plant LOs [21]. Mono- or dihydroxy HETEs may be acted upon successively by LOs in other cell types, providing unique, potentially interesting products. For example, 5-HETE is metabolized in vitro by the 15-LO present in macrophages to diasteriomeric mixtures of 5,15diHETEs. The extent to which this type of collaboration between cells normally operates in vivo is uncertain, although obviously inflammatory processes do normally contain mixtures of different cell types, where such interactions would be possible.

While possible effects on enzyme activity during cell purification have to be kept in mind, the 12-LO in human platelets seems to be normally present in an activated form. Merely supplying the cell with exogenous AA leads to the formation of AA metabolites [22]. On the other hand with resting mature leukocytes at least, the 5-LOs seem to exist in the cell primarily in an inactive form and LO products are formed only if the cells are activated. The most effective form of activation is to add the divalent cation ionophore A-23187 in Ca^{2+}-containing medium to suspended cells. Once the cells are stimulated both exogenous and endogenous AA is utilized as substrates. While the mechanism of the ionophore activation is not completely clear, studies with purified 5-LO from RBL-1 cells indicate that at least one form of the enzyme exists as a monomer in its inactive state. In the presence of Ca^{2+} the enzyme undergoes dimerization and becomes active. A mechanism for activation involving binding to calcium would seem to correlate with the known influx of calcium into cells when leukocytes are activated by exogenous stimuli. Nonetheless, the concentrations of calcium required to activate the purified enzyme are high, and additional intracellular factors may be involved.

Following activation of cells, the formation of AA metabolites through the 5-LO pathway rapidly reaches a maximum (within a few minutes). Beyond 15 or 20 min very little or no additional products are formed. This is not due simply to the exhaustion of the free AA substrate since the addition of exogenous AA after enzyme activity has apparently ceased does not lead to further product formation. While the mechanism of this inactivation is not fully elucidated, contributing factors probably include inhibition of the enzyme by its own products, including 5-HETE and 5-HPETE, autoinactivation of the enzyme through hydroperoxides and reactive oxygen metabolites, and very possibly degradation of the enzyme by proteolysis [23, 59].

Two questions that remain unresolved are the degree of heterogeneity of 5-LOs in different tissues and whether or not they are subject to long-term regulatory influences affecting enzyme biosynthesis. The human granulocytic cell line H-60 shows a marked increase in 5-LO product foundation when induced to differentiate in vitro [24], but many other enzymes show increases in activity under these conditions. The production of LO metabolites by mature leukocytes may be markedly increased by sustained exposure to naturally occurring stimuli, including pathogenic microorganisms, raising the possibility of increased enzyme levels. For example, a recent study of macrophages from animals infected with *Leishmania donovani* indicates that exposure to the organism for 24 h in vitro is associated with a marked increase in the ability of the cells to produce LTC_4 when they are additionally stimulated by LPS or zymogen [25]. While this might suggest that more 5-LO is available in infected cells (as might occur due to increased biosynthesis), the production of metabolites through the CO pathway is also increased and activation of phospholipase may be occurring.

Another question that has not been fully explored is the extent to which 5-LOs may exist outside the animal kingdom or in lower forms within the animal kingdom. A recent study in cercariae from *Schistosoma mansoni*, the form of the organism which traverses the skin and leads to human infection, indicates that they are capable of producing substantial quantities of leukotrienes [26]. The formation of lipoxygenase products is stimulated in vitro by exposure to linoleic acid. It is postulated that linoleic acid and other fatty acids in skin may act on the organism after it enters the skin, leading to AA release and 5-LO activation in situ. The local release of mediators could then affect vascular reactivity and promote penetration by the organism into blood vessels as well as act on the organism itself.

Biologic Actions

Judging from the information available, LTB_4 may be a major mediator of leukocyte inflammation since it is capable of producing cell aggregation, lysosomal enzyme release, and chemotaxis. LTB_4 is a potent stimular of leukocyte aggregation, producing responses at concentrations in the nanomolar or high picomolar range; this makes it comparable to potent leukocyte activators such as F-Met-Leu-Phe in its biologic activity [27, 28]. On the other hand, it is important to keep in mind that inflammatory exudates may contain considerable amounts of serum protein which may bind LTB_4 and considerably lower its biologic effectiveness. LTB_4 also stimulates chemotaxis and chemokinesis but significantly higher concentrations of the mediator are needed. The effects of LTB_4 on lysosomal enzyme release are difficult to evaluate since LTB_4 is only effective at substantial concentrations of cytochalasins which themselves produce complex effects on leukocyte function. LTB_4 has also been reported to increase the number of surface receptors for C3b in polymorphonuclear leukocytes and eosinophils. Whether this is an effect on receptor availability or a result of increased receptor biosynthesis remains to be demonstrated.

In considering the possible mechanism of action of LTB_4 on leukocytes, there are apparent analogies with other activators of leukocyte function such as C5a, F-Met-Leu-Phe (F-MLP) LTB_4, PAF, and ATP. Like LTB_4, these agents all enhance aggregation, migration, and the release of granule enzymes extracellularly. While there is no doubt that different receptors mediate the responses to these different agents, there may be some commonality of the activation mechanisms [29]. For example LTB_4 and F-MLP both considerably enhance Ca^{2+} and Na^{+} influx in neutrophils [30], owing either to changes in membrane permeability, in transport, or in both, and both responses are inhibited by phorbol esters [31]. Moreover, the responses to F-MLP and LTB_4 show very similar time courses, although F-MLP produces a more marked response than LTB_4.

When the aggregating activity of LTB_4 for leukocytes from various species is compared with that of its diasteroisomers and metabolites hydroxylated or carboxylated at the C20 position, LTB_4 is more potent than the other agents by a factor of 10 or greater. This suggests that LTB_4 is acting on cells through specific receptors. Direct binding studies with radiolabeled LTB_4 with human leukocytes have confirmed the existence of saturable and reversible binding inhibited by excess unlabeled ligand [32, 33]. Because LTB_4 is rapidly metabolized at 37° C, the results of the binding studies are more easily interpreted at lower temperatures, particularly at 4° C. A detailed analysis of the binding curves with human polymorphonuclear leukocytes by several laboratories indicates the existence of at least two classes of binding sites of differing affinities [28, 33, 34]. The high affinity receptor is active in the concentration range at which LTB_4 produces cell aggregation. Chemokinetic and chemotactic responses occur at considerably higher LTB_4 concentrations and may involve the lower affinity receptor. Interestingly, rat peripheral blood leukocytes possess high affinity binding sites comparable to those on human cells but apparently lack the lower affinity binding sites. Rat cells aggregate readily in response to LTB_4, but fail to show a chemokinetic or chemotactic response even though they are highly responsive to other agents affecting cellular motility [28].

Very little is known about the factors controlling the number of LTB_4 receptors on cells or their possible variation in various disease states. LTB_4 receptors appear apparently de novo when the immature human monocyte cell line U937 is induced to differentiate but this is almost certainly due to cell maturation per se. Because their protein synthesizing activity is very limited there is considerable doubt whether mature polymorphonuclear leukocytes can regulate LTB_4 receptor levels by synthesizing new LTB_4 receptors, although down regulation through internalization or shedding remains a possibility. However, these cells turn over rapidly and the induction of new receptor molecules on less mature precursors in the bone marrow might rapidly alter receptor numbers on cells in the periphery.

LTB_4 is also currently attracting interest as a possible mediator of T-lymphocyte function. Studies some years ago with human peripheral T-lymphocytes indicated that nonspecific LO inhibitors such as eicosatetraynoic acid and nordihydroguaretic acid markedly decreased the DNA synthetic response to lectin and nonlectin mitogens [35]. It was subsequently shown that 15-HETE and 5-HETE or other hydroperoxides inhibited DNA synthesis in human and murine lymphocytes although relatively high concentrations were required [36]. Since these HETEs are LO inhibitors, these observations suggested indirectly that LO products might be necessary for the response. Subsequent studies have shown that 15-HPETE is a more effective inhibitor of DNA synthesis than 15-HETE and that LTB_4 is capable of stimulating transformation in OKT-8 positive (suppressor) human peripheral blood T-lymphocytes, whereas the response in OKT-4 positive (helper) T cells is suppressed [37, 38]. The significance of the changes in DNA synthesis is not altogether clear since the suppression or enhancement is seldom greater than 50% and detailed studies on the kinetics of the altered response have not been performed. Nonetheless, changes are seen at LTB_4 concentrations as low as 10^{-10} M, so that response could have physiologic significance. Taken as a whole these observations raise the possibility of a role of LTB_4 in regulating the balance between helper and suppressor T-lymphocytes, tipping the response toward the suppressor side, as has been suggested for other small molecular weight mediators such as histamine. Further elucidation of the basis for the LTB_4 suppression may be difficult since there is evidence that T cells, both helper and suppressor, are heterogeneous in regard to their ability to interact with LTB_4-albumin conjugates, with only about 10% of cells in each population showing binding activity [38].

In contrast to LTB_4, the predominant effects of the sulfidoleukotrienes are on smooth muscle contraction and vascular permeability [39, 40], although leukotriene effects on nerve cell activity [41, 42] and mucin production [43] have been described. In addition to the work with LTB_4 receptors described above, studies have been done on possible cellular receptors for LTC_4, LTD_4 and LTE_4. Aside from one study done in a smooth muscle cell line, these observations have been complicated by the use of heterogeneous tissues, such as the lung or heart muscle, which makes it difficult or even impossible to correlate binding with the biologic response of the tissue. Even considering this limitation, evidence is emerging to indicate that there are primarily two types of receptor for this group of mediators, one which binds much better to LTC_4 than to other leukotrienes and another with binding activity primarily for LTD_4 and LTE_4 [44].

Inhibitors of Leukotriene Formation or Action

Work is in progress attempting to identify selective inhibitors of 5-LOs which might permit this group of enzymes to be suppressed without other AA metabolizing enzymes being affected. Among the agents currently under study are aryloxymethylacetophenones [45], AA analogs methylated at C-7 and C-10 [46], a diphenylimino, epoxy prostaglandin [47], butylated hydroxytoluene and its congeners [48], 7-thia-arachidonic acid [49], 5-hydroxy-6-thio-substituted carboxylic acids [50], 5-HETE, 15-HETE and their congeners [23, 51, 53, 59]. In addition to agents which act directly on the LO, the formation of LTC_4 can be markedly decreased without concomitant changes in 5-HETE or LTB_4 biosynthesis by lowering the intracellular concentration of reduced glutathione [52]. While it might be argued that substantial reductions in intracellular glutathione concentrations would produce too much toxicity for therapeutic application in man, inhibitors of glutathione-metabolizing enzymes are well tolerated in rats over considerable periods. A more promising approach might be to inhibit the S-transferase enzyme involved in transferring glutathione to LTA_4 [12], particularly if further studies bear out early indications that this conjugation is mediated by a unique enzyme not involved in the usual forms of drug detoxification by S-transferase enzymes. Still another approach might involve the administration of a thiol which would compete intracellularly with glutathione for LTA_4 and perhaps also provide a biologically inactive sulfidopeptide analogue of the C, D, and E leukotrienes. While unpleasant to take, thiols have been used successfully in the treatment of acute acetoaminophen poisoning. Penicillamine has been used on a chronic basis in the treatment of Wilson's disease and chronic inflammatory arthritis but has significant toxicity. Various inhibitors of the end-organ action of leukotrienes are also being studied [54].

One question currently of considerable interest is the possibility of using simple dietary manipulations to alter the balance of the inflammatory mediators in chronic inflammatory diseases of immunologic origin, such as systemic lupus erythematosus (SLE). Based on studies in experimental animals it appears that the diet can be supplemented with long chain fatty acids such as eicosapentaenoic acid (C20 fatty acid with 5, 8, 11, 14, 17 double bonds), leading to a marked enrichment of intracellular lipids with this fatty acid and, in some instances, to a decrease in the cellular content of AA. When circulating leukocytes from such animals are recovered and treated in vitro with A-23187, substantial amounts of LTB_5 are formed whereas LTB_4 production may be decreased [55]. Since LTB_5 is 10- to 30-fold less potent than LTB_4 in assays of leukocyte function, this provides a possible means of decreasing an ongoing inflammatory response. Evidence has already been presented that inflammatory changes in murine SLE may be partially controlled on such diets. Similar diets have been shown to produce less striking changes in the lipid content of circulating leukocytes in man [56], although it remains to be demonstrated that these changes can be sustained over prolonged periods or what the eventual consequences for inflammation or the possible undesirable effects would be.

The metabolites of AA represent a diverse array of highly reactive lipids, some of which are intrinsically highly unstable or are rapidly metabolized. Others are apparently stable, at least in vitro, for considerable periods, although it should be kept in mind that in inflammatory responses in tissue the activity of a mediator may be considerably limited by dilution, binding to extracellular protein, or removal due to the flow of blood or extracellular fluid. While it might appear that the lipid mediators more or less duplicate the actions of other mediators of hypersensitivity, such as histamine, a more careful analysis of the various biologic effects indicates differences in time course and spectrum of reactivity in various smooth muscle preparations which provide for considerable subtlety of action. Moreover the various mediators may affect the biosynthesis or action of one another, and thus considerably potentiate or antagonize a response. For example, through their effects on intracellular cyclic AMP concentrations, prostacyclin and PGE_2 tend to neutralize the lipid-contracting effects of other agents as well as to inhibit their biosynthesis. These effects are not limited to CO products. Hydroperoxides may affect the biosynthesis of potent unstable lipid mediators obtained through the CO pathway such as thromboxane A_2 [57] or even unrelated products such as cyclic GMP. LTB_4 may affect PAF biosynthesis [58]. Among the mediators which have to be considered in a given situation are histamine, leukotrienes, prostaglandins, thromboxane A_2, the kinins, PAF, active complement fragments (particularly C5a and C3a), fragments produced by clotting enzymes such as the fibrinopeptides, and serotonin. While much of the emphasis has centered primarily on the effects of mediators on vascular reactivity and smooth muscle contraction as may relate to immediate hypersensitivity responses, many mediators can regulate long-term leukocyte function with effects at the level of expression of macrophage surface antigens such as Ia and on relative reactivities of suppressor and helper T cells [6]. Actions of this general nature may help provide a mechanism for the overall regulation of immune responsiveness.

References

1. Samuelsson B (1983) Leukotrienes: mediators of immediate hypersensitivity reactions and inflammation. Science 220:568
2. Samuelsson B (1984) Lipoxins: a novel series of compounds formed from arachidonic acid. In: Pike JE, Morton DR (eds) Advances in prostaglandin, thromboxane, and leukotriene research, vol 14. Raven, New York, p 45
3. Goetzl EJ (1980) Oxygenation products of arachidonic acid as mediators of hypersensitivity and inflammation. Med Clin North Am 65:809
4. Lewis RA, Austen KF (1981) Mediation of local homeostasis and inflammation by leukotrienes and other mast cell-dependent compounds. Nature 293:103
5. Parker CW (1983) Immunopharmacology of slow reacting substances. In: Newball HH (ed) Immunopharmacology of the lung. Dekker, New York, p 25
6. Parker CW (1984) Mediators: release and function. In: Paul WE (ed) Fundamental immunology Raven, New York, p 697
7. Vliegenthart JFG, Veldink GA, Verhagen J, Slappendel S (1983) Lipoxygenases from plant and animal origin. In: Sund H, Ullrick V (eds) Biological oxidations, Springer, Berlin Heidelberg New York, p 203
8. Stenson WF, Parker CW (1983) Metabolites of arachidonic acid. Clin Rev Allergy 1:369
9. Wei Y, Evans RW, Morrison AR, Sprechert H, Jakschik BA (1985) Double bond requirement for the 5-lipoxygenase pathway. Prostaglandins 29:537
10. Reddy CC, Rao MK, Mastro AM, Egan RW (1984) Measurement of glutathione requiring enzymes involved in arachidonic acid cascade of rat basophilic leukemia cells. Biochem Int 9:755
11. Stenson W, Parker CW (1980) Monohydroxyeicosatetraenoic acids (HETEs) induce degranulation of human neutrophils. J Immunol 124:2100
12. Bach MK, Brasher JR, Morton DR Jr (1984) Solubilization and characterization of the leukotriene C4 synthetase of rat basophil leukemia cells: a novel particulate glutathione S-transferase. Arch Biochem Biophys 230:455
13. Kuo CG, Lewis MT, Jakschik A (1984) Leukotriene D_4 and E_4 formation by plasma membrane bound enzymes. Prostaglandins 28:929
14. Abe M, Kawazoe Y, Tsunematsu H, Shigematsu N (1985) Peritoneal macrophages of guinea pig possibly lack LTC_4 synthetase. Biochem Biophys Res Commun 127:15
15. Clark RA, Szot S (1982) Chemotactic factor inactivation by stimulated human neutrophils mediated by myeloperoxidase-catalyzed methionine oxidation. J Immunol 128:1507
16. Parker CW, Koch D, Huber MM, Falkenhein SF (1980) Formation of the cysteinyl form of slow reacting substance (Leukotriene E_4) in human plasma. Biochem Biophys Res Commun 97:1038
17. Koller M, Schonfeld W, Knoller J, Bremm K-D, Konig W, Spur B, Crea A, Peters W (1985) The metabolism of leukotrienes in blood plasma studied by high-performance liquid chromatography. Biochim Biophys Acta 833:128
18. Yokata K, Shono F, Yamamoto S, Kominami E, Katunuma N (1983) Transformation of leukotriene D_4 catalyzed by lysosomal cathepsin H of rat liver. J Biochem 94:1173
19. Hammarstrom S (1981) Metabolism of leukotriene C_3 in the guinea pig. J Biol Chem 256:9573
20. Radmark O, Shimizu T, Fitzpatrick F, Samuelsson B (1984) Hemoprotein catalysis of leukotriene formation. Biochim Biophys Acta 792:324
21. Frankel EN (1982) Volatile lipid oxidation products. Prog Lipid Res 22:133
22. Parker CW (1982) The chemical nature of slow-reacting substances. In: Weissmann I (ed) Advances in inflammation research, vol 4. Raven, New York, p 1
23. Parker CW (1985) 5-Lipoxygenases. In: Hayaishi O, Yamamoto S (eds) Advances in prostaglandin, thromboxane, and leukotriene research. Kyoto Conference on Prostaglandins, vol 15. Raven, New York, p 167
24. Agins AP, Hollmann AB, Agarwal KC, Wiemann MC (1985) Detection of a novel cyclooxygenase metabolite produced by human promyelocytic leukemia (HL-60) cells. Biochem Biophys Res Commun 126:143

25. Reiner NE, Malemud CJ (1985) Arachidonic acid metabolism by murine peritoneal macrophages infected with *Leishmania donovani:* evidence for parasite-induced alterations in cyclooxygenase and lipoxygenase pathways. J Immunol 134:556
26. Fusco AC, Salafsky B, Kevin MB (1985) *Schistosoma mansoni:* eicosanoid production by cercariae. Exp Parasitol 59:44
27. Goldman DW, Goetzl EJ (1984) Heterogeneity of human polymorphonuclear leukocyte receptors for leukotriene B_4. J Exp Med 159:1027
28. Kreisle R, Parker CW, Griffin GL, Senior RM, Stenson WF (1985) Studies of leukotriene B_4-specific binding and function in rat polymorphonuclear leukocytes: absence of a chemotactic response. J Immunol 134:3356
29. Ford-Hutchinson AW, Bray MA, Doig MV, Shipley ME, Smith MJH (1980) Leukotriene B, a potent chemokinetic and aggregating substance released from polymorphonuclear leukocytes. Nature 286:264
30. Shaafi RI, Naccache PH, Molski TFP, Borgeat P, Goetzl EJ (1981) Cellular regulatory role of leukotriene B_4: its effects on cation homeostasis in rabbit neutrophils. J Cell Phys 108:401
31. Naccache PH, Molski TFP, Borgeat P, White JR, Shaafi RI (1985) Phorbol esters inhibit the fMet-Leu-Phe- and leukotriene B-stimulated calcium mobilization and enzyme secretion in rabbit neutrophils. J Biol Chem 260:2125
32. Kreisle RA, Parker CW (1983) Specific binding of leukotriene B_4 to a receptor on human polymorphonuclear leukocytes. J Exp Med 157:628
33. Goldman DW, Goetzl EJ (1982) Specific binding of leukotriene B_4 to receptors on human polymorphonuclear leukocytes. J Immunol 129:1600
34. Lin AH, Ruppel PL, Gorman RR (1984) Leukotriene B_4 binding to human neutrophils. Prostaglandins 28:837
35. Kelly JP, Johnson MC, Parker CW (1979) Effect of inhibitors of arachidonic acid metabolism of mitogenesis in human lymphocytes. Possible role of thromboxanes and products of the lipoxygenase pathway. J Immunol 122:1563–1571
36. Bailey JM, Bryant RW, Low CE, Pupillo MB, Vanderhoek JY (1982) Role of lipoxygenases in regulation of PHA and phorbol ester-induced mitogenesis In: Samuelsson B, Paoletti R (eds) Leukotrienes and other lipoxygenase products. Raven, New York, p 341
37. Gualde N, Atluru D, Goodwin JS (1985) Effect of lipoxygenase metabolites of arachidonic acid on proliferation of human T cells and T cell subsets. J Immunol 134:1125
38. Payan DG, Missirian-Bastian A, Goetzl EJ (1984) Human T-lymphocyte subset specificity of the regulatory effects of leukotriene B_4. Proc Natl Acad Sci USA 81:3501
39. Drazen JM, Austen KF, Lewis RA, Clark DA, Goto G, Marfat A, Corey EJ (1980) Comparative airway and vascular activities of leukotrienes C-1 and D in vivo and in vitro. Proc Natl Acad Sci USA 77:4354
40. Hanna CJ, Bach MK, Pare PD, Schellenberg RR (1981) Slow reacting substances (leukotrienes) contract human airway and pulmonary vascular smooth muscle in vitro. Nature 290:343
41. Palmer MP, Mathews R, Murphy RC, Hoffer B (1980) Leukotriene C elicits a prolonged excitation of cerebellar Purkinje neurons. Neurosci Lett 18:173
42. Richardson PS, Peatfield AC, Jackson DM, Piper PJ (1982) The effect of leukotrienes on the output of mucins from the cat trachea. In: Piper PJ (ed), Leukotrienes and other lipoxygenase products, Raven, New York, p 178
43. Marom Z, Shelhamer JH, Kaliner M (1981) Effects of arachidonic acid, monohydroxyeicosatetraenoic acid and prostaglandins on the release of mucous glycoproteins from human airways in vitro. J Clin Invest 67:1695
44. Hogaboom GK, Mong S, Stadel JM, Crooke ST (1985) Characterization of guinea pig myocardial leukotriene C_4 binding sites. Mol Pharmacol 27:236
45. Dillard RD, Carr FP, McCullough D, Haisch KD, Rinkema LE, Fleisch JH (1985) New aryloxymethylacetophenones: antagonists of LTD_4-induced contractions of guinea pig ileum. Fed Proc 44:471
46. Welton AF, Hope WC, Fiedler-Nagy C, Batula-Bernardo C, Coffey JW (1984) Analogs of arachidonic acid methylated at C-7 and C-10 inhibit leukotriene biosynthesis and phospholipase A_2 activity. Prostaglandins 28:649

47. Robinson C, Holgate ST (1984) Modulation of arachidonic acid metabolism in dispersed human cells by the inhibitor of leukotriene formation U-60. Prostaglandins 28:648
48. Jung G, Yang D-C, Nakao A (1985) Modulation of 5- and 15-lipoxygenase activities in human polymorphonuclear leukocytes (PMN) by A23187, butylated hydroxytoluene (BHT) and SKF-525A. Fed Proc 44:578
49. Corey EJ, Cashman JR, Eckrich TM, Corey DR (1985) A new class of irreversible inhibitors of leukotriene biosynthesis. J Am Chem Soc 107:713
50. Baker SR, Boot JR, Ross WJ, Todd A (1984) Some β-hydroxy-sulphides as leukotriene D_4 antagonists. Prostaglandins 28:655
51. Marone G, Hammarstrom S, Lichtenstein LM (1980) An inhibitor of lipoxygenase inhibits histamine release from human basophils. Clin Immunol Immunopathol 17:117
52. Parker CW, Fischman CM, Wedner HJ (1980) Relationship of slow reacting substance biosynthesis to intracellular glutathione levels. Proc Natl Acad Sci USA 77:6870
53. Bailey JM, Bryant RW, Low CE, Pupillo MB, Vanderhoek JY (1982) Role of lipoxygenases in regulation of PHA and phorbol ester-induced mitogenesis. In: Samuelsson B, Paolett R (eds) Leukotrienes and other lipoxygenase products. Raven, New York, p 341
54. Toda M, Arai Y, Hayashi M (1985) Analogs of leukotrienes and related lipoxygenase products. In: Pike JE, Morton DR (eds) Advances in prostaglandin, thromboxane, and leukotriene research, vol 14. Raven, New York, p 427
55. Terano T, Salmon JA, Moncada S (1984) Effect of orally administered eicosapentaenoic acid (EPA) on the formation of leukotriene B_4 and leukotriene B_5 by rat leukocytes. Biochem Pharmacol 33:3071
56. Strasser T, Fischer S, Weber PC (1985) Leukotriene B_5 is formed in human neutrophils after dietary supplementation with eicosapentaenoic acid. Proc Natl Acad Sci USA 82:1540
57. Engineer DM, Morris HR, Piper PJ, Sirois P (1978) The release of prostaglandins and thromboxanes from guinea-pig lung by slow reacting substance of anaphylaxis and its inhibition. Br J Pharmacol 64:211
58. Hopkins NK, Lin AH, Gorman RR (1983) Evidence for mediation of acetyl glyceryl ether phosphorylcholine stimulation of adenosine 3',5'-(cyclic) monophosphate levels in human polymorphonuclear leukocytes by leukotriene B_4. Biochim Biophys Acta 763:276
59. Parker CW (1985) 5-Lipoxygenases In: Hayaishi O, Yamamoto S (eds) Advances in Prostaglandin, Thromboxane, and Leukotriene Research. Kyoto Conference on Prostaglandins, vol. 15, Chapter 45. Raven Press, New York, pgs 167–168

Lipoxygenase Activity in Cutaneous Inflammation

T. Ruzicka

Dermatologische Klinik der Ludwig-Maximilians-Universität München, 8000 Munich, Federal Republic of Germany

Abstract

The molecular basis of cutaneous inflammation – immunologic or non-immunologic – is largely unknown. Mediators of inflammation such as histamine may play a certain role in itching dermatoses such as atopic eczema, however, the interest has recently focused on metabolites of arachidonic acid (eicosanoids). The assumption of their involvement in the pathophysiology of cutaneous inflammation is based on several observations:

- extraordinary biological activities of eicosanoids on blood vessels and cellular constituents of inflammatory reactions;
- generation of proinflammatory eicosanoids by granulocytes, macrophages and epidermis;
- recovery of eicosanoids from inflamed skin;
- effects of antiinflammatory drugs on eicosanoid production.

In involved skin in atopic eczema, normal levels of histamine and cyclooxygenase metabolites of arachidonic acid were measured, although increased histamine release was observed upon immunological stimulation of biopsy specimens. In contrast, markedly elevated levels of immunoreactive leukotriene B_4 (LTB_4) were recovered from suction blister fluid taken from involved atopic eczema skin. The immunoreactive material showed chromatographic properties of LTB_4 on HPLC analysis. These findings may not be unique to atopic eczema and may be encountered in other inflammatory dermatoses as well. The lack of specificity of leukotriene elevation does not, however, argue against its pathophysiological importance: various inflammatory dermatoses may have similar pathobiochemical changes in common. The specific characteristics of these diseases, however, may be due to factors unrelated to arachidonic acid metabolism.

Since enhanced "releasability" of inflammatory mediators is assumed to play a key role in various clinical manifestations of atopy, an attempt was made to measure the generation of lipoxygenase- and cyclooxygenase-derived eicosanoids by peripheral blood mononuclear cells. Measurable levels of prostaglandin E_2 and leukotrienes B_4 and C_4 were detected in supernatants of cells challenged with Ca-ionophore A23187, anti-IgE and C5a. The release of eicosanoids was dependent on the dose of the stimulants. An attempt was made to evaluate quantitative and qualitative differences in eicosanoid releasability between healthy and atopic subjects.

Biological Effects of Eicosanoids

The biochemical mediators causing immunological or nonimmunological inflammation in skin have not yet been clearly identified. In recent years, research interest has focused on eicosanoids, i.e. mediators derived from arachidonic acid [8]. This surge in interest has been due to their potent pro- and anti-inflammatory properties [reviewed in 3, 7].

Skin itself possesses a high capacity to transform arachidonic acid into oxygenated products [reviewed in 5]. The main metabolic pathway of arachidonic acid in skin is the 12-lipoxygenase pathway, leading to the formation of 12-hydroxyeicosatetraenoic acid (12-HETE), which thus represents the major eicosanoid in skin of all species so far examined, including man. Cyclooxygenase activity is also expressed in skin, with PGE_2 and PGD_2 as major products. Both 12-lipoxygenase and cyclooxygenase enzymes are localized mainly in the epidermal layer of the skin; the dermis exhibits only low enzyme activities. Only very low activities of 5-lipoxygenase are present in normal skin. This situation may, however, change in inflammatory conditions since the main producers of the 5-lipoxygenase metabolites 5-HETE and the leukotrienes LTB_4 and LTC_4, i.e., neutrophil and eosinophil granulocytes and macrophages, can frequently be encountered in inflammatory infiltrates in great numbers.

Besides the formation of eicosanoids in skin, their biological effects in this tissue is deserving interest. Eicosanoids exert the following effects in skin [5], which might be of pathophysiological relevance in a variety of skin diseases:

1. They can lead to vasodilation, erythema, and wheal and flare.
2. They enhance vascular permeability and thus cause edema formation.
3. They cause pain and hyperalgesia. (Hyperalgesia is a sensation observed, for example, in sunburn reaction, where a light touch on the skin is perceived as painful.)
4. They exert potent chemotactic actions on leukocytes and lead to their activation.
5. They play a role in immune regulation, where they predominantly act as negative feedback regulators [2]; in addition, LTB_4 has recently been reported to activate suppressor T-lymphocytes.
6. They lead to enhanced proliferation of keratinocytes and thus may be involved in hyperproliferative disorders such as psoriasis [9].
7. Their synthesis is inhibited by glucocorticosteroids, which are the mainstay of anti-inflammatory therapy in dermatology and allergy. While these drugs inhibit the formation of all leukotrienes, HETEs, and prostaglandins, nonsteroidal anti-inflammatory drugs (NSAIDs) such as indomethacin or aspirin act predominantly as inhibitors of prostaglandin synthesis and influence to a lesser degree lipoxygenase-catalyzed arachidonate transformations. This and the fact that very few skin diseases are amenable to treatment with NSAIDs,

in contrast to glucocorticosteroids, makes a major role of the classic prostaglandins in cutaneous inflammation unlikely and has led to the focus on the lipoxygenase products HETEs and particularly LTB_4.

Studies in Skin Diseases

For several years our group has been pursuing research into the mechanisms involved in atopic eczema, a common skin disease characterized by chronic cutaneous inflammation and numerous immunological abnormalities which thus appears particularly suited to analysis in terms of arachidonic acid metabolism. We measured the concentrations of arachidonic acid-derived mediators and histamine (which can be suspected of being involved in atopic eczema owing to the prominent itch accompanying the disease) in suction blister fluid obtained from involved and uninvolved skin of patients with atopic eczema. On lesional skin, intact blisters can rarely be raised, but the interstitial fluid accumulates in the vacuum bell of the suction blister apparatus. For comparison, samples were obtained from corresponding body sites of healthy controls and lesional and healthy appearing skin of patients with psoriasis.

Concentrations of the mediators histamine, PGE_2, PGD_2 and leukotriene B_4 were measured in suction blister fluid using specific radioimmunoassays [for experimental details, see 6]. PGD_2 could not be detected in any suction blister sample using two radioimmunoassays with different specificities, one directed against a stable catabolite of PGD_2 and another against native PGD_2. This finding is in agreement with the experiences of others in PGD_2 determination in suction blister fluid from other skin diseases such as cold urticaria (Greaves 1985, personal communication).

In addition, no significant differences were observed between PGE_2 concentrations in control skin and those in involved and uninvolved skin from patients with atopic eczema or psoriasis. Likewise, histamine concentrations were not significantly different in suction blister fluids obtained from patients with atopic eczema, patients with psoriasis, and healthy subjects. This result is in accord with our previous findings of normal histamine concentrations in whole skin biopsies in atopic eczema, although higher histamine releasability was observed from skin slices upon immunological stimulation [4]. Since histamine is the only mediator known to cause itch, its normal levels in atopic eczema in the two studies appear surprising at first glance. However, it is conceivable that its release precedes the development of established lesions in this disease.

In contrast to the above findings, marked elevation of LTB_4 was found in both inflammatory conditions: whereas LTB_4 concentrations were very low or undetectable in most samples from healthy control skin, high concentrations ranging up to 1524 pg/ml (mean value 426 ± 85 pg/ml) were found in lesional atopic eczema skin. There was no correlation between severity of disease, serum IgE levels, and LTB_4 concentrations. In psoriatic skin, LTB_4 levels were even higher, although not strikingly, with a mean of 649 ± 102 pg/ml.

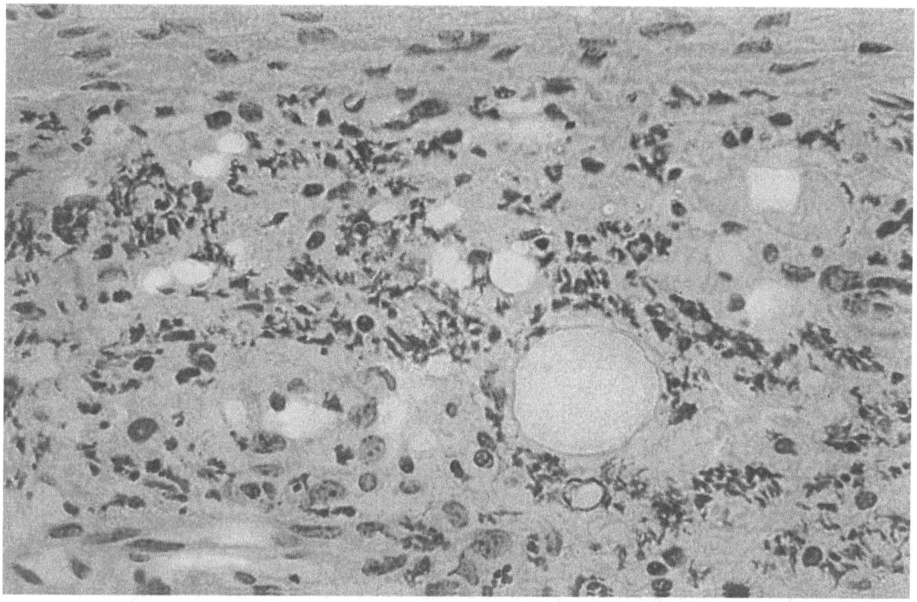

Fig. 1. Effect of chronic LTB_4 administration in skin: dense, perivascular inflammatory infiltrate with prominent leukocytoclasia

Therefore, of those mediators which we measured there is a selective elevation of the 5-lipoxygenase metabolite LTB_4 in atopic eczema and psoriasis. In addition, it is conceivable that an amplification mechanism might be operative in these disorders which might even enhance the biological effects of LTB_4, since increased responsiveness toward the chemotactic action of LTB_4 was found in atopic eczema and psoriasis monocytes [1]. Therefore, these diseases are characterized both by elevated levels and by enhanced effects of LTB_4.

LTB_4 in Guinea Pig Skin

In order to investigate the biological effects of LTB_4 in skin, we injected guinea-pig ears twice daily for 5 days with LTB_4 in saline or with saline alone, and examined the effects histologically. LTB_4 dose per injection was 100 ng. Leukotriene injections led to some increase in epidermal thickness; however, the acanthotic epidermis showed no change in structure. Specifically, little spongiosis, no intraepidermal infiltrate, and no alteration in the keratinization pattern could be observed. On the other hand, there was a massive inflammatory infiltrate and edema in the dermis. The infiltrate was predominantly perivascular and composed of granulocytes, histiocytes, and a conspicuously high number of eosinophils. Another prominent feature was the presence of nuclear fragments in the perivascular space (Fig. 1). The changes on the whole corresponded to those which one observes in leukocytoclastic vasculitis.

In summary, LTB_4 may play an important role in inflammatory skin diseases such as atopic eczema and psoriasis. However, it does not reproduce all the aspects of these diseases, and additional pathogenetic factors must be postulated. Furthermore, LTB_4 might be involved in various forms of cutaneous vasculitis and in all those skin diseases characterized by tissue eosinophilia.

Acknowledgments. The results reported herein were obtained in cooperation with Prof. B. A. Peskar and Dr. T. Simmet, Bochum, and Profs. J. Ring and G. Burg, Munich. The technical assistance of Ms. C. Trautwein is gratefully acknowledged. This work was supported by Deutsche Forschungsgemeinschaft (Ru 292/2-1).

References

1. Czarnetzki B (1983) Increased monocyte chemotaxis towards leukotriene B_4 and platelet activating factor in patients with inflammatory dermatoses. Clin Exp Immunol 54:486–492
2. Goldyne ME, Stobo JD (1981) Immunoregulatory role of prostaglandins and related lipids. CRC Crit Rev Immunol 189–233
3. Lewis RA, Austen KF (1981) Mediation of local homeostasis and inflammation by leukotrienes and other mast cell-dependent compounds. Nature 293:103–108
4. Ruzicka T, Glück S (1983) Cutaneous histamine levels and histamine releasability from the skin in atopic dermatitis and hyper-IgE syndrome. Arch Dermatol Res 275:41–44
5. Ruzicka T, Printz MP (1984) Arachidonic acid metabolism in skin: a review. Rev Physiol Biochem Pharmacol 100:121–160
6. Ruzicka T, Simmet T, Peskar BA, Ring J (1985) Skin levels of arachidonic acid-derived inflammatory mediators and histamine in atopic dermatitis and psoriasis. J Invest Dermatol 86:105–108
7. Samuelsson B (1983) Leukotrienes: mediators of immediate hypersensitivity reactions and inflammation. Science 220:568–575
8. Voorhees JJ (1983) Leukotrienes and other lipoxygenase products in the pathogenesis and therapy of psoriasis and other dermatoses. Arch Dermatol 119:541–547
9. Voorhees JJ (1985) Eicosanoids in the pathogenesis and therapy of psoriasis. Presentation at 2nd Annual symposium, Skin Pharmacology Society, Boston

Methods in Eicosanoid Determination

T. Simmet

Institut für Pharmakologie und Toxikologie, Ruhr-Universität Bochum, Im Lottental, 4630 Bochum 1, Federal Republic of Germany

Abstract

The very low concentrations of eicosanoids present in most biological systems require extremely sensitive detection methods. The determination of eicosanoids is further complicated by the structural similarity among the different types of cyclooxygenase and lipoxygenase products of polyunsaturated fatty acid metabolism calling for high specificity of the detection technique employed. Basically three different methods for eicosanoid determination have been commonly used. Bioassays reveal moderate sensitivity, specificity and precision but have been crucial for the discovery of short-lived compounds such as thromboxane A_2 and prostaglandin I_2. Combined gaschromatography/mass spectrometry (GC/MS), on the other hand, is the only method allowing formal identification of the compounds to be measured, provides good sensitivity, very good specificity and precision, but is rather time-consuming and expensive. Finally, immunoassays provide very good sensitivity and speed of sample processing together with good specificity and precision. The commercial availability of radiolabeled eicosanoids and of specific antibodies in combination with the simple principle of radioimmunoassay has contributed to the wide-spread use of these techniques in quantitative eicosanoid determination. However, to fully utilize the advantages radioimmunoassays may offer and in order to avoid pitfalls, several basic points have to be considered. Thus, standards and unknowns must be identical in such parameters as pH, temperature, ionic strength of buffers, protein content, anticoagulants etc. The only difference between standards and unknowns should be the amount of eicosanoid to be measured. Furthermore, immunoassay values should correlate to values obtained by unrelated methods e.g. bioassay or GC/MS, and addition of known quantities of exogenous standard material should result in the expected increment in immunoassay values. In addition, the immunoreactive material should cochromatograph with authentic standard, preferably in several solvent systems. Cross-reacting compounds present in the biological sample should be separated by appropriate techniques such as column/thin-layer-chromatography or high performance liquid chromatography before radioimmunoassay. In conclusion, radioimmunoassays properly validated provide a valuable, economical and rapid method for eicosanoid determination.

Introduction

Owing to the short chemical and/or biological half-life of most eicosanoids, one of the initial decisions to be made is whether to determine a primary eicosanoid or a more long-lived metabolite. In the bloodstream, for example, the biological half-lives of PGE_2 and $PGF_{2\alpha}$ are very short, less than 1 min, suggesting that the circulating levels are very low [30]. Therefore, it might be appropriate to determine metabolites of these compounds [9], which have also been identified in incubates from human gastrointestinal tissue [15, 22]. Another important issue to be addressed concerns sample collection and processing. Especially the collection and handling of blood samples might easily induce production of large amounts of eicosanoids, which could then obscure the true in vivo levels [27, 30, 32]. Favorable conditions for removal, preparation, and storage of human plasma have recently been published [33]. Extraction during sample processing, on the other hand, might result in loss or deterioration of some components [2, 18], indicating the necessity to establish the recovery during such procedures.

In most biological systems eicosanoids are present in very low concentrations that call for extremely sensitive detection techniques. The determination of eicosanoids is further complicated by the structural similarity between the different types of cyclooxygenase and lipoxygenase products of polyunsaturated fatty acid metabolism; the detection method employed must therefore have a high specificity. Basically three different methods for eicosanoid determination have been commonly used.

Assays for Eicosanoid Determination

The only method allowing formal identification of the compound to be measured is combined gas chromatography-mass spectrometry, which provides good sensitivity and very good specificity and precision [10, 17, 28, 31, 37]. This technique is based on the addition to the sample of a comparatively large amount of deuterium-labelled compound to be measured. This acts as a carrier during the chromatographic purification steps and as an internal standard during the final mass spectrometry [7]. The recent improvement of gas chromatographic-mass spectrometric profiling with negative-ion chemical ionization detection of prostaglandins now allows the simultaneous determination of several cyclooxygenase-derived products of arachidonic acid metabolism in the same sample, with a detection limit similar to that of radioimmuno assays [21, 32]. The major drawbacks of the method are the complexity of the technique and instrumentation and the very high costs. Furthermore, sample processing is rather time consuming. Thus, sample workup and analysis by gas chromatography-negative-ion chemical ionization mass spectrometry has been reported to take 10 days for six samples [21].

Bioassays, having been crucial for the discovery of short-lived compounds such as thromboxane A_2 [11, 25] and PGI_2 [19, 36], represent the only method permitting direct determination of these unstable but biologically highly active eicosanoids [20, 26, 36]. The method is based on the fact that the different eicosanoids exhibit both quantitative and qualitative differences on smooth muscle preparations obtained from different organs of various species. Starting out from the ordinary organ bath technique, the bioassay sensitivity was increased by the reduction of the bath volume, finally resulting in the superfusion technique. The introduction of superfusion of several tissues in cascade [35], resulting in a whole pattern of mechanical smooth muscle responses as well as the use of specific antagonists against other biologically active substances such as histamine, serotonin, bradykinin, and catecholamines, has allowed the establishment of quite specific assay systems made of suitable organs with different reactions to various compounds [20, 36]. However, any biological effect which can be quantitated, e.g., promotion or inhibition of platelet aggregation by thromboxane A_2 or PGI_2 respectively, is to be called a bioassay. Besides their obvious advantages, bioassays reveal moderate sensitivity, specificity, and precision.

The commercial availability of radiolabelled eicosanoids and of specific antisera in combination with the simple principle of immunoassay has contributed to the widespread use of these techniques in quantitative eicosanoid determination. Numerous radioimmunoassays have been developed for many products of the cyclooxygenase or lipoxygenase pathway of polyunsaturated fatty acid metabolism [8]. The basic principle of an immunoassay, as established by Yalow and Berson [40], is that in a reversible reaction the competition of a labelled antigen (usually radioactive labelled), or a so-called tracer, with an unlabelled antigen for a limited number of antibody binding sites results in two groups of antigen-antibody complexes, an unlabelled and a labelled group. The amount of labelled complex is a function of the concentration of unlabelled antigen present and the concentration of antigen in the unknown samples is calculated by comparison with standard samples containing known amounts of the antigen [38]. Due to the sigmoidal shape of most standard curves, logit plot, which also applies when the antibody is not completely saturated, has been shown to be the most versatile method for data calculation [29]. In a typical radioimmunoassay standards or unknown samples are mixed with a fixed amount of labelled antigen to which an antiserum dilution is finally added. After an appropriate incubation time the free and antibody-bound fractions of the antigen are separated and the radioactivity of one or both of the fractions measured.

Thus, for a radioimmunoassay a suitable labelled antigen, a specific antiserum, and a standardized method for separating antibody-bound and free fractions of antigen are required. Labelled eicosanoids are usually tritiated tracers from commercial sources but the use of iodinated derivatives has also been described [5, 24, 34]. High specific activity of labelled antigen increases the sensitivity of the radioimmunoassay, but highly iodinated molecules are often liable to enhanced radiodegradation [39].

Recently, enzymes have been used to label eicosanoid molecules such as PGD_2, $PGF_{2\alpha}$ thromboxane B_2, and a stable degradation product of the circulating PGE_2 metabolite [12, 13, 15, 41]. These enzyme immunoassays reveal a significantly enhanced sensitivity while avoiding the use of radioactive material. For the production of specific antisera the haptenic eicosanoids need to be coupled to a high molecular weight carrier molecule such as bovine serum albumin. Several coupling procedures have been described [1, 6]. Immunization is usually done by intradermal, intramuscular, or subcutaneous injection of the antigen emulsified with complete Freund's adjuvant. Usually rabbits are used for immunization, even though monoclonal antibodies against eicosanoids have recently been described [3, 4, 16]. A large number of methods for the separation of antibody-bound and free antigen have been described [38, 39]. Those commonly used are the absorption of free antigen to charcoal, the precipitation of antigen-antibody complexes with polyethylene glycol, or antibodies directed against the γ-globulin fraction of antiserum used in the immunoassay; because of its rapidity the charcoal method is often preferred. The critical point is that the antigen-antibody complexes are not supposed to dissociate during the process of separation. Extremely rapid separation is achieved by the use of solid phase radioimmunoassays where the antibody is bound to a solid phase such as polystyrene beads or tubes [23].

The immunoassay procedure provides very good sensitivity and rapid sample processing combined with good specificity and precision. However, to utilize fully the advantages radioimmunoassays may offer and in order to avoid pitfalls, proper validation is required for each experimental situation. Thus, Lands et al. [14] recommended a number of quality controls to help in validating immunoassays:

1. Particularly in the early stage of assay development it is helpful to demonstrate that immunoassay values in tissue correspond to those obtained by other methods (e.g., bioassay, gas chromatography-mass spectrometry).
2. Addition of known quantities of exogenous standard material should produce the expected increment in the immunoassay.
3. Immunoreactive antigen in the samples should co-chromatograph with trace amounts of radio-labelled antigen as well as authentic standard, preferably in more than one chromatographic system.
4. If an enzyme capable of destroying antigen in the sample is available, it should reduce the immunoreactivity of the sample to low levels.
5. Quantities of cross-reacting antigens known to be present in the samples should be shown not to influence the assay or be removed by a suitable fractionation procedure such as column or thin layer chromatography or high performance liquid chromatography before radioimmunoassay.
6. Every sample must be handled as comparably as possible to avoid spurious effects of pH or ionic strength in the assay. All stimulatory agents must be evaluated in the absence of tissue for non-specific effects in the assay. Furthermore, the only difference between standards and unknowns should be the amount of eicosanoids to be measured.

In conclusion, immunoassays properly validated provide valuable, economical, and rapid methods for eicosanoid determination.

References

1. Axen U (1974) *N,N*-Carbonyldiimidazole as coupling reagent for the preparation of bovine serum conjugates. Prostaglandins 10:45–47
2. Borgeat P (1984) Reversed phase HPLC profiling and quantitation of lipoxygenase products. Prostaglandins 27:356–358
3. Brune K, Busse WD, Grützmann R, Wyss T (1982) Monoclonal antibodies against $PGF_{2\alpha}$ and 6-keto-$PGF_{1\alpha}$. V. International Conference on Prostaglandins, 18–21 May, Florence, Italy, Abstractbook, p 48
4. David F, Sommé G, Provost-Wisner A, Roth C, Astoin M, Dray F, Thèze J (1985) Characterization of monoclonal antibodies against prostaglandin E_2: fine specificity and neutralization of biological effects. Mol Immunol 22:339–346
5. Dray F (1982) Iodinated derivatives as tracers for eicosanoid radioimmunoassays. Methods enzymol 86:297–306
6. Erlanger BF (1973) Principles and methods for the preparation of drug protein conjugates for immunological studies. Pharmacol Rev 25:271–280
7. Granström E (1980) Assay methods for prostaglandins and thromboxanes. In: Samuelsson S, Ramwell PW, Paoletti R (eds) Advances in prostaglandin and thromboxane research, vol 6. Raven, New York, pp 69–76
8. Grandström E, Kindahl H (1978) Radioimmunoassay of prostaglandins and thromboxanes. In: Frölich JC (ed) Advances in prostaglandin and thromboxane research, vol 5. Raven, New York, pp 119–210
9. Granström E, Kindahl H (1984) Circulating and urinary metabolites of PGE_2 and $PGF_{2\alpha}$. Prostaglandins 27:350–352
10. Gréen K, Hamberg M, Samuelsson B, Smigel M, Frölich JC (1978) Measurement of prostaglandins, thromboxanes, prostacyclin and their metabolites by gas liquid chromatography-mass spectrometry. In: Fröhlich JC (ed) Advances in prostaglandin and thromboxane research, vol 5. Raven, New York, pp 39–94
11. Hamberg M, Svensson J, Samuelsson B (1975) Thromboxanes: a new group of biologically active compounds derived from prostaglandin endoperoxides. Proc Natl Acad Sci USA 72:2994–2998
12. Hayashi Y, Yamamoto S (1982) Enzyme immunoassay of $PGF_{2\alpha}$. Methods enzymol 86:269–273
13. Hayashi Y, Ueda N, Yokota K, Kawamura S, Ogushi F, Yamamoto Y, Yamamoto S, Nakamura K, Yamashita K, Miyazaki H, Kato K, Terao S (1983) Enzyme immunoassay of thromboxane B_2. Biochem Biophys Acta 750:322–329
14. Lands WEM, Hammarström S, Parker CW (1976) Limitations of prostaglandin assays. J Invest Dermatol 67:658–660
15. Lange K, Simmet T, Peskar BM, Peskar BA (1985) Determination of 15-keto-13,14-dihydro-prostaglandin E_2 and prostaglandin D_2 in human colonic tissue using a chemiluminescence enzyme immunoassay with catalase as labeling enzyme. In: Hayaishi O, Yamamoto S (eds) Advances in prostaglandin, thromboxane, and leukotriene research, vol 15. Raven, New York pp 35–38
16. Lee JY, Chernov T, Goetzl EJ (1984) Characteristics of the epitope of leukotriene B_4 recognized by a highly specific mouse monoclonal antibody. Biochem Biophys Res Commun 123:944–950
17. Maas RL, Lawson JA, Brash AR, Oates JA (1983) Derivatization and analysis of leukotrienes by desorption-chemical ionization mass spectrometry at subnanomole level. In: Samuelsson B, Paoletti R, Ramwell P (eds) Advances in prostaglandin, thromboxane and leukotriene research, vol 11. Raven, New York, pp 229–234
18. Mitchell MD, Brunt JD, Webb R (1981) Instability of 6-keto-prostaglandin $F_{1\alpha}$ when subjected to normal extraction procedures. Prostaglandins Med 6:437–440
19. Moncada S, Gryglewski R, Bunting S, Vane JR (1976) An enzyme isolated from arteries transforms prostaglandin endoperoxides to an unstable substance that inhibits platelet aggregation. Nature 263:663–665

20. Moncada S, Ferreira SH, Vane JR (1978) Bioassay of prostaglandins and biologically active substances derived from arachidonic acid. In: Frölich JC (ed) Advances in prostaglandin and thromboxane research, vol 5. Raven, New York, pp 211–237
21. Pace-Asciak CR, Micallef S (1984) Gas chromatographic-mass spectrometric profiling with negative-ion chemical ionization detection of prostaglandins and their 15-keto- and 15-keto-13,14-dihydro catabolites in rat blood. J Chromatogr 310:233–242
22. Peskar BM, Peskar BA (1976) On the metabolism of prostaglandins by human gastric fundus mucosa. Biochem Biophys Acta 424:430–438
23. Peskar BA, Peskar BM (1977) Advances in hapten immunoassays. Eur J Drug Metabol Pharmacokin 4:163–170
24. Peskar BA, Anhut H, Kröner EE, Peskar BM (1979) Development, specificity and some applications of radioimmunoassays for prostaglandins and related compounds. In: Tillement JP (ed) Advances in pharmacology and therapeutics. Pergamon, Oxford, pp 275–286 (Biochemical clinical pharmacology, vol 7)
25. Piper PJ, Vane JR (1969) Release of additional factors in anaphylaxis and its antagonism by antiinflammatory drugs. Nature 223:29–35
26. Podium Discussion, moderation: Peskar BA (1985) Methods of measurement of eicosanoids. In: Schrör K (ed) Prostaglandins and other eicosanoids in the cardiovascular system. Karger, Basel, pp 29–39
27. Podium Discussion, moderation: Sinzinger H (1985) Sample processing – the "normal" value of eicosanoids. In: Schrör K (ed) Prostaglandins and other eicosanoids in the cardiovascular system. Karger, Basel, pp 40–55
28. Rigaud M (1984) Glass capillary-gas chromatography-mass spectrometry analysis of hydroxy and hydroxy-epoxy polyunsaturated fatty acids. Prostaglandins 27:358–361
29. Rodbard D, Bridson W, Rayford PL (1969) Rapid calculation of radioimmunoassay results. J Lab Clin Med 74:770–781
30. Samuelsson B, Granström E, Gréen K, Hamberg M, Hammarström S (1975) Prostaglandins. Annu Rev Biochem 44:669–695
31. Sautebin L, Caruso D, Galli G (1984) Analysis of cyclooxygenase and lipoxygenase products in incubation media. Prostaglandins 27:361–363
32. Schweer H, Kammer J, Seyberth HW (1985) Simultaneous determination of prostanoids in plasma by gas chromatography-negative-ion chemical ionization-mass spectrometry. J Chromatogr 338:273–280
33. Sinzinger H, Reiter S, Peskar BA (1985) Removal, preparation, and storage of human plasma for radioimmunological detection of prostaglandins. In: Schrör K (ed) Prostaglandins and other eicosanoids in the cardiovascular system. Karger, Basel, pp 62–67
34. Sors H, Maclouf J, Pradelles P, Dray F (1977) The use of iodinated tracers for a sensitive radioimmunoassay of 13,14-dihydro-15-keto-prostaglandin $F_{2\alpha}$. Biochem Biophys Acta 486:553–564
35. Vane JR (1964) The use of isolated organs for detecting active substances in the circulating blood. Br J Pharmacol 23:360–373
36. Vane JR (1983) Adventures and excursions in bioassay: the stepping stones to prostacyclin. Br J Pharmacol 79:821–838
37. Vesterqvist O, Gréen K (1984) Development of a GC-MS method for quantitation of 2,3-dinor-6-keto-$PGF_{1\alpha}$ and determination of the urinary excretion rates in healthy humans under normal conditions and following drugs. Prostaglandins 28:139–154
38. Yalow RS (1973) Radioimmunoassay methodology: application to problems of heterogeneity of peptide hormones. Pharmacol Rev 25:161–178
39. Yalow RS (1973) Radioimmunoassay. Practices and pitfalls. Circ Res [Suppl I] 32/33:I-116-I-128
40. Yalow RS, Berson SA (1960) Immunoassay of endogenous plasma insulin in man. J Clin Invest 39:1157–1175
41. Yamamoto S (1984) Enzyme immonoassay. Prostaglandins 27:366–367

Chemotactic Factors as Mediators of Allergy

B. M. Czarnetzki
Universitäts-Hautklinik Münster, 4400 Münster, Federal Republic of Germany

Abstract

Mast cells are the central effector cells of acute allergic reactions. Besides histamine which has no significant chemotactic activity of its own, mast cells release other inflammatory mediators into their environment. Several of these factors have neutrophil or eosinophil chemotactic activities, such as leukotriene B_4 (LTB_4), platelet activating factor (PAF) and neutrophil chemotactic factor (NCF). Enzymes of mast cells can also activate the complement casade, resulting in the production of the potent chemotactic peptide C5a. Once inflammatory leukocytes have entered the site of allergic reaction, they can generate the same chemotactic mediators that are produced by mast cells. Chemotactic mediators serve to amplify and perpetuate mast cell-dependent allergic processes, and they induce chronic inflammatory changes and tissue damage in persistent, severe allergic reactions.

Introduction

Chemotaxis is one of the most basic functions of living cells. It enables unicellular organisms to obtain food through migration toward chemical signs that diffuse from the source of food. In multicellular organisms, chemotaxis enables the body to defend itself against noxious foreign substances. The penetrating agents give off chemicals that cause the influx of leukocytes which are to kill and eliminate the foreign material. Alternatively, the invading agents cause the generation of chemotactic factors at the site of penetration, either by stimulating the resident cells to secrete such mediators or through the activation of complement.

Allergic reactions occur in response to the invasion of foreign substances via the skin, the respiratory, or the gastrointestinal route in individuals whose immune system has previously come into contact with and responded to the same substances. In common thinking, allergy is associated with immediate-type, IgE-dependent, mast cell-mediated, fleeting reactions. Mediators like histamine or slow-reacting substances (SRS) cause the smooth muscle contracting, vasospastic, and edematous tissue responses which give these reactions their transient features.

On closer scrutiny of the clinical reactions, however, it becomes apparent that mast cell-dependent reactions can be more prolonged, and recently good evidence has been provided as to the mechanism of these latter reactions:

1. Leukocytic and, more recently, mononuclear infiltrates have been demonstrated in mast cell-dependent, delayed allergic reactions [24].
2. Mononuclear perivascular infiltrates have also been observed in chronic urticaria [27].
3. Mixed infiltrates, at times with some eosinophils, are found in pressure urticaria [13].
4. Eosinophils, neutrophils, macrophages, and plasma cells have been shown to accumulate in the bronchial mucosa of patients who had died in status asthmaticus [22].
5. A vasculitis with eosinophils, plasma, and other mononuclear cells has been found in the lungs of patients with hypersensitivity pneumonitis [12].

In order to explain these leukocytic infiltrates, one must postulate the chemotactic factors are operative in the pathophysiology of allergic reactions.

Chemotactic mediators have been found in acute but more so in delayed allergic reactions. The major pathological reaction types involved include (a) mast cell-dependent processes (Table 1), (b) immune complex- and complement-dependent reactions, (c) cytotoxic reactions, and (d) the classical lymphocyte/macrophage-dependent, delayed-type hypersensitivity reactions.

Mast Cell-Dependent Reactions

Mast cells or basophils participate in some way in almost all types of allergic reactions. This is suggested by the demonstration of histamine in the tissue and by the frequently associated pruritus. In the immediate-type reactions, tissue mast cells are able to induce the often massive clinical reactions through potent mediators which are either stored in their cytoplasmic granules in a preformed state or generated de novo from the membrane lipids on stimulation of the cells (Fig. 1).

A few of these mast cell mediators have primarily smooth muscle-contracting and edema-producing properties. They include histamine, bradykinin, SRS, platelet-activating factor (PAF), and several of the prostaglandins. The increased local blood flow, the vasodilatation, and the increased capillary permeability that is mediated by these agents prepare the tissue for the emigration of leukocytes from the bloodstream in response to the chemotactic factors which are also released from the mast cells. Some of the mast cell mediators have both SRS and chemotactic properties. This is most obvious for PAF, which is a moderately potent chemoattractant for neutrophils, and in some patients also for monocytes [7, 10] (Table 2). PAF is best known for one additional biological property, its platelet activating activities.

Table 1. The most important pathomechanisms in allergic reactions. Examples of the associated clinical picture and the presumptive chemotactic mediators involved in these reactions are also shown

Pathomechanisms	Clinical picture	Chemotactic mediators
1. Mast cell dependent	Anaphylaxis Asthma Urticaria	LTB_4, PAF NCF, IF-A ? Histamine?
2. Complement dependent	Vasculitis Pneumonitis	C5a, C5a-des-arg
3. Cytotoxic	Vasculitis Purpura	C5a, C5a-des-arg
4. Lymphocyte/macrophage dependent	Contact eczema Atopic eczema	LDCF MDCF

Abbreviations: LTB_4, leukotriene B_4; PAF, platelet-activating factor; NCF, neutrophil chemotactic factor; IF-A, inflammatory factor of anaphylaxis; LDCF, MDCF, lymphocyte- and monocyte-derived chemotactic factor

Table 2. Listing of the comparative activities of the most common chemotactic factors on different cell types in allergic reactions

Target cells	Chemotactic factors			
	C5a (C5a-des-arg)	LTB_4 (ECF)	PAF (AGEPS)	LDCF, MDCF
Neutrophils	++	++	+	+
Eosinophils	++	++	–	+
Monocytes/macrophages	++	+	+	+
Lymphocytes	+	–	–	+
Basophils	+	–	–	+
Fibroblasts	+	+	–	+

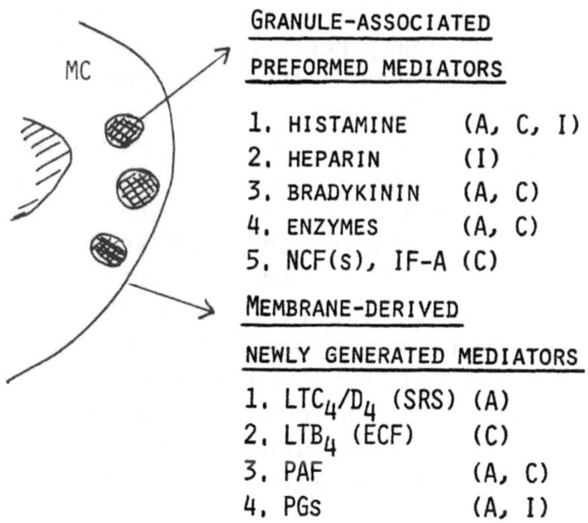

Fig. 1. The most important mast cell mediators. The *letters in parenthesis* indicate whether these factors have anaphylatoxic (*A*), chemotactic or chemotaxogenic (*C*), and inhibitory (*I*) effects

The role of histamine as a chemoattractant is controversial. Clark et al. [4] observed a chemotactic response of cells from patients with hypereosinophilic syndrome at low concentrations of histamine. H_1 or H_2 receptors were not involved. We have been unable to reproduce these findings in patients with eosinophilia due to other causes, but have observed that neutrophils from some patients with allergic dermatoses respond to histamine with a chemotactic and chemokinetic response, as proven by so-called checkerboard analyses.

If one disrupts mast cells and places the extracts in test chambers, one can also observe neutrophil chemotactic activity. In contrast, one never finds preformed eosinophil chemotactic factors (ECFs) in mast cells of unsensitized animals [16]. Peptide neutrophil chemotactic factors (NCFs) have also been identified in the venous blood of patients with cold urticaria after cold challenge [33] and in patients with asthma after bronchial provocation with a specific allergen [26]. While these latter plasma factors have never been proven to be of mast cell origin and their true chemotactic nature is even questioned [3], further evidence for peptide leukotactic activity has been provided by the injection of mast cell extracts into rat skin [28]. A histological examination of the injection sites revealed a leukocytic infiltrate similar to that observed in IgE-dependent, late cutaneous reactions.

One of the most potent chemotactic mediators produced by mast cells is the arachidonate-derived, lipoxygenase-dependent, 5,12-dihydroxyeicosatetraenoic acid (HETE), leukotriene B_4 (LTB_4). This factor corresponds to the activity formerly called ECF [4, 12]. It is released rapidly into tissue sites after stimulation of neutrophils, eosinophils, and monocytes [12, 32]. The 20-OH-metabolite of LTB_4 is about one-tenth as active as LTB_4, and the 20-COOH-LTB_4 has barely any activity at all [14]. 5-HETE, and less so 12-HETE, also has neutrophil chemotactic activity, but is about 100 times less potent than LTB_4 [29].

Bradykinin is not a chemotactic factor on its own, but it activates the complement system, causing the generation of chemotactic C5a. In addition, bradykinin induces the release of histamine from mast cells [21]. Enzymes from mast cell granules share both of these properties with bradykinin. Mast cell enzymes and bradykinin can thus be classified with the chemotaxinogens, i.e., with agents that generate chemotactic factors. PAF, which has been shown to induce LTB_4 secretion from neutrophils [19], is thus both a chemotactic factor on its own and a chemotaxinogen.

Considering that mast cells release several chemotactic factors immediately after their stimulation, it is surprising that infiltrating leukocytes are detected only in late allergic reactions. There are several possible reasons for this phenomenon. One of them may be related to the time sequence in which mast cell mediators are released. Histamine diffuses readily from the cell after stimulation, and the lipid mediators are also released very rapidly, reaching peak levels even before histamine. Simultaneously with the chemotactic signals of LTB_4 and PAF, the inhibitory effect of high concentrations of histamine on leukocyte migration would counteract the inhibition of a migratory response of the leukocytes. Furthermore, PGE_2, which increases the cAMP level of cells, would also prevent the diapedesis of cells through the vessel walls toward tissue sites [9].

Heparin, which is released more slowly than histamine from the membrane matrix of mast cells, binds a number of mediators very readily by means of its high charge. Such binding has so far been shown for ECF (LTB_4) and for lymphocyte-derived migration inhibitory factor (MIF) [15]. The release of inflammatory factor of anaphylaxis (IF-A) from the granular matrix, on the other hand, is slow and requires high ionic concentrations [28]. The delay in the release of IF-A from the granule matrix is thus another possible reason why leukocytic infiltrates are seen only in very intense, mast cell-dependent release reactions and only after several hours of cell stimulation.

An additional explanation for the delayed influx of leukocytes to sites of allergic reactions relates to the time it takes for cells to migrate from the endothelial cell wall through the tissue to the site of high concentrations of the stimulus. Lymphocytes and macrophages respond more sluggishly than neutrophils to the same chemotactic factors (Table 2). Their predominance in older reaction sites where neutrophils are missing is not well understood but might be due to an inhibitor from mononuclear cells.

Chemotactic Factors in Other Types of Allergic Reaction

In allergen-dependent reactions, but also in drug reactions, complement activation is a central pathogenetic mechanism (Table 1). Immune complexes containing IgG_{1-3} or IgM activate the classical pathway while IgA-containing complexes as well as a wide variety of nonspecific agents [LPS, zymosan, $F(ab)_2$, dextran sulfate, and allergens] activate the alternative complement pathway [2]. Both classical and alternative complement activation result in the formation of the anaphylatoxins C3a, C4a, and C5a. These mediators fulfill the same role that is played by histamine and SRS in mast cell-dependent reactions, causing vasodilatation and increased capillary permeability. This in turn facilitates the action of the potent leukotactic factors C5a and C5a-des-arg. The infiltrating leukocytes can secrete more prostaglandins, leukotrienes, PAF, and lysosomal enzymes, resulting in further complement activation, more anaphylatoxin generation, and an amplification of the inflammatory process.

Cytotoxic reactions present themselves clinically as purpura and vasculitis. The pathomechanisms involved are poorly understood, and the reactions are probably relatively rare. Cytotoxic reactions may, however, be a minor component in other types of allergic reactions, primarily through the terminal components of complement activation which are potent lytic factors for cells. In the past, killed cells have been injected into animals, and by a so-called process of necrotaxis, leukocytes could be shown to accumulate at the injected sites. Complement activation by cellular constituents may be the major mechanism of chemotactic mediator generation in this situation. It provides a model for what may occur in cytotoxic reactions.

Contact eczema and atopic eczema are characterized by a lymphocytic, a monocytic, and occasionally an eosinophilic cellular infiltrate. In the acute eczematous reaction, an immigration of neutrophils or basophils may be observed as well. Chemotactic factors that regulate the development of this infiltrate are poorly defined. LTB_4 has been identified in atopic eczema lesions [31], but it is uncertain whether this mediator derives from mast cells or basophils, from the infiltrating leukocytes, or from resident cells like keratinocytes [20, 32]. Histamine is elevated in eczematous skin, and one must therefore assume a contribution of mast cells and basophils to these reactions. Macrophages and monocytes can also secrete arachidonate-derived mediators [5, 6, 32], PAF [30], and peptides with chemotactic activities [23]. It has been suggested that the recently described monocyte-derived chemotactic factor is identical to the chemotactic lymphokine LCDF, which was described several years ago [1].

Lymphocyte-derived factors have also been described to cause the accumulation of neutrophils, eosinophils, and basophils [1], cells which are seen in early and acute lesions of contact allergy. The exact nature of these mediators and their relative significance with regard to complement-derived and lipid-type mediators at tissue sites is, however, uncertain.

General Biological Properties of Chemotactic Factors

Most of what we know about the in vivo activities of chemotactic factors has become apparent through in vitro studies of purified mediators. Table 2 shows the spectrum of target cell specificities and the relative potencies of the most important chemotactic factors in allergic reactions. C5a and C5a-des-arg are potent chemoattractants with a wide range of target cell specificity. LTB_4 is as potent a chemotactic factor as C5a for granulocytes, but it is inactive toward lymphocytes and basophils. PAF is a relatively weak chemoattractant, with a narrow spectrum of activities, while lymphokines and monokines have a weak but protracted effect on a wide spectrum of cells. At present it is uncertain whether the lymphokine and monokine chemotactic activities for different cell types are due to several chemical entities or to one factor with several target cell specificities.

Migrating cells have specific membrane receptors for chemotactic factors. The number of receptors on cells can be increased or decreased in different pathological states. Contact of the chemotactic molecule with its receptor in the cell membrane initiates a complex sequence of events within the membrane and the cytosol, resulting in an increased ability of the cells to stick to each other and to endothelial cells, and thus allowing them to follow the chemotactic signal via the vessel wall into the tissue more readily (Fig. 2). The general, undirected mobility of the cells (chemokinesis) is also increased by the stimulus, and the same holds for the oxidative metabolism and the secretory capabilities of the cells. High concentrations of the chemotactic factor in the environment of the cell will, on the other hand, inhibit its chemotactic response. This so-called process of deactivation is important to keep the cell at the site of maximal factor concentration where phagocytic and cytotoxic activities must be exerted [9].

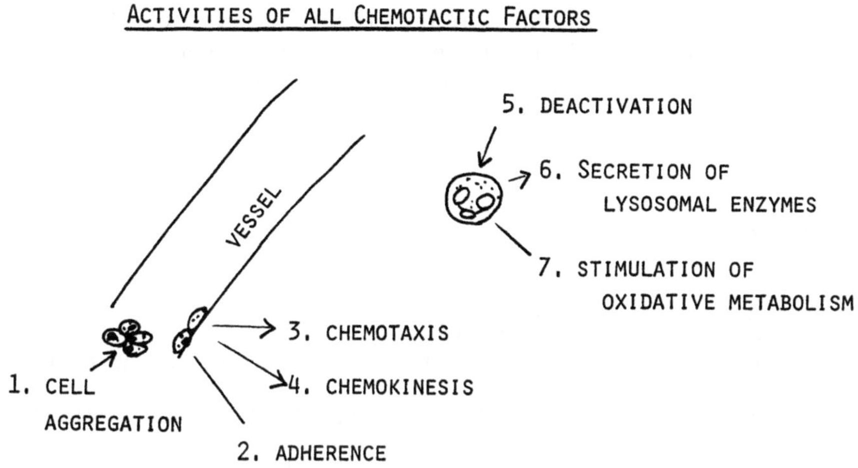

Fig. 2. Schematic presentation of the biological effects of most chemotactic factors

Some factors have specific biological effects in addition to their chemotactic properties. The anaphylatoxic and platelet-aggregating activities of C5a and PAF, and the immunomodulatory properties of LTB_4 are some prominent examples.

The combination of several chemotactic factors in vitro can have inhibitory as well as stimulatory, synergistic effects on migrating cells [8]. Since one must assume that in most allergic reactions more than one mediator is generated from cells or plasma, the interaction of factors with each other should be considered when one measures individual mediators in different pathological tissues.

Conclusion

With the recent discovery of new groups of mediators and with the availability of tools to measure these factors in cellular extracts and fluids, our understanding of the role of chemotactic factors in allergic reactions has deepened considerably. There is now a broad range of data which show that the biological effects of the factors, as studied in vitro, can be reproduced in vivo. This holds not only for histamine, bradykinin, prostaglandins, and the complement-derived anaphylatoxins, but also for the more recently identified leukotrienes and for PAF. Leukotrienes have been identified in a variety of allergic tissue reactions, such as in bullous drug eruptions, urticarial lesions, and atopic eczema [29, 31]. Studies with specific inhibitors of the mediators should provide an insight into which factors are truly clinically relevant. This has so far even failed for antihistamines in allergic asthma. Much remains thus to be done to show which factors predominate and are the primary initiators of allergic reactions and to what extent the different chemotactic and nonchemotactic factors augment or inhibit each other, to perpetuate or to terminate allergic reactions.

References

1. Altman LC (1978) Chemotactic lymphokines: a review. In: Gallin JI, Quie PG (eds) Leukocyte chemotaxis. Raven, New York, pp 267–267
2. Berrens L (1981) Struktur und Eigenschaften der atopischen Allergene. Hautarzt [Suppl 54] 32:83–85
3. Cundell DR, Moodley I, Davies RJ (1984) Properties of a high molecular weight neutrophil chemotactic factor, possibly derived from mast cells: evidence for chemokinetic rather than chemotactic activity. Agents Actions 14:384–387
4. Clark AF, Gallin JI, Kaplan AP (1975) The selective eosinophil chemotactic activity of histamine. J Exp Med 142:1462–1476
5. Czarnetzki BM (1980) Low molecular weight eosinophil chemotactic factor (ECF) production by rat peritoneal mononuclear phagocytes. Immunobiology 157:62–66
6. Czarnetzki BM (1981) In vitro generation of eosinophil chemotactic factor (ECF) from human and murine mononuclear phagocytes. Scand J Immunol 13:511–516
7. Czarnetzki BM (1983) Increased monocyte chemotaxis towards leukotriene B_4 and platelet activating factor in psoriasis and atopic eczema. Clin Exp Immunol 54:486–492
8. Czarnetzki BM (1985) Combined effect of chemotactic factors on in vitro leukocyte chemotaxis. J Invest Dermatol 84:444 (Abstract)
9. Czarnetzki BM (1985) Chemotaktische Mediatoren. Allergologie 8:63–68
10. Czarnetzki BM, Benveniste J (1981) Effect of synthetic PAF-acether in human neutrophil leukocytes. I. Analysis of the in vitro migration of human neutrophils. Chem Phys Lipids 29:317–326
11. Czarnetzki BM, Frosch PJ, Mardin M (1983) Leukotriene B_4 and neutrophil-derived eosinophil chemotactic factor: Comparison of their biological activities. Monogr Allergy 18:193–195
12. Czarnetzki BM, König W, Lichtenstein LM (1975) Release of eosinophil chemotactic factor from human polymorphonuclear neutrophils by calcium ionophore A23187 and phagocytosis. Nature 258:725–726
13. Czarnetzki BM, Meentken J, Kolde G, Bröcker EB (1985) Morphology of the cellular infiltrate in delayed pressure urticaria. J Am Acad Dermatol 12:253–259
14. Czarnetzki BM, Mertensmeier R (1985) In vitro and in vivo chemotaxis of guinea pig leukocytes towards leukotriene B_4 and its ω-oxidation products. Prostaglandins 30:5–12
15. Czarnetzki BM, Panneck W, Frosch PJ (1980) Inhibitory effect of heparin on leukocyte chemotactic factors. Clin Exp Immunol 39:526–531
16. Czarnetzki BM, Zimmermann RE, Fischer N (1981) Further characterization of the neutrophil-derived eosinophil chemotactic factor and comparison to eosinophil chemotactic activity from mast cells. Int Arch Allergy Appl Immunol 66 (S):172–173
17. Fink JN (1985) Allergic bronchopulmonary aspergillosis. Chest 87:81 S–84 S
18. Ford-Hutchinson AW (1984) Leukotriene involvement in pathological processes. J Allergy Clin Immunol 74 (S):437–440
19. Gorman EE, Morton DR, Hopkins NK, Lin AH (1983) Acetyl glyceryl ether phosphorylcholine stimulates leukotriene B_4 synthesis and cyclic AMP accumulation in human polymorphonuclear leukocytes. In: Samuelsson B, Paoletti R, Ramwell P (eds) Advances in prostaglandin, thromboxane, and leukotriene research, vol 12. Raven, New York, pp 57–63
20. Grabbe J, Czarnetzki BM, Mardin M (1984) Release of lipoxygenase products of arachidonic acid from freshly isolated human keratinocytes. Arch Dermatol Res 276:128–130

21. Ishizaka T, Iwata M, Ishizaka R (1985) Release of histamine and arachidonate from mouse mast cells induced by glycosylation-enhancing factor and bradykinin. J Immunol 134:1880–1887
22. Kaliner M (1985) Mast cell mediators and asthma. Chest 87:2S–5S
23. Kownatzki E, Kapp A, Uhrich S (1985) Novel neutrophil chemotactic factor derived from human monocytes. J Invest Dermatol 84:444 (Abstract)
24. Lemanske RF, Guthman DA, Kaliner M (1983) The biologic activity of mast cell granules. VII. The effect of anti-neutrophil antibody-induced neutropenia on rat cutaneous late phase reactions. J Immunol 131:929–933
25. Mensing H, Czarnetzki BM (1984) Leukotriene B_4 induces in vitro fibroblast chemotaxis. J Invest Dermatol 82:9–12
26. Nagy L, Lee TH, Kay AB (1982) Neutrophil chemotactic activity in antigen-induced late asthmatic reactions. N Engl J Med 306:497–501
27. Nathbony SF, Phillips ME, Elias JM, Godfrey HP, Kaplan AP (1983) Histologic studies of chronic idiopathic urticaria. J Allergy Clin Immunol 71:177–183
28. Oertel HL, Kaliner M (1981) The biologic activity of mast cell granules. III. Purification of inflammatory factors of anaphylaxis (IF-A) responsible for causing late-phase reactions. J Immunol 127:1398–1402
29. Rosenbach T, Grabbe J, Möller A, Schwanitz HJ, Czarnetzki BM (1985) Generation of leukotrienes from normal epidermis and their demonstration in cutaneous disease. Br J Dermatol 113 (285) 157–167
30. Roubin R, Mencia-Huerta JM, Benveniste J (1982) Release of platelet-activating factor (PAF acether) and leukotrienes C and D from inflammatory macrophages. Eur J Immunol 12:141–146
31. Ruzicka T, Simmet T, Peskar BA, Braun-Falco O (1984) Leukotrienes in skin of atopic dermatitis. Lancet 1:222–223
32. Samuelsson B (1982) The leukotrienes. An introduction. In: Samuelsson B, Paoletti R (eds) Leukotrienes and other lipoxygenase products. Raven, New York, pp 1–17
33. Wassermann SI, Soter NA, Center DM, Austen KF (1977) Cold urticaria: recognition and characterization of a neutrophil chemotactic factor which appears in serum during experimental cold challenge. J Clin Invest 60:189–196

Complement-Derived Mediators: Induction of Vascular Changes and Cellular Triggering Reactions by Anaphylatoxins

M. Meurer

Dermatologische Klinik der Ludwig-Maximilians-Universität, 8000 Munich 2, Federal Republic of Germany

Abstract

During complement activation two types of mediators are generated by enzymatic cleavage of complement proteins: those which attach to the target of complement activation and those that are released into the fluid-phase as biologically active peptides.

Among these mediators, the low-molecular peptides C3a and C5a have been shown to increase vascular permeability and to promote smooth muscle contraction. C3a and C5a also serve as ligands for specific receptors present on polymorphonuclear leukocytes, eosinophils, monocytes and macrophages, mast cells and lymphocytes.

These ligand-receptor interactions stimulate multiple cellular responses: The binding of C3a and C5a to specific C3a and C5a receptors on basophils and mast cells stimulates these cells to secrete the contents of their granules including histamine. Interaction of C5a with the C5a receptor on neutrophils promotes chemotaxis and adhesion to endothelial cells, induces the expression of C5b receptors on the cell membrane and probably stimulates the generation and release of leukotrienes.

C5a is also chemotactic for monocytes and induces slow secretion of glycolytic and proteolytic enzymes by these cells and may also promote production of interleukin 1 by macrophages.

Neutrophils also possess receptors for the low molecular peptide C3e (LMF) which causes leukocytosis and may therefore contribute to the availability of neutrophils for localization at sites of inflammation.

Recent findings indicate that different fragments of C3 have selective effects on various lymphocyte populations and can modulate recirculation, antigen processing, proliferation and differentiation of these cells.

Thus, complement-derived mediators play a profound role in regulating both humoral immune functions and the cellular immune response.

Introduction

The human complement system consists of more than 20 different components that participate in host defense and inflammation by direct killing or lysis of microorganisms and by the generation of peptides with phlogistic activities [1]. These activities are produced by a complex sequence of reactions involving limited proteolysis and specific protein interactions which follow two principal modes, termed the classical and the alternative pathway of complement activation [2]. The most important step in both pathways is the enzymatic cleavage and activation of C3 and C5, whereby two types of mediators are generated: large particles like C3b that bind to nonspecific acceptor sites on the activating surface and small diffusible peptides which are immediately released into the fluid phase and which can bind to specific receptors on a variety of cells [3]. The most active of these hormone-like mediators of the complement system are the anaphylatoxins C3a and C5a [4]. The C4a fragment of C4 has also been found to have anaphylactic activity, but this biological function of C4a may not be relevant in vivo [5].

C3a and C5a Anaphylatoxins

C3a is a 77-residue polypeptide with a molecular weight of 10000; C5a is a 74-residue glycopolypeptide of 10000–15000 daltons (depending on the species-specific carbohydrate content) (Table 1). Both peptides are cleaved from the N-terminal portions of the α-chains of their parent molecules by specific C3/C5-convertases formed during complement activation. In addition, other enzymes in the blood, such as plasmin and thrombin [6] and even cellular proteases like mast cell tryptase [7], have the potential to generate C3a and C5a. The anaphylatoxins are controlled by the regulator protein carboxypeptidase N, a kininase-like enzyme endogenous to serum [8]. Under natural conditions, this anaphylatoxin inhibitor removes short arginyl residues from the C-terminal portion of C3a and C5a almost as rapidly as these peptides are generated. The resulting des-Arg derivates are devoid of most of their biological activities. Human C3a des-Arg is functionally inactive whereas C5a des-Arg retains its chemotactic activity but functions poorly as an anaphylatoxin. C5a des-Arg is

Table 1. C3a and C5a anaphylatoxins [4]

	C3a	C5a
Molecular weight	10000	10000–15000
Amino acid composition	77	74
Carbohydrate content	–	+
Serum concentration	152±69 ng/ml	~20 ng/ml

probably the physiological form of this mediator. In fact, the classical anaphylatoxin – discovered in 1913 by Friedberger [9] – has now been identified as C5a des-Arg [10]. The mean C3a serum level in normal persons as assessed by a radioimmunoassay described by Chenoweth and Hugli [11] was found to be 152 ± 69 ng per milliliter [12]. Maximal C3a concentrations of 10000–70000 ng/ml have been measured in patients with acute serum sickness [13]. The physiological serum concentration of C5a is approximately 20 ng per milliliter [11].

Cutaneous Vascular Effects of Anaphylatoxins

Both anaphylatoxins promote smooth muscle contraction and increase vascular permeability [4]. The effects of C5a on the cutaneous vasculature were recently reexamined by Yancey et al. [14]: Intradermal injections of nanomolar concentrations of purified C5a into the skin of healthy volunteers produced dose-dependent immediate wheal and flare reactions that lasted for 60–75 min; purpura, blistering, or late phase reactions were not observed. C5a was 50 times more potent than C3a and about 25 times more potent than histamine in producing these reactions. Histological examination of the injection site demonstrated a superficial and mid-dermal perivascular infiltrate of neutrophils and eosinophils that was most prominent 20 min after injection of C5a. Mast cell degranulation and endothelial swelling were other histological features (Table 2).

The H_1-antihistamine hydroxyzine reduced erythema but did not affect the whealing reaction or the histological changes. Björk et al. [15] directly demonstrated the microvascular response to human C3a and C5a in hamster cheek pouches prepared for in vivo microscopy: topical application of nanomolar concentrations of C3a or C5a resulted in arteriolar vasoconstriction with transient platelet aggregation, leakage of postcapillary venules, and marked extravasation of plasma proteins. Perivascular leukocyte accumulation was observed only after application of C5a. The histamine inhibitor mepyramine did not affect the spasmogenic and chemotactic activities of C5a but reduced the initial phase of C5a-induced vascular leakage (which was significantly longer than that observed with C3a). The late phase of vascular changes, however,

Table 2. Intradermal effects of anaphylatoxins [14, 15]

Clinical:	Erythema, edema (pruritus)
Histological:	Arteriolar vasoconstriction Endothelial swelling Vascular leakage Mast cell degranulation PMN accumulation (C5a only)

when leukocytes attracted by C5a may be involved, is independent of histamine. These observations support the view that the various tissue effects of anaphylatoxins are not accomplished by a single or even a common mechanism [4].

Inflammatory Effects of Anaphylatoxins

C3a and C5a from all species studied stimulate the release of histamine from mast cells and basophils [16]. Complement-induced histamine release follows a different time course from IgE-mediated histamine liberation in human basophils, occurring much faster and resulting only in incomplete degranulation of basophils [17]. Also, indomethacin, an inhibitor of the cyclooxygenase pathway of arachidonic acid, has been shown to inhibit the C5a-induced but not the IgE-mediated basophil degranulation [18, 19]. Thus, there seem to be both qualitative and pharmacological differences in the regulation of the two mechanisms of basophil histamine release.

The two anaphylatoxins are also different in their ability to interact with peripheral blood cells other than basophils. Binding studies with radiolabeled C3a and C5a indicate that C3a binds preferentially to basophils and possibly to eosinophils whereas C5a binds primarily to neutrophils and monocytes [20] (Table 3). Neither C3a nor C5a, however, bind to lymphocytes or erythrocytes. A biological function of C5a that is not associated with the C3a molecule is its ability to attract neutrophils and macrophages. This chemotactic activity of C5a is mediated through specific receptors for this anaphylatoxin which have been identified on human neutrophils [21], on monocytes, and more recently also on murine macrophages [22] (Table 4). Human C5a des-Arg is

Table 3. Cellular receptors for anaphylatoxins [20–22]

Cell type	C3a receptors	C5a receptors
PMNs	–	++
Monocytes	–	++
Lymphocytes	–	–
Basophils	+	+
Mast cells	+	+
Macrophages	–	+

Table 4. Cellular triggering reactions of anaphylatoxins [4, 16]

Chemotactic migration (C5a and C5a des Arg):
Neutrophils, eosinophils, macrophages, monocytes

Mediator release (C3a, C5a, and C5a des Arg):
Vasoactive amines, constituents of platelet granules,
activated oxygen species, biologically active metabolites of arachidonic acid

also capable of binding to these cellular receptors, but with a 50- to 100-fold lower affinity than C5a [21].

Receptor-mediated interaction of neutrophils with C5a induces a range of cellular responses: increased stickiness that may promote adhesion of neutrophils to endothelial cells, release of lysosomal enzymes, enhanced superoxide production, and formation of thromboxane A_2 and platelet activating factor [16]. The possible biosynthesis of leukotrienes, including the potent chemotactic factor LTB_4 in neutrophils stimulated by C5a, is still controversial [23]. Recent results indicate that C5a cannot stimulate neutrophils to metabolize endogenous arachidonic acid into LTB_4 [24]. However, LTB_4 and other metabolites of the lipoxygenase pathway of arachidonic acid may be generated from exogenous arachidonic by C5a-stimulated (and not be resting) neutrophils [24]. Thus, in vivo, C5a-stimulated neutrophils may utilize arachidonic acid that is derived from stimulated platelets, from monocytes, or from damaged tissue cells in order to amplify the local inflammatory response.

Immunoregulatory Effects of Anaphylatoxins

Cellular responses occurring after C5a binds to specific receptors are not limited to acute phase reactions. It was recently shown that the binding of C5a to macrophages triggers the chemotactic migration of these cells and the production of interleukin-l, which can act to stimulate antigen-specific antibody production in vitro [25].

Additional immunoregulatory effects of anaphylatoxins on cells other than macrophages have also been reported: Incubation of highly purified C3a with cultures of human peripheral blood lymphocytes that were challenged with sheep red blood cells resulted in suppression of the anti-sheep erythrocyte antibody response [26]. In addition, C3a was found to suppress polyclonal antibody production induced by Fc fragments of immunoglobulin. C3a des-Arg was nonsuppressive in both experiments. It is postulated that C3a acts via generation of suppressor T cells which then interfere with the action of T helper cells [27]. In contrast to C3a, human C5a enhanced both the anti-sheep erythrocyte and the Fc-fragment-mediated polyclonal antibody response of human peripheral lymphocytes [28] (Table 5). C5a and C5a des-Arg were equally effective. When in

Table 5. In vitro immunoregulatory effects of anaphylatoxins [26–28]

Immune response	C3a	C5a
Polyclonal antibody production	▼	▲
Specific antibody production	▼	▲
B cell proliferation	–	–
Antigen-induced T cell proliferation	▼	▲
Natural killer activity	–	–

these experiments C3a and C5a were tested simultaneously, the immunopotentiating properties of C5a overrode the suppressive effects of C3a [27]. The exact mechanism by which C3a and C5a interact with peripheral blood lymphocytes devoid of specific receptors for both peptides is, however, not clear at present. Also, it is not known whether the C3a- and C5a-mediated immunoregulation has a physiological significance since in vivo C3a is rapidly converted to its inactive des-Arg form and C5a, once generated, immediately binds to its specific receptors on peripheral neutrophils.

Conclusion

The interaction of C3a and C5a with inflammatory cells occurs via specific receptors and triggers the release or synthesis of mediators which in most cases amplify or reinforce processes already initiated by the anaphylatoxins.

In addition to its chemotactic activity, C5a seems to have the potential to augment the primary humoral immune response in vitro by triggering interleukin-l secretion from macrophages and by enhancing the responsiveness of T-lymphocytes to antigen-specific stimuli. C3a, in contrast, exhibits an immunosuppressive effect that possibly involves direct interaction with T suppressor cells.

References

1. Gigli I (1979) The complement system in inflammation and host defense. Clin Exp Dermatol 4:271–289
2. Reid KBM, Porter RR (1981) The proteolytic activation systems of complement. Ann Rev Biochem 50:433–464
3. Vogt W (1983) Activation of the complement system. Agents Action 113:391–397
4. Hugli TE, Müller-Eberhard HJ (1978) Anaphylatoxins C3a and C5a. Adv Immunol 26:1–53
5. Gorski JP, Hugli TE, Müller-Eberhard HJ (1979) The third anaphylatoxin of the human complement system. Proc Natl Acad Sci USA 76:5299–5302
6. Gerard C, Hugli TE (1981) C5a: A mediator of chemotaxis and cellular release reactions. In: Becker EL, Simon AS, Austen KF (eds) Biochemistry of the acute allergic reactions. Liss, New York, pp 147–160
7. Schwartz LB, Kawahara MS, Hugli TE, Vik D, Fearon DT, Austen KF (1983) Generation of C3a anaphylatoxin from human C3 by human mast cell tryptase. J Immunol 130:1891–1895
8. Bokisch WA, Müller-Eberhard HJ (1970) Anaphylatoxin inactivator of human plasma: its isolation and characterization as a carboxypeptidase. J Clin Invest 49:2427–2436
9. Friedberger E, Mita S, Kumagai T (1913) Die Bildung eines akut wirkenden Giftes (Anaphylatoxin) aus Toxinen (Tetanus, Diphtherie, Schlangengift). Z Immunforsch 17:506–520
10. Gerard C, Hugli TE (1981) Identification of classical anaphylatoxin as the des-Arg form of the C5a molecule: evidence for a modulator role for the oligosaccharide unit in human des-Arg C5a. Proc Natl Acad Sci USA 78:1833–1837

11. Hugli TE, Chenoweth DE (1980) Biologically active peptides of complement: techniques and significance of C3a and C5a measurements. In: Nakamura RM (ed) Future perspectives in clinical laboratory immunoassays. Liss, New York, pp 443–460
12. Wagner JL, Hugli TE (1984) Radioimmunoassay for anaphylatoxins: a sensitive method for determining complement activation products in biological fluids. Anal Biochem 136:75–88
13. Lawley TJ, Bielory L, Gascon P, Yancey KB, Young NS, Frank MM (1984) A prospective clinical and immunological analysis of patients with serum sickness. N Engl J Med 22:1407–1413
14. Yancey KB, Hammer CH, Harvath L, Renfer L, Frank MM, Lawley TJ (1985) Studies of human C5a as a mediator of inflammation in normal human skin. J Clin Invest 75:486–495
15. Björk J, Hugli TE, Smedegard G (1985) Microvascular effects of anaphylatoxins C3a and C5a. J Immunol 134:1115–1119
16. Bult H, Herman AG (1983) Inflammatory mediators released by complement-derived peptides. Agent Actions 13:405–414
17. Dvorak AM, Lett-Brown M, Thueson D, Grant JA (1981) Complement-induced degranulation of human basophils. J Immunol 126:523–528
18. Farnam J, Grant JA, Lett-Brown MA, Hunt C, Thueson DO, Giclas PC (1985) Complement- and IgE-mediated release of histamine from basophils in vitro. V. Differential effects of drugs modulating arachidonic acid metabolism. J Immunol 134:541–547
19. Ring J, Walz U (1985) Indomethacin enhances in vitro histamine release induced by anti-IgE and Ca-ionophore but inhibits C5a-induced release reactions from basophils of atopics and normals. Int Arch Allergy Appl Immunol 77:225–227
20. van Epps DE, Chenoweth DE (1984) Analysis of the binding of fluorescent C5a and C3a to human peripheral blood leukocytes. J Immunol 132:2862–2867
21. Chenoweth DE, Hugli TE (1978) Demonstration of specific C5a receptor on intact human polymorphonuclear leukocytes. Proc Natl Acad Sci USA 75:3043–3947
22. Chenoweth DE, Goodman MG, Weigle WO (1983) Demonstration of a specific receptor for human C5a anaphylatoxin on murine macrophages. J Exp Med 156:68–78
23. Pison U, Kunau WH, Damerau B, König W (1983) Induction of leukotriene formation by the anaphylatoxins C3a and C5a. Immunbiology 164:265 (A)
24. Clancy RM, Dahinden CA, Hugli TE (1983) Arachidonate metabolism by human polymorphonuclear leukocytes stimulated by *N*-formyl-Met-Leu-Phe or complement component C5a is independent of phospholipase activation. Proc Natl Acad Sci USA 80:7200–7204
25. Goodman MG, Chenoweth DE, Weigle WO (1982) Induction of interleukin 1 secretion and enhancement of humoral immunity by binding of human C5a to macrophage surface C5a receptors. J Exp Med 1156:912–917
26. Morgan EL, Weigle WO, Hugli TE (1982) Anaphylatoxin-mediated regulation of the immune response. A Exp Med 155:1412–1426
27. Morgan EL, Weigle WO, Hugli TE (1984) Anaphylatoxin-mediated regulation of human and murine immune responses. Fed Proc 43:2543–2547
28. Morgan EL, Thoman ML, Weigle WO, Hugli TE (1983) Anaphylatoxin-mediated regulation of the immune response. II. C5a-mediated enhancement of human humoral and T cell-mediated immune response. J Immunol 130:1257–1261

Paf-acether (Platelet-activating Factor)

J. Benveniste

INSERM U.200, Université Paris-Sud, 32 rue des Carnets, 92140 Clamart, France

Abstract

Platelet-activating factor was first described as originating from IgE-sensitized rabbit basophils challenged with the specific allergen. When its structure, 1-O-alkyl-2-acetyl-*sn*-glyceryl-3-phosphorylcholine was unveiled in 1979, it was thus named "Paf-acether", given the ether linkage at position 1 and the acetyl group at position 2 of glycerol. Paf-acether is synthesized by rabbit basophils, murine peritoneal macrophages, human alveolar macrophages, blood neutrophils and monocytes. Its release from human and rabbit platelets suggests that it could be the mediator of the third pathway of platelet aggregation. Paf-acether biosynthesis takes place in two steps:

1. the intervention of a phospholipase A_2 on membrane etherphospholipids results in the formation of the non-acetylated compound, 2-lyso Paf-Ether;
2. activation of a short-chain fatty-acid specific acyl transferase.

Alveolar macrophages from asthmatic patients but not from normal donors release Paf-acether when stimulated with the specific pneumallergens. This, joined to the potent bronchomotor effect of Paf-acether, may represent a new pathway (platelet-dependent?) in the pathophysiology of human asthma. Paf-acether is also a potent neutrophil activator, inducer of vascular permeability in various organs and constrictor of the coronary bed. Also the intrication between arachidonate-derived agonists and Paf-acether metabolism and action is under active investigation in a number of laboratories. Therefore this mediator possesses two types of effects:

1. cell to cell interaction e.g. neutrophil/neutrophil/platelet; macrophage/platelet; platelet/platelet;
2. direct effects on the vasculature.

The variety of the sources and targets of this mediator makes it a candidate as an instrumental agent in various lung diseases such as asthma and acute respiratory distress syndrome.

Introduction

Paf-acether is the first example of a phospholipid being a mediator of inflammation. Besides the platelets, it acts on various cell types such as neutrophils and macrophages. As an in vivo agonist, it is capable of inducing major pathological changes in lung and heart functions, and of increasing skin vascular permeability. It exhibits antihypertensive properties. Recently, Paf-acether has been shown to cause the release of secondary mediators, leukotrienes (LTs) and prostaglandins (PGs), from various cell types and organs.

Definition and Assay

In 1972, the release of Paf-acether from immunoglobulin E-sensitized rabbit basophils was demonstrated [11]. It was then named platelet-activating factor (Paf). Its human origin [7], its effect on human platelets [12], and some of its physicochemical characteristics, including its phospholipid nature [13], were unveiled thereafter. The procedure for its purification was described [54], its structure was elucidated as being 1-*O*-alkyl-2-acetyl-*sn*-glycero-3-phosphorylcholine [14, 17, 27] – hence the new name Paf-acether – and its chemical synthesis was achieved [31] (Fig. 1). Several criteria are used to distinguish Paf-acether from other platelet agonists: (a) platelet aggregation (or release of labeled serotonin) in the presence of aspirin or indomethacin and of ADP scavengers, (b) an elution pattern identical to that of synthetic Paf-acether during high pressure liquid chromatography, (c) inactivation by phospholipases A_2, C, and D, and resistance to lipase from *Rhizopus arrhizus* [13], and (d) mass spectrometry characteristics when enough of the mediator can be recovered.

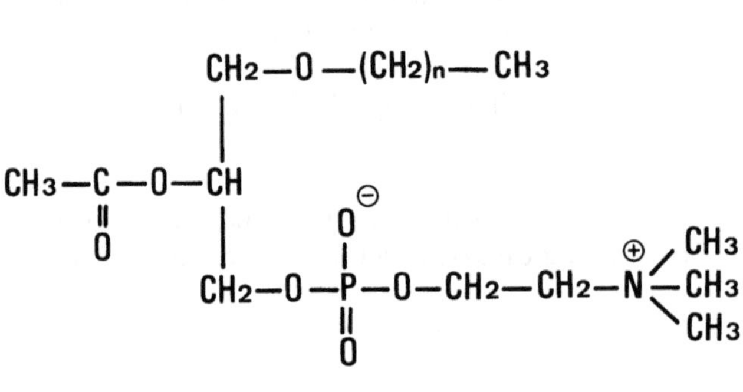

n = 15,17...

Fig. 1. Structure of Paf-acether

Origin of Paf-acether

Circulating basophils are a source of Paf-acether, at least in the rabbit [11]. Release of Paf-acether was obtained in murine macrophages and murine bone marrow-derived mast cells [40], whereas rat peritoneal mast cells do not form the mediator [38]. Paf-acether is also released by the platelets themselves, by rat, rabbit, and human alveolar macrophages [4], by human blood monocytes, and, in high amounts, by neutrophils but not from 100% pure lymphocyte preparations [33, 36].

Both in its formation and in its action on platelets, Paf-acether is independent from the arachidonate-cyclooxygenate pathway. This is well recognized for rabbit platelets [21], but several authors have claimed that in man the effect of Paf-acether is abolished by a cyclooxygenase blocker. In fact it is well demonstrated that this blockade occurs only at low Ca^{2+} concentration, such as in citrated platelet-rich plasma where platelet/platelet contacts are favored, resulting in stimulation of the arachidonate cascade (reviewed in [23]).

Paf-acether Metabolism

A series of enzymatic steps appear to be involved in the formation of Paf-acether upon stimulation of the cells. Through the activity of several substrates and enzymes, including acyl-CoA and acyltransferase, the substrate for phospholipase A_2 is eventually formed, namely 1-alkyl-2-acyl-*sn*-glycero-3-phosphorylcholine, an analogue of phosphatidylcholine. The PLA_2 is then capable of hydrolyzing this product to form 1-alkyl-2-lyso-glycerophosphorylcholine (2-lyso Paf-acether), which in turn serves as a substrate for an acetyltransferase yielding Paf-acether upon acetylation of lyso Paf-acether from acetyl-CoA. It is important to realize that activation of phospholipase A_2 leads to the freeing of both the precursor of Paf-acether and of fatty acids, among them arachidonic acid. Therefore interaction of the same phospholipid – 1-alkyl-2-acyl-*sn*-glycero-3-phosphorylcholine – and the same enzyme – PLA_2 – can result in the triggering of the main pathways of biosynthesis of inflammatory mediators. The inactivation of Paf-acether depends on acetylhydrolase and acyltransferase activities. Together these two enzymatic systems in activated cells are responsible not only for the formation of the inactive form of Paf-acether but also for the overall rate of biosynthesis of both intracellular and extracellular Paf-acether. The basis for this system has been derived from the experimental evidence gathered in membrane preparations from various cells, namely peritoneal and alveolar macrophages, neutrophils, and platelets [1, 2, 10, 25, 34, 43, 59].

Effects of Paf-acether

The effects of Paf-acether are reviewed in references 8, 51, and 55.

Cells

Paf acether is the most potent platelet aggregating agent so far described since it activates washed rabbit platelets at concentrations of 10–100 pM. Sixty times more is needed to trigger aggregation of rabbit platelets suspended in plasma. There are also variations in sensitivity in different species, the most responsive being the platelets of guinea pigs, followed by rabbits, dogs, and humans.

Intravenous injection of Paf-acether causes thrombocytopenia but also neutropenia with formation of neutrophil aggregates. Paf-acether is a very potent in vitro neutrophil-activating factor, since it induces aggregation, lysosomal enzyme release, chemotaxis, and release of superoxide anions [20, 26, 44, 49].

Lung

In various species intravenous injection of Paf-acether induced acute and reversible pulmonary and circulatory alterations, similar to those observed during IgE anaphylactic shock in rabbits. In the guinea pig, injection of 60 ng/kg induced a bronchoconstriction which was platelet dependent since it was inhibited by prior platelet removal [56]. Those mechanisms involved in the bronchoconstriction due to Paf-acether have not been clearly elucidated. However, there appears to be a relationship between the route of administration of this factor and the primary sites of action, that is, either cyclooxygenase dependent [57] or via a lipoxygenase activity [19]. Using a platelet radiolabeling technique, the trapping of platelets by the lung was observed in the guinea pig 30 s after bronchoconstriction [45], again suggesting a relationship between bronchoconstriction and platelet activities. Similar anaphylactic effects of Paf-acether were observed in the rabbit [37]. Intratracheal administration of Paf-acether (60 μg/kg) to premedicated baboons provoked an immediate bronchomotor effect determined as an increase of the peak inspiratory pressure [28]. Oxygen blood pressure (PaO_2) and blood platelet and neutrophil counts decreased a few minutes after injection. The bronchomotor effect was not inhibited by pretreatment with aspirin or atropine but was partially inhibited by intravenous injection of a β-adrenergic drug (salbutamol 0.5 mg i.v.). Acute pulmonary effects of Paf-acether have also been described in the primate *Macaca mulatta* [46].

A preliminary report of the biological effects of Paf-acether in comatous (cerebral death) patients has recently been published [30]. In these experiments Paf-acether induced an increase in peak inspiratory pressure as well as changes in blood cell and blood gas values. We also observed significant cardiac modifications, such as a severe drop in left ventricle stroke work index.

All these pulmonary and circulatory modifications mimic human asthma disease. In keeping with the release of Paf-acether by human alveolar macrophages and particularly upon stimulation with the sensitizing allergen in asthmatic patients [5, 32], our results suggest that Paf-acether might play a role in the pathogenesis of human asthma.

Heart and Vessels

The structure of Paf-acether is exactly that of the antihypertensive polar renomedullary lipid [19, 41, 42], i.e., Paf-acether is an hypotensive agent. This effect of Paf-acether can be observed in guinea pigs, baboons, and rats, independently from platelet aggregation. We described recently a dramatic negative inotropic effect and decrease in coronary flow induced by Paf-acether administered in the nM range to guinea pig isolated perfused heart [9]. This effect has also been described in the pig [29]. In dog Paf-acether induces an acute circulatory collapse [15]. However, the only in vitro vascular response to Paf-acether stimulation has been observed in the rat portal vein preparation [52]. There is no effect on isolated vascular muscle preparations ([22] and R. Santamaria, unpublished observations).

When Paf-acether was intradermally administered to the rat or humans it induced edema and in the latter case hyperalgesia [3, 16, 18, 47, 48, 53]. This effect appears to be independent of the cyclooxygenase pathway [16, 47, 48] and of platelet and neutrophil activation [16, 48]. A dual response – early and late – was reported in human skin [3].

Arachidonate Derivatives and Paf-acether

In several cell systems and organs Paf-acether has been shown to induce the generation of secondary mediators. Interaction of its action with the lipoxygenase pathway was demonstrated in neutrophils [20, 35, 44]. Release of leukotrienes B_4 from Paf-acether-stimulated neutrophils is observed with concentrations as low as 20 nM in the presence of cytochalasin B [24]. However, the amount of leukotriene B_4 released upon Paf-acether stimulation represents only 1% of that released upon ionophore A23187 stimulation, questioning the relevance of Paf-acether-induced leukotriene production under pathophysiologic circumstances [39].

When Paf-acether is administered intratracheally to guinea pigs, the resulting bronchoconstriction is blocked by indomethacin alone, demonstrating that cyclooxygenase products and most probably thromboxane A_2 are involved; this contrasts with results obtained using the intravenous route [56, 57]. For other authors the release of leukotrienes may play an important role during

Paf-acether-induced bronchoconstriction [19]. These discrepant results may be partially due to the procedures used in the experimental protocols, namely anesthesia, antagonist medication, or the quantity of Paf-acether injected. The direct demonstration that Paf-acether induces the generation of leukotrienes (C_4 and D_4) in perfused rat lung was achieved recently [58]. Paf-acether-induced release of leukotrienes C_4, D_4, and E_4 from rat lung has also been demonstrated [6]. The decrease in coronary flow and in contractile force induced by Paf-acether (see above) was inhibited by the cyclo- and lipoxygenase blocker BW755c, whereas aspirin and indomethacin were without effect. Interestingly, the inhibitory effect of BW766c was more pronounced when high doses of Paf-acether were used, suggesting that recruitment of leukotrienes may depend upon the concentration of the mediator. In addition, FPL 55712, an antagonist of the effect of leukotrienes, markedly inhibited the Paf-acether-induced decrease in coronary flow and contractile force (M. Pretolani et al., unpublished results). Further studies are required to determine precisely the role of every component of the inflammatory and allergic reactions. The lack of specific inhibitors both of the enzymes involved in the biosynthetic pathway of these lipid mediators and of their effect on various cell types and organs at present impairs the determination of their precise role.

Conclusion

Paf-acether can be detected in a variety of cell types activated with specific agents, in association with the onset of various signs of inflammatory states. Thus the contribution of Paf-acether to the inflammatory process seems considerable in the light of its in vitro effects. However, it is too soon to define precisely its role in in vivo inflammatory states. Moreover, there appears to be a complex relationship between arachidonate metabolites and Paf-acether formation or effects. Important efforts are now being made to search for molecules capable of inhibiting Paf-acether metabolism, release, and biological effects.

References

1. Albert DH, Snyder F (1983) Biosynthesis of 1-alkyl-2-acetyl-*sn*-glycero-phosphocholine by rat alveolar macrophages. J Biol Chem 258:97–102
2. Alonso F, Garcia Gil M, Sanchez-Crespo M, Mato JM (1982) Activation of 1-alkyl-2-lyso-glycero-3-phosphocholine: acetyl-CoA transferase during phagocytosis in human polymorphonuclear leukocytes. J Biol Chem 257:3376–3378
3. Archer CB, Page CP, Paul W, Morley J, McDonald DM (1984) Inflammatory characteristics of platelet-activating factor (Paf-acether) in human skin. Br J Dermatol 110:45–50
4. Arnoux B, Duval D, Benveniste J (1980) Release of platelet-activating factor (Paf-acether) from alveolar macrophages by the calcium ionophore A23187 and phagocytosis. Eur J Clin Invest 10:437–441

5. Arnoux B, Simoes-Caeiro MH, Landes A, Mathieu M, Duroux P, Benveniste J (1982) Alveolar macrophages from asthmatic patients release platelet-activating factor (Paf-acether) and lyso Paf-acether when stimulated with the specific allergen. Am Rev Respir Dis 125:70 (abstract)
6. Beaubien BB, Tippins JR, Morris HR (1984) Platelet-activating factor stimulation of peptido-leukotriene release: inhibition by vasoactive polypeptide. Biochim Biophys Res Commun 125:105–108
7. Benveniste J (1974) Platelet-activating factor, a new mediator of anaphylaxis and immune complex deposition from rabbit and human basophils. Nature 249:481–583
8. Benveniste J, Arnoux B (eds) (1983) Platelet-activating factor and structurally-related ether-lipids. INSERM symposium n° 23. Elsevier, Amsterdam
9. Benveniste J, Boullet C, Brink C, Labat C (1983) The actions of Paf-acether (Platelet-activating factor) on guinea-pig isolated heart preparations. Br J Pharmacol 80:81–83
10. Benveniste J, Chignard M, Le Couedic JP, Vargaftig BB (1982) Biosynthesis of platelet-activating factor (Paf-acether). II. Involvement of phospholipase A_2 in the formation of Paf-acether and lyso-Paf-acether from rabbit platelets. Thromb Res 25:375–386
11. Benveniste J, Henson PM, Cochrane CG (1972) Leukocyte-dependent histamine release from rabbit platelets: the role of IgE, basophils and a platelet-activating factor. J Exp Med 136:170–171
12. Benveniste J, Le Couedic JP, Kamoun P (1975) Aggregation of human platelets by platelet-activating factor. Lancet 1:344
13. Benveniste J, Le Couedic JP, Polonsky J, Tencé M (1977) Structural analysis of purified platelet-activating factor by lipases. Nature 269:170–171
14. Benveniste J, Tencé M, Varenne P, Bidault J, Boullet C, Polonsky J (1979) Semi-synthèse et structure proposée du facteur activant les plaquettes (Paf): Paf-acéther, un alkyl-éther analogue de la lysophosphatidylcholine. C R Acad Sci (Paris) 289 D:1037–1040
15. Bessin P, Bonnet J, Apffel D, Soulard C, Desgroux L, Pelas I, Benveniste J (1983) Acute circulatory collapse caused by platelet-activating factor (Paf-acether) in dogs. Eur J Pharmacol 86:403–413
16. Björk J, Smedegard G (1983) Acute microvascular effects of Paf-acether, as studied by intravital microscopy. Eur J Pharmacol 96:87–94
17. Blank ML, Snyder F, Byers LW, Brooks B, Muirhead EE (1979) Anti-hypertensive activity of an alkyl ether analog of phosphatidylcholine. Biochim Biophys Res Commun 90:1194–1200
18. Bonnet J, Loiseau AM, Orvaen M, Bessin P (1981) Platelet-activating factor (Paf-acether) involvement in acute inflammatory and pain process. In: Russo-Marie F, Vargaftig BB, Benveniste J (eds) Pharmacology of inflammation and allergy: lipids and cells, vol 100. INSERM, Paris, pp 111–118
19. Bonnet J, Thibaudeau D, Bessin P (1983) Dependency of the Paf-acether-induced bronchospasm on the lipoxygenase pathway in the guinea-pig. Prostaglandins 26:457–466
20. Camussi G, Tetta C, Bussolino F, Caligaris-Cappio F, Coda R, Masera C, Segoloni G (1981) Mediators of immune-complex-induced aggregation of polymorphonuclear neutrophils. II. Platelet-activating factor as the effector substance of immune-induced aggregation. Int Arch Allergy Appl Immunol 64:25–41
21. Cazenave JP, Benveniste J, Mustard JF (1979) Aggregation of rabbit platelets by platelet-activating factor is independent of the release reaction and the arachidonate pathway and inhibited by membrane-active drugs. Lab Invest 41:275–285
22. Cerrina J, Raffestin B, Labat C, Boullet C, Bayol A, Gateau O, Brink C (1983) Effects of Paf-acether on isolated muscle preparations from the rat, guinea-pig and human lung. In: Benveniste J, Arnoux B (eds) Platelet-activating factor and structurally-related ether-lipids. INSERM symposium n° 23. Elsevier, Amsterdam, pp 205–212
23. Chignard M, Coëffier E, Benveniste J (1985) Role of Paf-acether and related ether-lipid metabolism in platelets. In: Westwick J, Scully HF, McIntyre DD, Kakar VV (eds) Advances in medicine and biology. Mechanisms of stimulus response coupling in platelets. Plenum, New York (to be published)
24. Chilton FM, O'Flaherty JT, Walsh CE, Thomas MJ, Wykle RL, DeChatelet LR, Waite BM (1982) Platelet-activating factor. Stimulation of the lipoxygenase pathway in poly-

morphonuclear leukocytes by 1-*O*-alkyl-2-*O*-acetyl-*sn*-glycero-3-phosphocholine. J Biol Chem 257:5402–5407
25. Chilton FH, O'Flaherty J, Marshall Ellis J, Swendsen CL, Wykle RL (1983) Selective acylation of lyso platelet-activating factor by arachidonate in human neutrophils. J Biol Chem 258:7268–7271
26. Czarnetzki MB, Benveniste J (1981) Effect of 1-*O*-octadecyl-2-*O*-acetyl-*sn*-glycero-3-phosphorylcholine (Paf-acether) on leukocytes. I. Analysis of the in vitro migration of human neutrophils. Chem Phys Lipids 29:317–326
27. Demopoulos CA, Pinckard RN, Hanahan DJ (1979) Evidence for 1-*O*-alkyl-2-*O*-acetyl-*sn*-glyceryl-3-phosphorylcholine as the active component (a new class of lipid chemical mediators). J Biol Chem 254:9355–9359
28. Denjean A, Arnoux B, Masse R, Lockhart A, Benveniste J (1983) Acute effects of intratracheal administration of platelet-activating factor (Paf-acether) in baboons. J Appl Physiol 55:799–804
29. Feurstein G, Boyd LM, Ezra D, Goldstein RE (1984) Effect of platelet-activating factor on coronary circulation of the domestic pig. Am J Physiol 246:H466–H471
30. Gateau O, Arnoux B, Deriaz H, Benveniste J (1984) Acute effects of intratracheal administration of Paf-acether (platelet-activating factor) in humans. Am Rev Respir Dis 129:A3 (abstract)
31. Godfroid JJ, Heymans F, Michael E, Redeuilh C, Steiner F, Benveniste J (1980) Platelet-activating factor (Paf-acether): total synthesis of 1-*O*-octadecyl-2-*O*-acetyl-*sn*-glycero-3-phosphorylcholine. FEBS Lett 116:161–164
32. Joseph M, Tonnel AB, Torpier G, Capron A, Arnoux B, Benveniste J (1983) The involvement of IgE in the secretory processes of alveolar macrophages from asthmatic patients. J Clin Invest 71:221–230
33. Jouvin-Marche E, Ninio E, Beaurain G, Tencé M, Niaudet P, Benveniste J (1984) Biosynthesis of Paf-acether (platelet-activating factor). VII. Precursors of Paf-acether and acetyltransferase activity in human leukocytes. J Immunol 133:892–898
34. Lee T-C, Malone B, Wasserman SI, Fitzgerald V, Snyder F (1982) Activities of enzymes that metabolize platelet-activating factor (1-alkyl-2-acetyl-*sn*-glycero-3-phosphocholine) in neutrophils and eosinophils from humans and the effect of a calcium ionophorese. Biochem Biophys Res Commun 105:1303–1308
35. Lin AH, Morton DR, Gorman RR (1982) Acetyl-glyceryl-ether-phosphorylcholine stimulates leukotriene, B_4 synthesis in human polymorphonuclear leukocytes. J Clin Invest 70:1058–1065
36. Lotner GZ, Lynch JM, Betz SJ, Henson PM (1980) Human neutrophil-derived platelet-activating factor, J Immunol 124:676–684
37. McManus LM, Hanahan DJ, Demopoulos CA, Pinckard RN (1980) Pathobiology of the intravenous infusion of acetyl-glyceryl-ether-phosphorylcholine (AGEPC), a synthetic platelet-activating factor (Paf) in the rabbit. J Immunol 124:2919–2934
38. Mencia-Huerta JM, Benveniste J (1979) Platelet-activating factor and macrophages. I. Evidence for the release from rat and mouse peritoneal macrophages and not from mastocytes. Eur J Immunol 9:409–415
39. Mencia-Huerta JM, Lee CW, Lee TH, Razin E, Corey EJ, Lewis RA, Austen KF (1983) Platelet-activating factor (Paf-acether): generation from a mast cell subclass by an IgE-dependent mechanism. In: Benveniste J, Arnoux B (eds) Platelet-activating factor and structurally-related ether-lipids. INSERM symposium n° 23. Elsevier, Amsterdam pp 101–108
40. Mencia-Huerta JM, Lewis RA, Razin E, Austen KF (1983) Antigen-initiated release of platelet-activating factor (Paf-acether) from mouse bone marrow-derived mast cells sensitized with monoclonal IgE. J Immunol 130:2958–2964
41. Muirhead EE, Byers LW, Desiderio DM, Brooks B, Brosius WM (1981) Antihypertensive lipids from the kidney: alkyl ether analogs of phosphatidylcholine. Fed Proc 40:2285–2290
42. Muirhead EE, Stirman JA (1958) Dietary proteins and hypertension in the dog: protection by ureterocaval anastomosis with a study of the kidney so treated. Am J Pathol 34:561 (abstract)

43. Ninio E, Mencia-Huerta JM, Heymans F, Benveniste J (1982) Biosynthesis of platelet-activating factor (Paf-acether). I. Evidence for an acetyltransferase activity in murine macrophages. Biochim Biophys Acta 710:23–31
44. O'Flaherty JT, Wykle RL, Miller CH, Lewis JC, Waite M, Bass DA, McGall MD, DeChatelet LR (1981) 1-*O*-alkyl-*sn*-glyceryl-3-phosphorylcholines. A novel class of neutrophil stimulants. Am J Pathol 103:70–78
45. Page CP, Paul W, Douglas GJ, Casals-Stenzel J, Morley J (1983) Paf-acether, platelets and bronchospasm. In: Benveniste J, Arnoux B (eds) Platelet-activating factor and structurally-related ether-lipids. INSERM symposium n° 23. Elsevier, Amsterdam, pp 327–334
46. Patterson R, Harris KE (1983) The activity of aerosolized and intracutaneous synthetic platelet-activating factor (AGEPC) in rhesus monkeys with IgE-mediated airway responses and normal monkeys. J Lab Clin Med 102:933–938
47. Pinckard RN, Kniker WT, Lee L, Hanahan DJ, McManus LM (1980) Vasoactive effects of 1-*O*-alkyl-2-acetyl-*sn*-glyceryl-3-phosphorylcholine (AcGEPC) in human skin. J Allergy Clin Immunol 65:196–202
48. Pirotzky E, Page CP, Roubin R, Pfister A, Paul W, Bonnet J, Benveniste J (1984) Paf-acether-induced plasma exudation in rat skin is independent of platelets and neutrophils. Microcirc Endothel Lymph 1:107–122
49. Poitevin B, Roubin R, Benveniste J (1984) Paf-acether generates chemiluminescence in human neutrophils in the absence of cytochalasin B. Immunopharmacology 7:135–144
50. Roubin R, Mencia-Huerta JM, Benveniste J (1982) Release of platelet-activating factor (Paf-acether) and leukotrienes C and D from inflammatory macrophages. Eur J Immunol 12:141–146
51. Roubin R, Tencé M, Mencia-Huerta JM, Arnoux B, Ninio E, Benveniste J (1983) A chemically defined monokine-macrophage-defined platelet-activating factor. In: Pick E (ed) Lymphokines, vol 8. Academic, New York, pp 249–276
52. Santamaria R, Pourrias B, Benveniste J (1983) Effet du Paf-acéther sur la veine porte du rat. J. Pharmacol. 14 (Suppl.): 83 (abstract)
53. Stimler NP, Bloor CM, Hugli TE, Wykle RL, McCall CE, O'Flaherty JT (1981) Anaphylactic actions of platelet-activating factor. Am J Pathol 105:64–69
54. Tencé M, Polonsky J, Le Couedic JP, Benveniste J (1980) Release, purification and characterization of platelet-activating factor. Biochimie 62:251–259
55. Vargaftig BB, Chignard M, Benveniste J, Lefort J, Wal F (1981) Background and present status of researchs on platelet-activating factor (Paf-acether). Ann NY Acad Sci 370:119–137
56. Vargaftig BB, Lefort J, Chignard M, Benveniste J (1980) Platelet-activating factor induces a platelet dependent bronchoconstriction unrelated to the formation of prostaglandin derivatives. Eur J Pharmacol 65:185–192
57. Vargaftig B, Lefort J, Rotilio D (1983) Route-dependent interactions between Paf-acether and guinea-pig bronchopulmonary smooth muscle: relevance of cyclooxygenase mechanisms. In: Benveniste J, Arnoux B (eds) Platelet-activating factor and structurally-related ether-lipids. INSERM symposium n° 23. Elsevier, Amsterdam, pp 307–316
58. Voelkel NF, Worthen S, Reeves JT, Henson PM, Murphy RC (1982) Non-immunological production of leukotrienes induced by platelet-activating factor. Science 218:286–288
59. Wykle RL, Malone B, Snyder F (1980) Enzymatic synthesis of 1-alkyl-2-acetyl-*sn*-glycero-3-phosphocholine, a hypotensive and platelet-aggregating lipid. J Biol Chem 255:10256–10260

Atopic Eczema and Food Allergy

Itch and Endorphins

Ö. Hägermark
Department of Dermatology, Karolinska Sjukhuset, 104 01 Stockholm, Sweden

Abstract

Knowledge of the neurochemistry of pruritus is incomplete and as yet there are no drugs available with a specific antipruritic effect. The classical antihistamines are widely used as antipruritic drugs. The rationale for this is mainly based upon the fact that histamine is a potent pruritogen when injected into the skin and that histamine can easily be released from the mast cells in acute inflammation. Still there is very little evidence that histamine is involved in any pruritic disease other than urticaria. The beneficial effect of antihistamines in pruritic diseases may thus very well be ascribed to their sedative action and to placebo effects. Although pain and itch are related anatomically and physiologically, it is interesting to note that non-narcotic analgesics, such as aspirin, do not alleviate itch, and narcotic analgesics, such as morphine, tend to aggravate the sensation of itch. This has been ascribed to the histamine-releasing capacity of morphine, but in fact morphine is a weak histamine liberator and more recent observations, discussed in this presentation, indicate that other processes than histamine release are involved in opiate-induced itching.

Research on opiates has made great advances during the last 10 years after the discovery in 1975 of the endorphins, i.e. endogenous peptides with morphine-like antinociceptive activity. These neurogenic peptides are believed to be involved in the endogenous control of pain. However, when applied to itch they enhance itching both at a peripheral and at a central level.

After intradermal injection, pruritogenic agents evoke a sensation of itch at the injection site lasting for several minutes. The duration of the itch response is dose-related and can be used for quantitative determination of the itch. This method has been used at our department for many years for investigating the pruritogenic effect of various inflammatory mediators and neurogenic peptides. Morphine and the endorphins enkephalin and β-endorphin were weak pruritogens per se when injected alone but caused a marked enhancement of histamine-induced itch. This potentiation was neither influenced by local pretreatment with compound 48/80 to deplete local stores of mast-cell bound histamine, nor by oral pretreatment with indomethacine to inhibit prostaglandin formation in the skin. Thus, the enhancement did not seem to be due to histamine release or prostaglandin formation. The specific morphine antagonist naloxone did not inhibit the potentiation, indicating that ordinary opiate receptors were not involved in this peripheral stimulatory effect.

It has been known for many years that intracisternal injection of morphine into the brains of laboratory animals can produce a violent scratching response. In recent years pruritus has proved to be an unexpected and unpleasant sequela to spinal opiate analgesia in man. This itching from spinal opioids is effectively inhibited by the opioid antagonist naloxone. These observations, when related to the discovery of endorphins in the central nervous system, make it conceivable that the endogenous morphine-like peptides are involved as central transmitters of the itch sensation. This hypothesis is supported by reports that naloxone may reduce both clinical and experimental itch, at least to some extent.

The pain-relieving endorphins increase pruritus both at peripheral and central levels. May be the future itch-relieving drugs are to be found among opioid antagonists?

Introduction

"Itch and endorphins" is a subject which might be of importance both for our understanding of the pathophysiology of itch and for indicating new possibilities for its pharmacological treatment. Itch is a symptom, sometimes very tormenting, occurring in many diseases, including several allergic conditions such as atopic eczema, contact eczema, and urticaria. As yet there are no drugs available with a specific antipruritic effect [19]. The anodynes used for treating pain have no effect in itch; morphine and other opiates even tend to aggravate the sensation of itch. In the absence of other drugs most doctors prescribe antihistamines as antipruritic drugs. The rationale for this is mainly based upon the facts that histamine is a potent pruritogen when injected into the skin and that histamine can easily be released from the mast cells in acute inflammatory reactions. Still, there is very little evidence that histamine is involved in any pruritic disease other than urticaria. For instance, I doubt that histamine is the main cause of itch in atopic eczema even if we know that histamine release is increased in these patients. The essential point for the atopic patient is the increased *sensitivity* to pruritogenic stimuli, including histamine itself. This can be shown in experiments where histamine is injected intradermally. Concentrations required to produce itch in atopic patients are weaker than in normal subjects. Much evidence indicates that the beneficial effects of antihistamines in pruritic diseases other than urticaria may be ascribed to their sedative action and to placebo effects [19]. Krause and Shuster [16] recently reported that the new nonsedative antihistamines terfenadine and astemizole relieve itch in urticaria but have a very poor antipruritic effect in eczema.

Endorphins (Endogenous Opioid Peptides)

Opiates have been used since ancient times but it is only during the last 10–15 years that we have begun to understand their molecular mechanism of action. In 1973 three research groups independently reported that there are specific receptors in the brain for the opiate drugs [18, 21, 24]. It was then logical to assume that there should exist some kind of endogenous ligand. The first attempts to isolate this ligand for the opiate receptors were unsuccessful due to the mistaken presumption that the endogenous opiates should have a chemical similarity to morphine. In 1975 Hughes and his colleagues [14] in Aberdeen isolated and characterized two pentapeptides from pig brain and named them enkephalins. The enkephalins acted as agonists at opiate receptor sites and could mimic morphine in most of its properties. In the next year, 1976, β-endorphin was identified [7]. This peptide is much larger and has 31 amino acids. To date more than 20 individual opioid peptides have been identified [5]. They belong to three opioid gene families [1]. Studies using various agonists and antagonists indicate that there are several receptors for the opiates. Morphine has high affinity for μ-receptors, the enkephalins for δ-receptors, β-endorphin for ε-receptors, and the newly detected compound dynorphin for $\varkappa$-receptors. The antagonist naloxone acts preferably on μ-receptors. However, there is a substantial cross-reactivity between agonists and antagonists for the different receptors [25].

The opioid peptides are recovered in the brain and peripheral nerves. Their functions seem to be involved in stress responses and they may be essential in the maintenance of homeostatis [1]. They take part in endogenous control of pain and in control of blood pressure. The evidence that endorphins have a role in human pain comes largely from studies in which the action of opioids have been blocked by naloxone. Naloxone is a pure opiate antagonist and has no detectable effect in normal man but consistently enhances postoperative pain. The explanation for this is that after surgical operation the endorphins are increased, which decreases the postoperative pain. Naloxone inhibits this effect.

Itch

There are several similarities between the anatomy and physiology of pain and itch. Both are unpleasant phenomena (warning signals) induced by noxious stimuli. Both are transmitted to the spinal cord by thin unmyelinated C-fibers. Some stimuli which at low intensity may induce itch may cause pain at a higher intensity. This is why it has been proposed that itch is a kind of mild cutaneous pain. However, itch differs from pain in many respects and there seems more reason to regard itch and cutaneous pain as distinct sensory experiences. Itch induces the compulsive need to scratch. It is always localized in the skin. Immersion of skin in water at 40 °C may relieve itching while it makes pain worse.

Pain is relieved by analgesics, whereas itch is not. Morphine and other opioids in fact may intensify itching [11]. This enhancement occurs both at a peripheral and at a central level.

Peripheral Effects

Ever since the 1920s when Lewis [17] demonstrated that intradermal injection of histamine causes a vascular triple response in the skin (redness, wheal, and flare) and itching, it has been debated whether or not histamine is the ultimate mediator that is always involved in pathological pruritus. Experimental itching induced by intradermal injection of histamine is always associated with a visible vascular response and is easily blocked by antihistamines. The itch in disease often occurs without whealing and erythema and antihistamines often have a poor antipruritic effect. It sems likely then that mediators other than histamine are involved in many itching diseases.

This aspect has been of great interest to us for many years and we have studied the pruritogenic effects of various inflammatory mediators and neurogenic peptides. Our results can be summarized as follows. Histamine released from dermal mast cells seems to be the cause of experimental itch induced by injection of proteases – such as trypsin and chymase [12] – and of neurogenic peptides – such as substance P, vasoactive intestinal peptide (VIP), and neurotensin [9]. Prostaglandins E_2 and H_2 produce virtually no itch when injected alone, but cause a marked enhancement of the itch response when given in combination with pruritogens [13]. This is similar to the observations concerning pain stimuli, which are also enhanced by prostaglandins.

More recently we extended our studies to opioids [10]. It has long been known that morphine is a histamine liberator and induces a triple response at the injection site when given intradermally [8]. It can also produce histamine release after subcutaneous injection, sometimes even after intravenous injection. Therefore the pruritogenic effect of morphine has been ascribed to its histamine-releasing capacity. However, we found that opioids can cause a potentiation of the itch response similar to that produced by prostaglandins [10]. Subthreshold doses of morphine, enkephalin and β-endorphin not producing any histamine release and itching when injected alone caused a marked enhancement of the histamine-induced itch when injected in a mixture with histamine. This potentiation was influenced neither by local pretreatment with compound 48/80 to deplete the local stores of mast cell bound histamine, nor by oral pretreatment with indomethacin to inhibit prostaglandin formation in the skin [10]. Thus, the enhancement did not seem to be due to histamine release or prostaglandin formation. It is interesting to note that *prostaglandins enhance* both pain and itch, whereas *opioids inhibit* pain and *enhance* itch at a peripheral level.

In our hands the morphine antagonist naloxone injected locally into the challenge site or given intravenously did not inhibit the opioid-induced potentiation, indicating that receptors of the μ-type are not involved in this peripheral stimulating effect [10]. However, somewhat contradictory results have been reported by Bernstein and collaborators [4], who found that systemically administered naloxone could inhibit histamine-induced itch. The discrepancy between our results might be explained by different techniques. Bernstein and collaborators induced itch by injecting increasing concentrations of histamine solutions and registered the sensory thresholds for itch, whereas we studied the duration of the itch response.

Central Effects

Almost 40 years ago Koenigstein [15] studied experimental itch in laboratory animals. He injected morphine into the fourth cerebral ventricle and the animals responded with violent scratching paroxysms. He concluded from his experiments that there is a scratching center in the lower part of the medulla oblongata. A similar center may exist in humans since patients with cerebral tumors infiltrating the floor of the fourth ventricle may suffer from a characteristic pruritus in the nostrils [2].

In recent years it has been found that intraspinal injection of opioids is a very effective way of obtaining segmental pain relief [26]. However, one of the most common side-effects of this treatment is pruritus, which sometimes can be very disabling [6]. The distribution of the itch is not confined to the segmental area of analgesia but occurs most frequently in the face, especially in the nostrils. There is no redness or whealing in the affected areas, indicating histamine release. It is not known why this pruritus is so often confined to the face and especially the nostrils, but it has been speculated that there might be an activation of an itching center in the medulla oblongata [20]. This facial itching from spinal opioids is effectively inhibited by naloxone.

Naloxone and Itch

From what I have said so far there seems much evidence that endogenous opioids could be involved in the transmission of the itch sensation both in the periphery and in the CNS. I mentioned that naloxone is very effective in stopping pruritus after spinal anesthesia and it would be natural to investigate the effect of opioid antagonists in pruritic diseases. However, very few such studies have been made. In 1979 Bernstein and Swift [3] reported on one patient with intractable pruritus due to cholestasis, who was relieved by naloxone. This patient was studied under double-blind conditions and relief was first noted 5 min after injection of naloxone and lasted for about 2 h. Saline provided no relief from itching. This is the only clinical investigation published by these authors, but as mentioned above they have studied experimental itch in volunteers and demonstrated that naloxone inhibits itch induced by histamine [4].

In 1980 Summerfield [22] reported a study of 20 patients with pruritus due to cholestatic liver disease. Naloxone and saline were given intravenously according to a double-blind, cross-over protocol at 6 p.m. Itching was assessed at 9 the following morning on a visual analog scale. When the whole group of patients was analyzed there was no difference between naloxone and placebo. However, the 11 patients who reported that itch improved after placebo (placebo responders), found that the itching became worse on naloxone. Conversely, placebo nonresponders reported less itch after naloxone. Thus, naloxone could either increase or decrease itching depending on the patients's response to placebo. These results differ somewhat from those obtained in pain studies, where the effect of naloxone is limited to placebo responders who report increased pain after naloxone, whereas a pain-decreasing effect of naloxone has not been observed in pain studies.

In 1981 Summerfield [23] stated that these preliminary results needed to be confirmed and extended. However, no such studies have been published. Over the years only a few uncontrolled cases have been reported in the literature with decreased pruritus after administration of naloxone. My personal impression is that naloxone has no obvious itch-relieving effect in pruritic diseases.

Conclusion

There is evidence that endorphins and opiate receptors could be involved in the transmission of pruritus both at peripheral and central levels. However, the itch-relieving effect of the opioid antagonist naloxone with high affinity for receptors of the μ-type remains to be established. New opioid antagonists with δ- and $\varkappa$-receptor activity are being developed. Clinical studies of these compounds are awaited with great interest and are required before we can tell whether or not the next generation of antipruritic drugs is to be found among the opioid antagonists.

References

1. Akil H, Watson SJ, Young E, Lewis ME, Khachaturian H, Walker JM (1984) Endogenous opioids: biology and function. Annu Rev Neurosci 7:223–255
2. Andreev VC, Petkov (1975) Skin manifestations associated with tumours of the brain. Br J Dermatol 92:675–678
3. Bernstein JE, Swift R (1979) Relief of intractable pruritus with naloxone. Arch Dermatol 115:1366–1367
4. Bernstein JE, Swift RM, Soltani K, Lorincz AL (1982) Antipruritic effect of an opiate antagonist, naloxone hydrochloride. J Invest Dermatol 78:82–83
5. Bloom FE (1983) The endorphins: a growing family of pharmacologically pertinent peptides. Annu Rev Pharmacol Toxicol 23:151–170
6. Bromage PR (1981) The price of intraspinal narcotic analgesia: basic constraints. Editorial. Anesthesia Analgesia 60:461–463

7. Cox BM, Goldstein A, Li CH (1976) Opioid activity of a peptide, β-lipotropin (61–69), derived from β-lipotropin. Proc Natl Acad Sci USA 73:1821–1823
8. Feldberg W, Paton WDM (1951) Release of histamine from skin and muscle in the cat by opium alkaloids and other histamine liberators. J Physiol (Lond) 114:490–509
9. Fjellner B, Hägermark Ö (1981) Studies on pruritogenic and histamine-releasing effects of some putative peptide neurotransmitters. Acta Derm Venereol (Stockh) 61:245–250
10. Fjellner B, Hägermark Ö (1982) Potentiation of histamine-induced itch and flare responses in human skin by the enkephalin analogue FK 33-824, β-endorphin and morphine. Arch Dermatol Res 274:29–37
11. Hägermark Ö (1983) Pruritus: pathogenesis and therapeutic trials. In: Kukita A, Seiji M (eds) Proceedings of the 16th international congress of dermatology. University of Tokyo Press, Tokyo, pp 61–67
12. Hägermark Ö, Rajka G, Bergqvist U (1972) Experimental itch in human skin elicited by rat mast cell chymase. Acta Derm Venereol (Stockh) 52:125–128
13. Hägermark Ö, Strandberg K, Hamberg M (1977) Potentiation of itch and flare responses in human skin by prostaglandins E_2 and H_2 and a prostaglandin endoperoxide analog. J Invest Dermatol 69:527–530
14. Hughes J, Smith TW, Kosterlitz H, Fothergill LA, Morgan BA, Morris HR (1975) Identification of two related pentapeptides from the brain with potent opiate agonist activity. Nature 258:577–579
15. Koenigstein H (1948) Experimental study of itch stimuli in animals. Arch Dermatol 57:828–849
16. Krause L, Shuster S (1983) Mechanism of action of antipruritic drugs. Br Med J 287:1199–1200
17. Lewis T (1927) The blood vessels of the human skin and their responses. Shaw, London
18. Pert CB, Snyder SH (1973) Opiate receptor: demonstration in nervous tissue. Science 179:1011–1014
19. Savin JA (1980) Do systemic antipruritic agents work? Br J Dermatol 102:113–118
20. Scott PV, Fischer HBJ (1982) Spinal opiate analgesia and facial pruritus: a neural theory. Postgrad Med J 58:531–535
21. Simon EJ, Hiller JM, Edelman I (1973) Stereospecific binding of the potent narcotic analgesics ^{3}H-etorphone to rat brain homogenate. Proc Natl Acad Sci USA 70:1947–1949
22. Summerfield JA (1980) Naloxone modulates the perception of itch in man. Br J Clin Pharmacol 10:180–183
23. Summerfield JA (1981) Pain, itch and endorphins. Br J Dermatol 105:725–726
24. Terenius L (1973) Characteristics of the receptor for narcotic analgesics in synaptic plasma membrane fraction from rat brain. Acta Pharmacol Toxicol 32:377–384
25. Terenius L (1985) Families of opioid peptides and classes of opioid receptors. Adv Pain Res Ther 9:463–477
26. Wang JK, Nauss LA, Thomas JE (1979) Pain relief by intrathecally applied morphine in man. Anesthesiology 50:149–151

Dry Skin (Sebostasis) and Inflammation: Heterogeneity of "Dry Skin" in Atopic Dermatitis

M. Uehara
Department of Dermatology, Shiga University of Medical Science, Seta, Otsu 520-21, Japan

Abstract

Uninvolved skin sites in 250 consecutive patients, 15 to 30 years old, with atopic dermatitis were observed during the winter months. Ichthyosis vulgaris occurred in 58 patients. Of the remaining patients, only 10 (5%) had generalized dry skin; 119 (62%) showed focal areas of dry skin; and 63 (33%) exhibited only normal-appearing skin.

Histologically, in 50 patients, dry skin associated with atopic dermatitis showed mild eczematous changes. Dry skin coexistent with ichthyosis in patients with atopic dermatitis revealed ichthyotic changes frequently superimposed on eczematous changes.

Immunohistochemically, in all biopsy specimens from dry skin of 20 patients with atopic dermatitis alone, the majority of the infiltrating lymphocytes were stained with Leu-3a antihelper/inducer T cell antibody. Leu-2a- reactive suppressor/cytotoxic cells formed a minor component of the infiltrating lymphocytes. The number of OKT6-positive Langerhans cells was increased in the slightly acanthotic epidermis and dermal infiltrates.

Thus, in patients with atopic dermatitis the presence of dry skin may reflect mild eczematous changes, a manifestation of concomitant ichthyosis vulgaris, or a mixture of both of these changes.

It is suggested that the histological and immunohistochemical pictures of dry skin in pure atopic dermatitis may show an intrinsic feature of this dermatosis, because the dry skin virtually is free from secondary effects due to topical remedies, scratching, or bacterial infections.

Introduction

There has been a common belief among dermatologists that the "uninvolved" skin of patients with atopic dermatitis (AD) is generally dry [1 – 3]. It is reported that the dry skin of AD patients shows a decrease in skin surface lipids [4 – 6], and that this reduction is mainly due to a decrease of sebaceous lipids [5,

6]. Sebaceous glands are atrophic in the dry skin [7, 8], suggesting that the atrophy of sebaceous glands is responsible for the dry skin in AD.

It it well known, however, that ichthyosis vulgaris is an important complication of AD [2, 9]. Ichthyosis vulgaris shows dry skin and atrophy of sebaceous glands [10, 11]. It is then natural that the primary characteristics of dry skin in AD are often modified by the concomitant ichthyosis.

Recently, Finlay et al. [12] and we [13] have demonstrated that the dry skin in AD histologically shows a mild eczematous change. This suggests that eczematous change is the cause of the dry skin in AD. On the other hand, it has been pointed out that some patients with AD have perfectly normal, smooth skin except where dry patches of lichenification are present [13, 14]. Thus, it appears that the "uninvolved" skins of AD patients are not homogeneous in nature.

This paper summarizes our recent studies on the clinical, histological, and immunohistological features of the dry skin in patients with AD who do not have ichthyosis vulgaris.

Clinical Observations

Prevalence of Ichthyosis Vulgaris in AD. A total of 300 consecutive patients, 10–35 years old, with AD were observed during winter months. In each patient the skins of the trunk, limbs, palms, and soles were closely examined. The diagnosis of ichthyosis vulgaris was established by both of the following two sets of criteria: (a) small polygonal scales symmetrically distributed on the extensor limbs and trunk, and (b) hyperlinearity of both palms and soles [15, 16]. These skin signs of ichthyosis vulgaris were seen in 49 (16%) of the 300 patients with AD examined.

Clinical Features of "Uninvolved" Skin in Patients with Pure AD. Of the 251 patients with AD who did not have ichthyosis vulgaris, only 9 (4%) patients showed generalized dry skin which covered 70% or more of the body surface. Sixty-eight (27%) patients revealed normal-appearing, smooth skin except where lichenified lesions existed. The remaining 174 (69%) patients had partial dry skin, i.e., coexistence of dry skin and normal-appearing skin.

In the dry skin of patients with pure AD, the degree of dryness was usually slight, while moderate to severe dryness was common in the dry skin of patients with AD and ichthyosis vulgaris (Figs. 1, 2).

Comment. Although the clinical examinations were all performed during the winter months when the dryness of the skin in AD is most prominent, generalized dry skin was observed in only a small number of patients with AD who did not have ichthyosis vulgaris. The majority of pure AD patients had partial dry skin or normal-appearing skin alone. These results indicate that general dryness of the skin is not an intrinsic feature of AD per se.

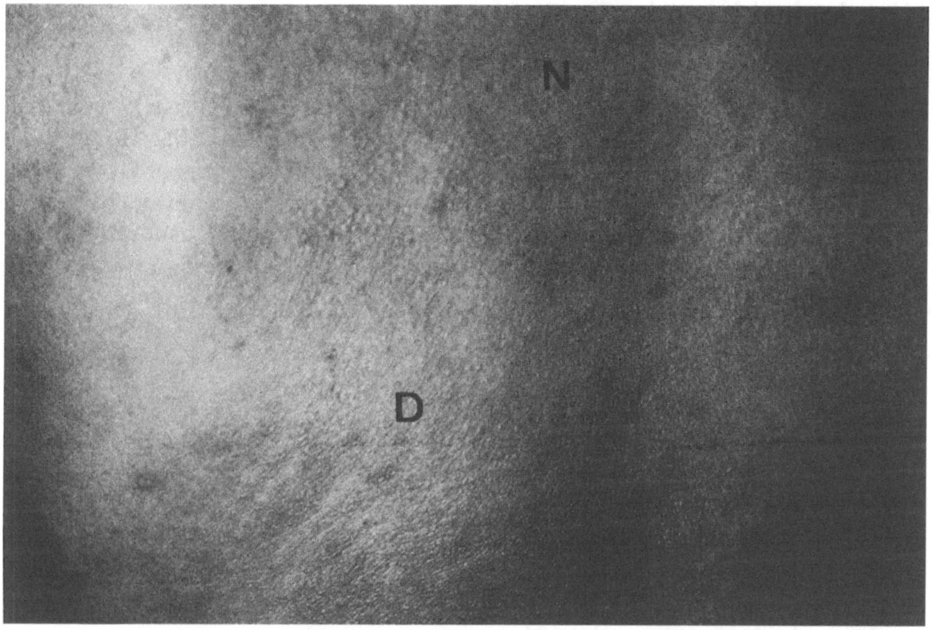

Fig. 1. Lower part of back of an 18-year-old patient with atopic dermatitis alone, showing coexistence of dry skin (*D*) and normal-appearing skin (*N*)

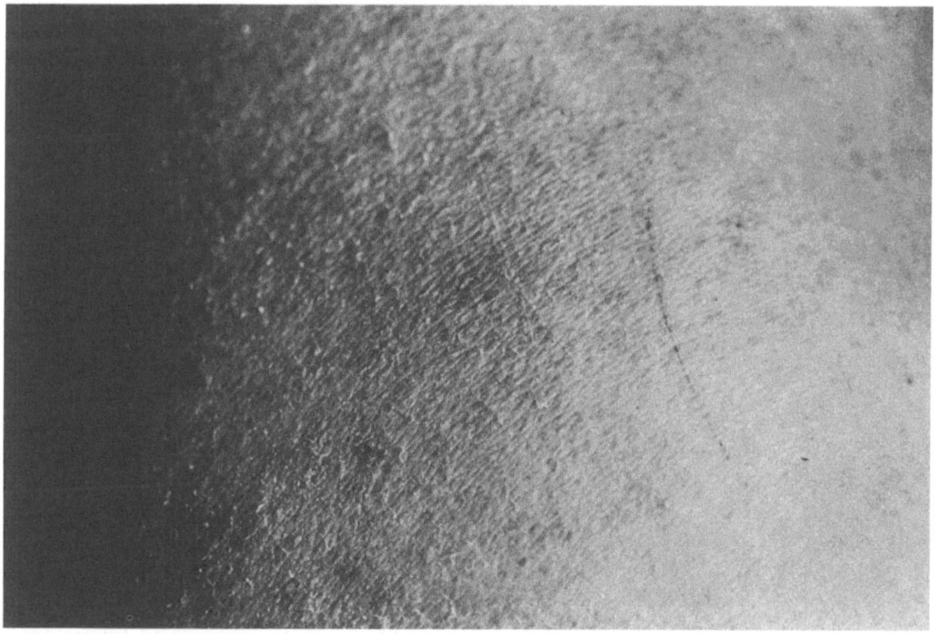

Fig. 2. Lower part of back of a 22-year-old patient with atopic dermatitis and ichthyosis vulgaris. Dryness of skin is more intense than that seen in pure atopic dermatitis (Fig. 1)

Histological Examination

Dry skin from 54 patients (22 with AD and ichthyosis vulgaris, 32 with AD alone) and normal-appearing skin from 14 patients (all with AD alone) were examined. In each patient, a 4-mm punch biopsy specimen was obtained from dry skin or normal-appearing skin on the lateral aspect of the buttock. The skin area examined had received no topical treatment for at least a month prior to biopsy. Each of the 68 biopsy specimens was serially sectioned and stained with hematoxylin-eosin.

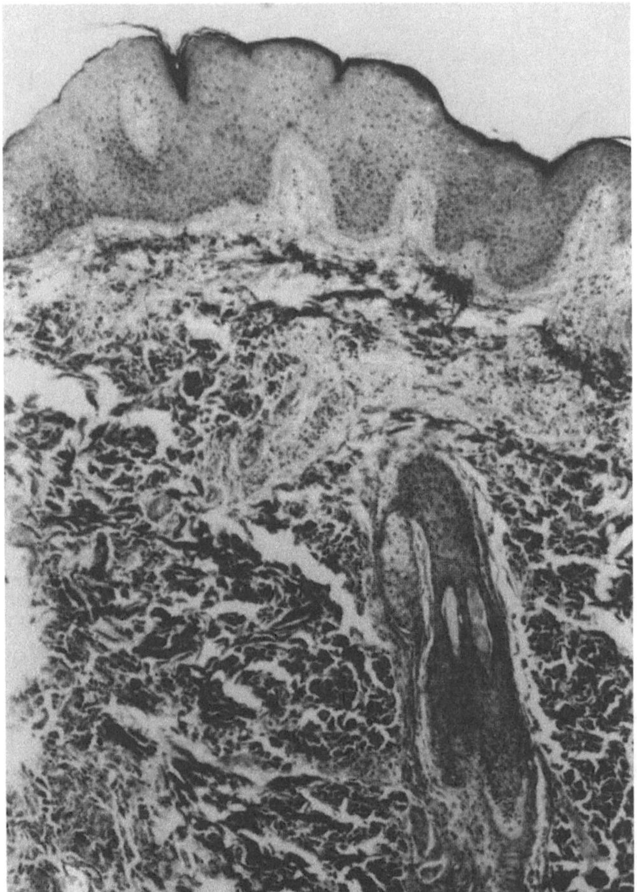

Fig. 3. Dry skin site biopsy specimen from patient with atopic dermatitis and ichthyosis vulgaris. Note hyperkeratosis, reduced thickness of the granular layer, atrophic sebaceous glands, and slight infiltrate of mononuclear cells

Histology of Dry Skin in Patients with AD and Ichthyosis Vulgaris. Of the 22 biopsy specimens, 20 showed atrophy of sebaceous glands (Fig. 3). Only two specimens had normally developed sebaceous glands. The granular layer was absent or reduced in all of the 22 biopsy specimens. In 15 specimens there were histopathological changes of mild eczema described below.

Histology of Dry Skin in Patients with Pure AD. In all of the 32 biopsy specimens, histological pictures of mild subacute eczema were regularly observed (Fig. 4). The epidermis showed patchy parakeratosis, slight acanthosis, and focal spongiosis with exocytosis of mononuclear cells. The dermis showed mononuclear cell infiltrates around the superficial blood vessels. Sebaceous glands were normally developed in 26 biopsy specimens. Atrophic sebaceous glands were observed in only six specimens.

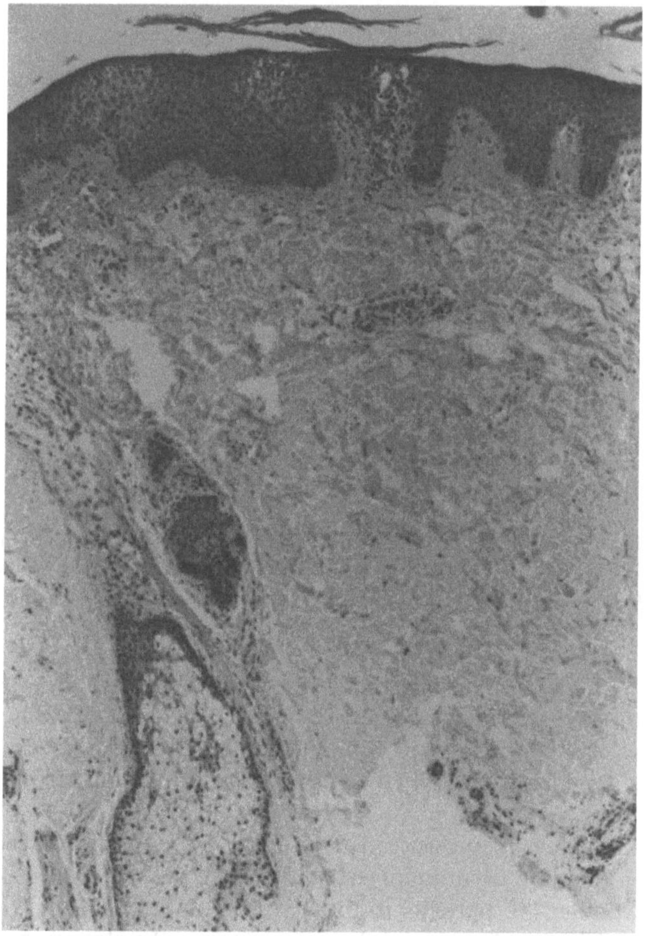

Fig. 4. Dry skin site biopsy specimen from patients with pure atopic dermatitis, showing parakeratosis, acanthosis, spongiosis, mononuclear cell infiltrate, and normally developed sebaceous glands

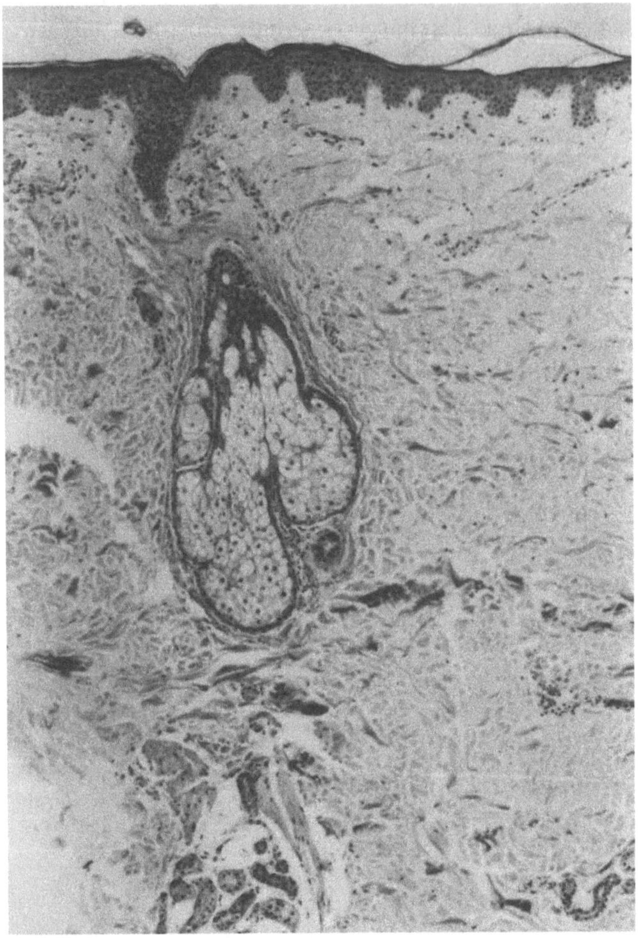

Fig. 5. Normal-appearing skin site biopsy specimen from patient with pure atopic dermatitis. No pathological changes except for slight infiltrate of mononuclear cells. Sebaceous glands are normally developed

Histology of Normal-Appearing Skin in Patients with Pure AD. In all of the 14 biopsy specimens, there were no pathological findings except for a mild perivascular infiltrate of mononuclear cells that were seen in the upper dermis in eight specimens (Fig. 5). Sebaceous glands were normally developed.

Comment. Previous studies [7, 8] described that sebaceous glands were atrophic in dry skin or uninvolved skin of patients with AD. It was not clear, however, whether the patients in these studies suffered from AD alone, or whether they had both AD and ichthyosis vulgaris. By classifying AD patients into those with pure AD and those with AD and ichthyosis vulgaris, the present study demonstrated that atrophy of sebaceous glands most commonly was seen in the dry skin of patients with AD who had ichthyosis vulgaris. Atrophic sebaceous glands occurred only rarely in the dry skin of patients with AD who did not have ichthyosis vulgaris. Normal-appearing skin of patients with pure AD showed normally developed sebaceous glands. It is, then, likely that the atrophic sebaceous glands often seen in dry skin of patients with AD are actually a manifestation of concomitant ichthyosis vulgaris. On the other hand, the dry skin in patients with pure AD consistently showed histological changes of mild, subacute eczema. Thus, we believe that the dry skin often seen in AD is heterogeneous in nature. The dry skin may be a manifestation of concomitant ichthyosis, or a mild eczematous change of AD per se, or a mixture of both of these changes.

Immunohistological Examinations

In 24 young adult patients with AD who did not have ichthyosis vulgaris, a 3-mm punch biopsy specimen from dry skin on the trunk or the buttock was obtained. The skin specimens were quick-frozen with liquid nitrogen. Serial cryostat sections, 5 μm thick, were prepared. Using the avidin-biotin complex method [17] with a panel of monoclonal antibodies, the cellular infiltrate in the cryostat sections was characterized. Monoclonal antibodies employed included Leu-1 (anti-pan T cell), Leu-2a (anti-T-suppressor/cytotoxic cell), Leu-3a (anti-T-helper/inducer cell), OKB-7 (anti-B cell), and OKT-6 (anti-Langerhans' cell) antibody.

In all biopsy specimens, the majority of infiltrating lymphocytes in the dermis showed positive staining with Leu-1 antibody. OKB-7 positive B-lymphocytes were virtually absent. Most of the dermal lymphocytes reacted with Leu-3a antibody (Fig. 6). Only a small number of the infiltrating lymphocytes were positively stained with Leu-2a antibody (Fig. 7). Most lymphocytes in spongiotic areas of epidermis also reacted with Leu-1 and Leu-3a antibodies. OKT-6 positive Langerhans' cells were increased in number in the slightly acanthotic epidermis and areas of spongiosis, and in the inflammatory infiltrate in the upper dermis (Fig. 8).

Comment. The immunohistological characteristics of inflammatory cells in lichenified lesions of AD have been studied by many authors. Willemze et al. [18] and Leung et al. [19] report that the infiltrating lymphocytes in the lichenified lesions are predominantly OKT-4 positive or Leu-3a positive T-lymphocytes possessing the helper/inducer phenotype. Contrarily, Rocha et al. [20] state that in lichenified lesions of AD, the mononuclear cells in the dermal infiltrate comprise primarily OKT-8 positive lymphocytes expressing the suppressor/cytotoxic phenotype. These conflicting opinions might be first of all due to the fact that the lichenified lesions from which biopsy specimens were taken were probably not homogeneous, since longstanding lichenified lesions are subjected to secondary damage superimposed by scratching, topical medications, and bacterial infections. For the purpose of establishing the cardinal

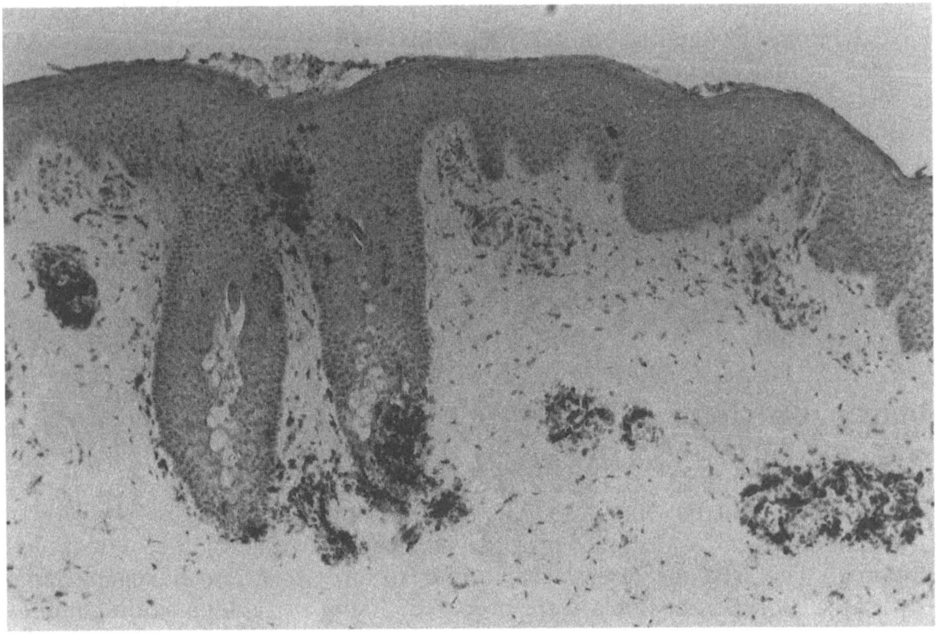

Fig. 6. Dry skin in pure atopic dermatitis. Leu-3a staining pattern. The majority of lymphocytes in the dermis and spongiotic areas of the epidermis are positive

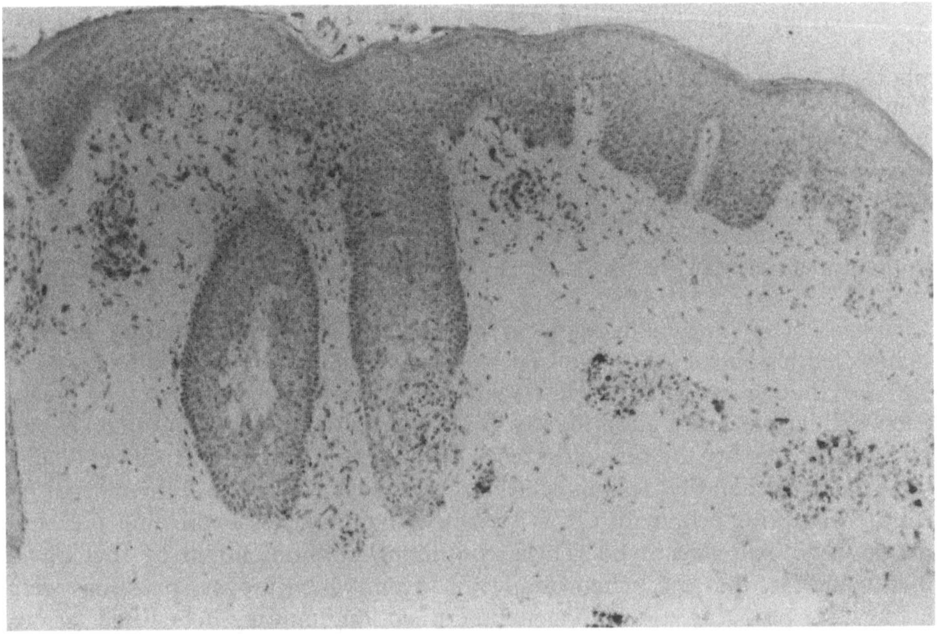

Fig. 7. Dry skin in pure atopic dermatitis. Leu-2a staining pattern. Scattered individual positive cells are seen in the dermal infiltrate and spongiotic areas of the epidermis

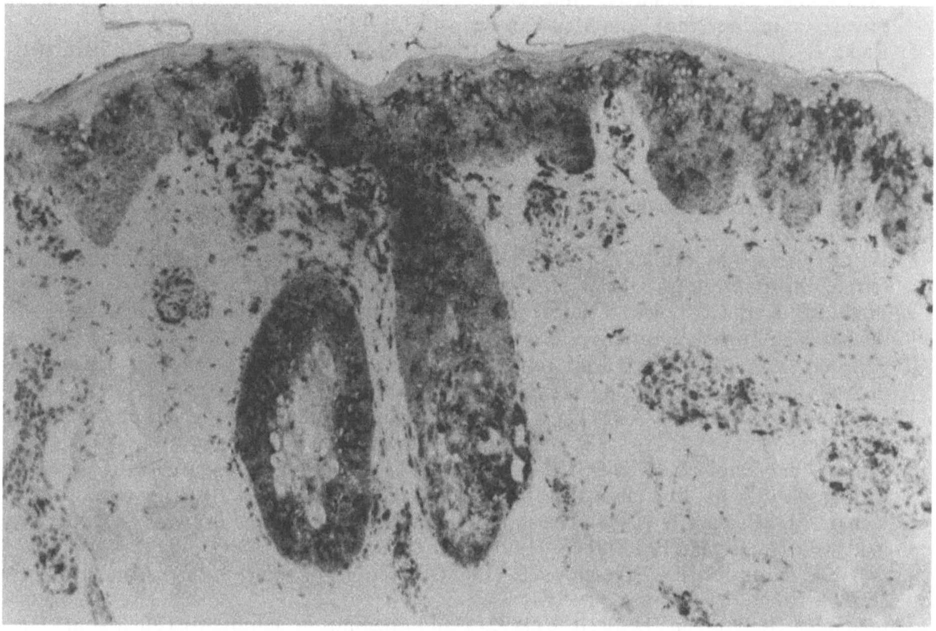

Fig. 8. Dry skin in pure atopic dermatitis. OKT-6 staining pattern. Increased numbers of positive cells are seen in the slightly acanthotic epidermis, in spongiotic areas, and in the dermal infiltrate

changes of AD, therefore, it is important to examine a skin lesion which has not incurred any secondary damage. The dry skin of pure AD patients examined in the present study was virtually free from mechanical trauma of scratching, topical remedies, and infections. It is, then, likely that the dry skin in pure AD represents a primary lesion of the disease. The present study demonstrated that in the dry skin of pure AD patients, the majority of infiltrating lymphocytes were stained with Leu-3a antibody. Leu-2a positive cells were scant. This finding indicates that the predominance of T helper/inducer cells over T suppressor/cytotoxic cells is characteristic of a probably primary, subacute lesion of AD.

In conclusion, we believe that the dry skin in patients with pure AD is a mild eczematous lesion of this disease.

References

1. Sulzberger MB (1971) Atopic dermatitis, part 3. In: Fitzpatrick T, Arndt KA, Clark WH (eds) Dermatology in general medicine. McGraw-Hill, New York, pp 687–697
2. Rajka G (1975) Atopic dermatitis. Saunders, Philadelphia, pp 105–130
3. Hanifin JM (1983) Clinical and basic aspects of atopic dermatitis. Semin Dermatol 6:5–19

4. Mustakallio KK, Kiistala U, Piha HJ, Nieminen E (1967) Epidermal lipids in Besnier's prurigo (atopic eczema). Ann Med Exp Fenn 45:323–325
5. Rajka G (1974) Surface lipid estimation on the back of the hands in atopic dermatitis. Arch Dermatol Forsch 251:43–48
6. Abe T, Ohkido M, Yamamoto K (1978) Studies on skin barrier functions. Skin surface lipids and transepidermal water loss in atopic skin during childhood. J Dermatol 5:223–229
7. Sulzberger MB, Hermann F, Morril SD, Pascher F, Miller K (1959) Studies of sweat, lipids, and histopathology in children with "dry skin" (xerosis). Int Arch Allergy 14:129–143
8. Wirth H, Gloor M, Stoika D (1981) Sebaceous glands in uninvolved skin of patients suffering from atopic dermatitis. Arch Dermatol Res 270:167–179
9. Wells RS, Kerr CB (1966) Clinical features of autosomal dominant and sex-linked ichthyosis in an English population. Br Med J 1:947–950
10. Feinstein A, Ackerman AB, Ziprkowski L (1970) Histology of autosomal dominant ichthyosis vulgaris and X-linked ichthyosis. Arch Dermatol 101:524–527
11. Ziprkowski L, Feinstein A (1972) A survey of ichthyosis vulgaris in Israel. Br J Dermatol 86:1–8
12. Finlay AY, Nicholls S, King CS, Marks R (1980) The 'dry' non-eczematous skin associated with atopic exzema. Br J Dermatol 102:249–256
13. Uehara M, Miyauch H (1984) The morphologic characteristics of dry skin in atopic dermatitis. Arch Dermatol 120:1186–1190
14. Hill LW, in discussion, Wheatley VR (1965) Secretions of the skin in eczema. J Pediatr 66:200–202
15. Leutgeb C, Bandmann HJ, Breit R (1972) Handlinienmuster, Ichthyosis vulgaris und Dermatitis atopica. Arch Dermatol Forsch 244:354–356
16. Uehara M, Hayashi S (1981) Hyperlinear palms – association with ichthyosis and atopic dermatitis. Arch Dermatol 117:490–491
17. Tayler CR, Horman FM, Modlin RL, Rea TH (1983) Immunoperoxidase techniques applied to dermatopathology. J Cutan Pathol 10:145–163
18. Willemze R, de Graaff-Reitsma CB, Cnossen J, Van Vloten WA, Meijer CJL (1983) Characterization of T-cell subpopulations in skin and peripheral blood of patients with cutaneous T-cell lymphomas and benign inflammatory dermatoses. J Invest Dermatol 80:60–66
19. Leung DYM, Bhan AK, Schneeberger EE, Geha RS (1983) Characterization of the mononuclear cell infiltrate in atopic dermatitis using monoclonal antibodies. J Allergy Clin Immunol 71:47–56
20. Rocha C, de Maubeuge J, Sarfati M, Song M, Delespesse G (1984) Characterization of cellular infiltrates in skin lesions of atopic eczema by means of monoclonal antibodies. Dermatologica 169:330–338

Food Allergy and Atopic Eczema

J. F. Soothill

Department of Immunology, Institute of Child Health, University of London, 30 Guilford Street, London WC1N 1EH, Great Britain

Allergic disease following quickly after ingestion of a single food has been recognized for centuries, established by Prauznitz and Küstner, and well handled largely by the patients themselves. IgE antibody levels to causative foods may be raised, but these are usually not needed diagnostically, and a pathogenetic role is not established for them. Slow responses to any combinations of any foods are much more difficult to diagnose, but treatment by antigen avoidance is possible and effective, so it is important. This has been established by double blind placebo-controlled trials in eczema, migraine and behaviour disorder, and the parallel recovery of many other symptoms in the same patients suggests a far wider range of application, which is being studied.

Infants with eczema have a wide range of disturbances of immunity, and the disease has apparently been transferred by bone marrow transplant in severe combined immunodeficiency, so the disease is probably an immunopathological one, though the mechanism is unknown. Some eczema is induced by contact agents and some by inhalants; complete avoidance of them, unlike foods, is impossible. With eczema, the case for immunopathogenesis is strong. For some other slow food allergies it is less so, but the combinations of foods causing illness in each individual suggests allergy rather than idiosyncrasy. Diets avoiding single foods, empirical diets, oligoantigenic diets and antigen-free feeding permit diagnosis and treatment but are difficult and dangerous. Exclusive breast feeding will probably reduce the prevalence of such disease, probably partly by antigen-non-specific mechanisms.

Drugs which influence the uptake of antigen in the gut (sodium cromoglycate) or which may have an anti-inflammatory effect in the gut (beclomethasone) also protect the sensitized subject from such diseases.

References

1. Atherton DJ, Sewell M, Soothill JF, Wells RS, Chilvers CED (1978) Lancet i:401–403
2. Businco L, Benicori N, Businco R, Infussi R, De Angelis M (1983) Double-blind crossover study with an oral solution of sodium cramoglycate in children with atopic dermitis due to food allergy. In: Proceedings of 2nd Fisions Food Allergy Workshop. Medicine Publishing Foundation, Oxford, p 116
3. Egger J, Carter CM, Wilson J, Turner MW, Soothill JF (1983) Lancet ii:865–869
4. Egger J, Carter CM, Gumley D, Soothill JF, Graham PF (1985) Lancet i:540
5. Heddle RJ, Soothill JF, Bulpitt CJ, Atherton DJ (1984) Br Med J 289:651–654

Intragastric Provocation under Endoscopic Control

H.-J. Reimann[1], U. Schmidt[1], J. Lewin[1], A. Zellmer[1], and J. Ring[2]

[1] II. Medizinische Klinik des Klinikums Rechts der Isar der Technischen Universität München, 8000 Munich, Federal Republic of Germany

[2] Dermatologische Klinik der Ludwig-Maximilians-Universität München, 8000 Munich, Federal Republic of Germany

Abstract

The symptoms of food allergy can occur in many organs and their intensity can vary from mild skin reactions to life-threatening anaphylactoid reactions.

Until now, diagnosis of food allergy can be difficult because of a lack of quantitative and objective provocation methods.

Using a fiberoptic gastroscope allergens were applied to mucosa of the gastrointestinal tract. Macroscopic changes of the mucosa were recorded and biopsies were taken for histological and biochemical analysis.

In patients with food allergy an increase in both tissue histamine and mast cell count was found. After allergen application a decrease of tissue histamine was measured. In some patients, significant increases in plasma histamine concentrations in peripheral venous blood were measured. Intragastral provocation under endoscopic control (IPEC) provides a means for objective and quantitative evaluation of gastrointestinal food allergy.

Introduction

For centuries physicians have been aware of food allergic reactions taking place in the gastrointestinal tract. The first physician to describe food allergy as a disease was Hippocrates [9]. It was mentioned again much later, at the end of the seventeenth century, by Hertod [8], and interest was once more aroused by Quincke [16], who postulated angioneurotic edema as a food allergic reaction (Table 1).

At the turn of the century Schlossmann and Moro [24] reported individual cases of food allergic reactions. In 1920 Schloss [23] investigated 120 children and thereby discovered the following food allergic reactions: diarrhea, vomiting, and skin irritation. Almost 50 years later Werner [28] and Siebels [25] proved that food allergic reactions can be observed in the gut. After application of milk Werner [28] X-rayed the gut. In some patients he found stasis in the duodenum and in others an increase in peristaltic movement of the small intestine.

Table 1. The discovery of food-allergic reactions and their symptoms in the gastrointestinal tract as described in historical medical works [2, 4, 6, 8, 9, 10, 11, 16, 17, 18, 22, 23, 24, 27, 28]

Date	Authors	Allergen	Symptoms
500 B.C.	Hippocrates	Cheese, wine	Abdominal pain
1684	Hertod	Bread	Vomiting
1735	Behrens	Mussels	Vomiting, diarrhea, exanthema
1773	Cullen	Eggs	Angioneurotic edema
1776	Planchon	Mussels, strawberries	Pain in stomach and gut
1835	Parreidt	Eggs	Pain in stomach and gut
1860	Salter	Milk, sugar	Asthmatic attack
1882	Quincke	Eggs	Angioneurotic edema
1885	Brunton	Egg white, biscuit	Vomiting, diarrhea
1888	Hutchinson	Eggs	Abdominal pain diarrhea
1905	Schlossmann and Moro	Milk	Abdominal pain
1914	Talbot	Eggs	Pain in stomach and gut
1919	Laroche, Richet Jr., Saint-Girons	Eggs	Anaphylactic reaction
1920	Schloss	Milk, vegetables	Abdominal pain, vomiting, diarrhea
1967	Werner	Protein	Stasis in the duodenum, increased bowel movements

Table 2. Symptoms induced by food allergens affecting the gastrointestinal tract

Epigastric pain	Inflammation
Regurgitation	Edema
Vomiting	Swelling
Stasis of the gut	Hemorrhagic lesions
Increased peristaltic movements	Bleeding

Table 3. Symptoms of food allergy other than in the gastrointestinal tract

Respiratory tract	*Cardiovascular*	*CNS*	*Skin*
Rhinitis	Arrhythmia	Migraine?	Urticaria/angioedema
Asthmoid symptoms	Tachycardia	Psychological changes?	Atopic eczema?
Laryngeal edema	Hypo-/hypertension		Exanthema?
	Shock		Flush

Today we know that symptoms of food allergy can vary and affect virtually any organ of the body; at the same time, we are becoming aware of more and more substances which are capable of functioning as allergens (Tables 2, 3) [26].

Symptoms brought on by food allergy in the gastrointestinal tract are often difficult to distinguish from those of other acute diseases [3, 5, 30, 31]. The oral application of allergens can lead not only to symptoms affecting the gastrointestinal tract but also to generalized reactions with erythema, conjunctivitis, rhinitis, bronchospasm, and even anaphylactic reactions [3, 5, 8, 12, 13, 28]. Apart from true allergies, pseudo-allergic reactions must also be taken into

Table 4. Substances which induce pseudo-allergic food reactions

Substances with:	*Substances which induce direct histamine release*
– A high histamine content	Strawberries
Cheese	Tomatoes
Tuna	Chocolate
Sauerkraut	Fish
Cooked pork	Pineapple
Sausages	Alcohol
– A high content of serotonin	
Bananas	
– A high content of tyramine	
Cheese	
Fish (herring)	
Chianti	
Yeast	
– A high content of phenylethylamine	
Chocolate	

account (Table 4). In the case of pseudo-allergic reactions, one should look upon substances such as colorings, preservatives, salicylic acid, and biogenic amines, e.g., histamine and serotonin, as being responsible for immediate reactions in the gastrointestinal mucosa (Table 4) [19, 20].

There have always been difficulties in the diagnosis of food allergy. The relevance of positive skin test reactions often remains unclear, similar to in vitro diagnostic rests such as RAST or histamine release [1, 5, 7, 12, 15, 21 b, 29]. Oral provocation tests must be performed under placebo-controlled conditions in order to be reliable and carry the risk of potential life-threatening anaphylactoid episodes [12, 21 b]. We have therefore introduced a method which enables us to apply measurable quantities of allergens under direct vision to the surface of the gastrointestinal mucosa.

Patients and Methods

Ten patients (seven female, three male, age 19–47 years) suffering from food allergy were examined allergologically; their histories were taken, skin prick tests were performed on the lower forearm, and specific IgE antibodies were determined [1, 21 a]. Informed consent was obtained prior to endoscopy. To prove that a food allergic reaction was taking place at the level of the gastrointestinal mucosa, we developed a method whereby allergen provocation on the mucosal surface of the gastrointestinal tract was carried out under endoscopic control. We call this technique intragastric provocation under endoscopic control, or IPEC (Fig. 1). Under endoscopic control 10 ml of the allergen extract dilution or solvent as control was applied to the mucosal surface of the dorsal part of the corpus ventriculi. The macroscopic mucosal reaction was visually monitored by two observers and graded according to its intensity [21]. Tissue and plasma histamine levels were determined using the fluorometric technique according to Lorenz et al. [13].

All patients were thoroughly examined prior to the allergen provocation in order to ensure that they were not suffering from any gastrointestinal disease. Via an endoscope biopsies were taken from certain parts of the stomach mucosa for histological, biochemical, and histochemical analysis. Biopsies were taken both before and after allergen provocation. Histamine levels in plasma were measured in peripheral veins. The histological assessments were carried out blind in the pathological institute.

If not mentioned otherwise, mean values and standard error of the mean were determined. The statistical significance between differences was evaluated using the parameter-free Wilcoxon test.

Results

After allergenic provocation definite reactions of the mucosa were observed (Table 5). Four patients showed stomach reactions, eight showed strong re-

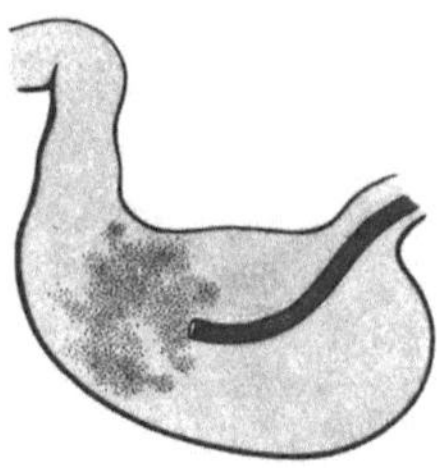

Fig. 1. Allergen provocation under endoscopic control (IPEC)

Table 5. Macroscopic reactions in the stomach and gut mucosa in ten patients with suspected food allergy who were provoked with their specific allergen

No.	Initials	Age	Allergen	Macroscopic reaction[a]	
				Stomach	Gut
1	P. M.	24	Celery	+	+ +
2	S. T.	27	Pork	+ +	+ +
3	H. K.	39	Milk	+	+ +
4	T. N.	20	Fish	+	+ +
5	G. M.	26	Tomatoes/Eggs	+ +	+
6	G. L.	33	Milk	+	+ +
7	J. D.	33	Eggs	+ +	+ +
8	A. D.	32	Fish	+	+ +
9	W. H.	24	Nuts	+ +	+
10	H. S.	36	Eggs	+	+ +

[a] Mucosal reactions were graded as follows: +, mild erythema (pink); + +, marked erythema plus swelling; + + +, dark red erythema plus petechial bleeding

Fig. 2. Macroscopic reaction after allergen provocation

actions in the small intestine, and two showed reactions in both. The following reactions were macroscopically observed after provocation: swelling (10), hemorrhagic lesions (10), and bleeding (5) (Fig. 2).

The microscopic reactions noted were mucosal edema, white cell infiltrations, hemorrhagic lesions, and bleeding.

In all patients tissue histamine was measured in biopsies. An increase in basic histamine levels was noted in all allergic patients, particularly in the stomach and even more so in the small intestine. After allergen provocation there was a noticeable decrease in tissue histamine concentrations in the gut (Fig. 3).

The number of mast cells, observed by way of the ortho-phthaldialdehyde (o-PD) method, correlated with the tissue histamine (Fig. 4), while the number of toluidine blue-stained mast cells remained constant.

After allergen provocation in the small intestine the plasma histamine concentration was measured in the peripheral venous blood. There was a significant increase in plasma histamine levels (Fig. 5). The levels returned to normal values approximately 30 min later. Two of the ten patients developed mild systemic symptoms (urticaria) which subsided spontaneously.

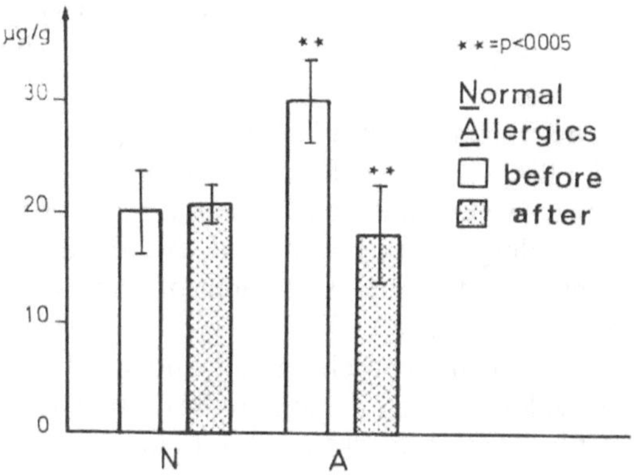

Fig. 3. Significant decrease in tissue histamine after allergen provocation

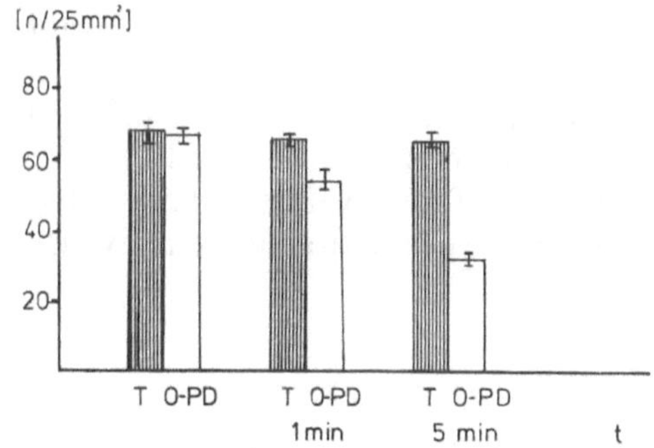

Fig. 4. Significant decrease in the count of o-PD treated mast cells. The number of toluidine blue-stained mast cells (*T*) remained constant

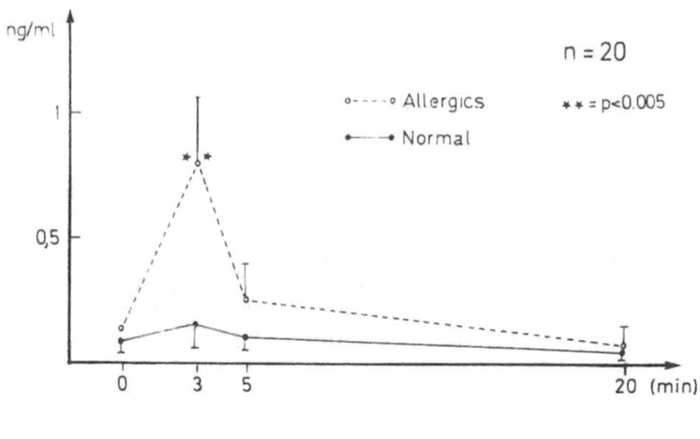

Fig. 5. Plasma histamine levels after provocation in the small intestine

Conclusions

The results show that patients suffering from food allergy have a significant increase in tissue histamine concentrations in their stomach. The reactions after provocation, such as swelling, hemorrhagic lesions, and even bleeding, can be explained by histamine liberation. Another histamine effect is disturbance of the permeability of the mucosa, so that allergens can pass into the blood stream, thus causing symptoms of food allergy in organs other than the gut (Table 3).

The introduction of IPEC could provide a new method in the diagnosis of food allergy [19] by offering the following possibilities:

- Objective evaluation of mucosal reactions after controlled provocation.
- The allergen can be applied to the surface of the mucosa under endoscopic control and direct assessment of local site of contact can be achieved by several observers.
- Histological, histochemical, and chemical analyses of biopsies taken from provoked as well as unprovoked areas is performed, allowing further investigations with regard to cellular changes and mediators released.
- By detection of immediate gross macroscopic changes a possible systemic reaction can be prevented.

There are, however, a number of disadvantages of IPEC:

- Stress for the patient.
- A certain personal and technical effort and a time requirement.
- Only few allergens can be tested.

IPEC will therefore never be suitable for screening purposes, but remains a possible tool in the evaluation of the relevance of other allergological test results.

References

1. Aas K (1978) The diagnosis of hypersensibility to ingested foods. Reliability of skin prick testing and the radioimmunosorbent test with different materials. Clin Allergy 8:39
2. Behrens RA (1735) Epistolica dissertatio pro spiceligo observationum de morbo maculoso haemorrhagico ex noxiis nonnullis mytulis perscripta. PhD dissertation, Braunschweig
3. Bleuminck E (1979) Food allergy and the gastrointestinal tract. In: Asquish P (ed) Immunology of the gastrointestinal tract. Churchill Livingstone, London
4. Brunton RA (1885) Lettsomian lectures on disorders of digestion: their consequences and treatment. Br Med J 1:163
5. Crook WG, Harrison WE, Crawford SE, Emerson BS (1961) Systemic manifestations due to allergy. Pediatrics 27:790
6. Cullen W (1789) A treatise of the materia medica, vol 1. Edinburgh, p 85
7. Gavani UD, Hyde JS, Moore BS (1971) Hypersensitivity to milk and egg white. Skin tests, RAST results and clinical intolerance. Ann Allergy 40:314
8. Hertod FM (1971) Panis antipathia. Misc Cur Dec 1, Ann 2, Obs 144, p 228
9. Hippocrates: Œuvres complètes d'Hippocrate. Hrsg. v. E. Littré. Paris 1839–1861. Hippokrates sämtliche Werke. Dtsch. Übers. v. R. Fuchs. München 1895–1900. Die Werke des Hippokrates. Stuttgart 1934–1938
10. Hutchinson J (1888) A case of summer eruption recurring with great severity for many years, but finally getting well (a form of Kaposi's disease). Clin Soc Trans 22:80
11. Laroche G, Richet C Jr, Saint-Girons F (1919) Anaphylaxie alimentaire. Paris
12. Lessoff MH, Wraith DG, Merrett TG, Merrett J, Buisseret PD (1980) Food allergy and intolerance in 100 patients – local and systemic effects. Q J Med 49:259
13. Lorenz W, Reimann H-J, Barth H, Kusche J, Meyer R, Doenicke A, Hutzel A, Hutzel M (1972) A sensitive and specific method for the determination of histamine in human whole blood and plasma. Hoppe-Seyler's Z Physiol Chem 353:911
14. Mackarness R (1979) The diagnosis and management of food allergy by dietary control and challenge. In: Pepys J, Edwards AM (eds) The mast cell. Pitman Medical, London, p 450

15. Merrett TG, Merrett J (1980) The RAST principle and the use of mixed allergen. RAST as screening test for IgE-mediated allergies. Methods Enzymol 70:276
16. Quincke HI (1882) Über akutes umschriebenes Hautoedem. Mh Prakt Derm 1:129
17. Parreidt FH (1835) Nonnulla de idiosyncrasiis. Dissertation, Halle
18. Planchon JB (1776) Extrait d'une lettré écrite de Tournay. Gaz Santé 30:117
19. Reimann HJ, Ring J, Wendt P, Lorenz R, Ultsch B, Swoboda K, Blümel G (1981) Der Histaminstoffwechsel des Magens bei Patienten mit Nahrungsmittelallergie. Verh Dtsch Ges Inn Med 87:823
20. Reimann HJ, Lewin J, Schmidt U (1984) Klinische Manifestation der Nahrungsmittelallergie außerhalb des Gastrointestinaltraktes. Allergologie 7 (8):295–299
21. Reimann HJ, Ring J, Ultsch B, Wendt P (1985) Intragastral provocation under endoscopic control (IPEC) in food allergy: mast cell and histamine changes in gastric mucosa. Clin Allergy 15:195–202
22. Salter HH (1890) On asthma: its pathology and treatment. London
23. Schloss OM (1920) Allergy in infants and children. Am J Dis Child 19:433
24. Schlossmann A, Moro E (1903) Zur Kenntnis der Arteigenheit der verschiedenen Eiweißkörper der Milch. Münch Med Wochenschr 14:397
25. Siebels H (1965) Diagnostische Methoden im Laboratorium und in der Röntgenologie bei allergischen Manifestationen am Magendarmtrakt. In: Letterer E, Gronemeyer W (eds) Allergie- und Immunitätsforschung I. Schattauer, Stuttgart, p 223
26. Soothill JF (1980) Food allergy. In: Pepys J (ed) The mast cell. Excerpta Medica, Amsterdam, p 367
27. Talbot FB (1916) Asthma in children. Its relation to anaphylaxis. Med Surg J 175:191
28. Werner M (1967) Krankheiten infolge peroraler Allergeninvasion (Allergische Manifestation der Verdauungsorgane). In: Hansen K (ed) Lehrbuch der klinischen Allergie. Thieme, Stuttgart
29. Wraith DG, Merrett J, Roth A et al. (1979) Recognition of food-allergic patients and their allergens by the RAST technique and clinical investigation. Clin Allergy 9:25
30. Zanussi C (1978) Allergenic potentials of food additives. In: Galli CL, Paoletti R, Vettorazzi G (eds) Chemical toxicology of food. Elsevier, Amsterdem, pp 271–285
31. Zanussi C (1982) Food allergy treatment. In: Brostoff J, Challacombe SJ (eds) Clinics in immunology and allergy, vol 2, part 1. Saunders, London, p 221

Allergy to Spices: Cross-reactivity to Other Allergens

C. Thiel[1], E. Fuchs[1], H.-J. Maasch[2], and R. Wahl[2]

[1] Stiftung Deutsche Klinik für Diagnostik, Fachbereich Allergologie, 6200 Wiesbaden, Federal Republic of Germany

[2] Firma Allergopharma, 2000 Hamburg, Federal Republic of Germany

Abstract

Since a few years we observed an increasing number of patients with rhinitis, asthma, urticaria and abdominal symptoms caused by allergens of plant origin like spices and some related vegetables.

A pilot study revealed a high incidence with pollen allergy – especially with a sensitization to herbs (mostly mugwort-pollen), more then with tree or grass pollen.

These results raised the question whether pollen-allergic individuals may have a special predisposition to acquire a sensitization to certain food-allergens – spices and related vegetables – if consumed more often as this happens nowadays regarding nutritional habits.

In a follow-up study a great number of spices and vegetables in patients with suspicion of food allergy have been investigated by skin test and again a high incidence of about 85% of sensitization in pollen-allergic individuals has been found compared with not pollen-allergic individuals, who only sometimes show a sensitization to spices (~ 15%).

Concerning these results we suggested possible cross-reacting allergens in both: pollen- and food-allergens as possible explanation for this phenomenon.

The presence of IgE antibodies could be demonstrated by Prausnitz-Küstner test and RAST for some spices in question.

By RAST-inhibition-test the presence of partly cross-reacting allergens, which are not yet identified, could be demonstrated for anis, celery and mixed spices (curry).

Analyzing more then 200 case histories including skin test and RAST a sensitization to the following spices and vegetables could be detected to be very frequent:

Camomile, soy, garlic, onion, celery, fennel, dill, coriander, caraway, mixed curry, parsley, peppermint, tomato, carrot and paprica beside some others of less importance.

The coincidence with a sensitization to herb-pollen was found to be about 70%.

Introduction

The incidence and clinical relevance of food allergies depend not only on the atopic state of the individual and the antigenic potency of food allergens but also on nutritional habits, which differ from continent to continent and from country to country. Wheat and peanut allergies, for example, seem to be of great importance in the United States while rye and hazelnut allergies occur more often in West Germany. On the other hand, the growth in international trade obviously influences nutritional habits and consequently the regional pattern and incidence of food allergies. These facts may explain some disagreements between allergists concerning statistics.

The following presentation will discuss developments in West Germany concerning allergies to spices, herbs, and vegetables, which seem to have been increasing recently for what we believe are special reasons.

Nutritional Habits in Germany

In order that the reader will understand the sense and results of our investigations and their possible relevance for the West German (and perhaps the broader European) population, some remarks are necessary on a new trend in nutritional habits. During and shortly after World War II food allergies were not regarded as of importance, a fact easily explained by the lack of various foodstuffs. The development of the economy, of supply and demand, and the increase in the import of foreign products have clearly influenced the nutritional habits of West German people, who have been converted into a population of consumers as regards the manifold foodstuffs and luxuries produced in Germany itself and imported from all over the world. More recently, fears of possible adverse effects of industrial treatment of foods has resulted in a new trend towards an "alternative way of living". Furthermore, there has been indoctrination towards some very curious eating habits, like the consumption of pure pollen grains, brews from various herbs, raw vegetables, etc.

As regards the medicinal value of herbs, German people have a long tradition in using camomile, anise, fennel, peppermint, coriander, and so on; in the past few years their use has undergone a renaissance in that extracts of plant origin are being used by people to treat bronchial asthma, rhinitis, bronchitis, gastrointestinal disorders, hepatic, gallbladder, and renal diseases, chronic eczema, etc. But spices, herbs, and vegetables are not only used for nutritional and medicinal purposes but also in cosmetics and alcoholic beverages, and for refining basic foodstuffs like breads, sweets, and cakes. The increase in the comsumption of spices and herbs is reflected by the increases in their import and production in West Germany from 1955 to 1983 (Fig. 1).

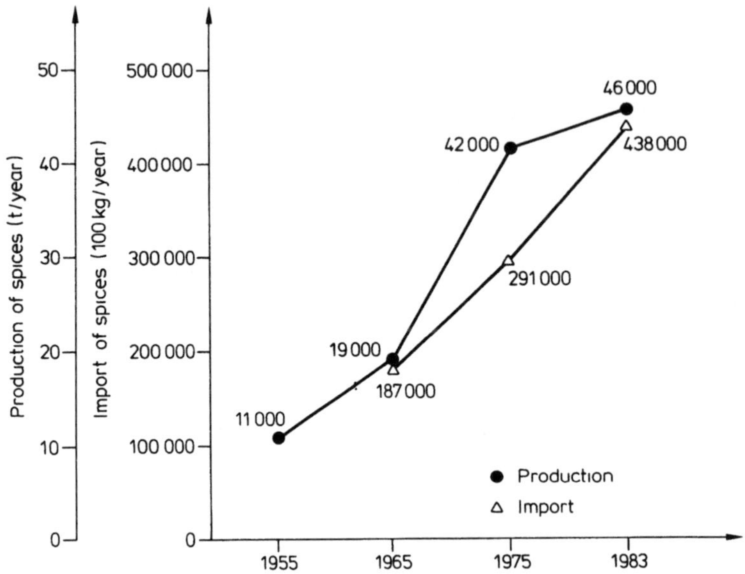

Fig. 1. Development of import (△) and production (●) of spices and herbs in West Germany between 1955 and 1983 (source: Statistisches Bundesamt)

Clinical Background

Since 1979 we have observed an increasing number of patients with sensitization to the pollen of herbs, especially of the artemisia group (mugwort and wermuth pollen), which in former times were only facultatively involved in hay fever. Apart from the typical symptoms of a seasonal hay fever, many patients have also suffered from perennial symptoms of the respiratory tract (which usually could not be referred to perennial allergens), gastrointestinal disorders, urticaria, Quincke's edema, and sometimes from life-threatening anaphylaxis induced by special meals, which gave us the impression that spices, herbs, and vegetables could be involved. Sensitization to these allergens was formerly regarded as of minor importance except in rare cases [3]. A possible relationship to a pollen allergy has not yet been taken into consideration. Hannuksela and co-workers reported in 1977 on positive skin tests with vegetables in patients with eczema [1], but the clinical relevance and specificity remained unclear. Positive skin tests to spices have mostly been regarded as an irritant effect.

In a pilot study published in 1981 [4] we were able to show in 50 patients a very close relation between sensitization to mugwort pollen and some herbs, spices, and vegetables by means of skin tests (Table 1). Most of the patients showed an almost equal pattern of positive skin tests with anise, celery, fennel, dill, coriander, caraway, parsley, carrot, and some other allergens of less importance.

Table 1. Results of skin prick, intradermal, and scratch tests with spices, herbs, and vegetables in 50 patients with sensitization to herb pollen

Allergen	Prick/intradermal (commercial extracts)	Scratch (natural material)
Anise	76%	
Celery	71%	
Fennel	64%	
Dill		64%
Coriander		63%
Caraway	62%	
Parsley		57%
Carrot		50%
Paprika	38%	
Chives		33%
Mustard	28%	
Pepper	26%	
Curcuma		19%

The results of this study, the increasing number of patients, follow up of nutritional habits, and further investigations posed a lot of questions and suggested some hypotheses:

- Spice and vegetable allergies are obviously often associated with sensitization to pollen of herbs – especially mugwort pollen, which seems to be a key allergen.
- Changing food habits, as mentioned above, seem to induce these allergies in pollen-allergic individuals but also sometimes in nonatopics; the allergens concerned are therefore autochthonous.
- The increase in sensitization may be due to the regular consumption of hot, exotic mixed spices and herbs which nowadays are used more and more by the food industry.
- Positive skin tests in pollen- and non-pollen-allergic individuals as well as negative skin tests in controls indicate a specific IgE-mediated reaction.
- Allergens involved do not necessarily need to stand in a botanical relationship to each other.

If these hypotheses are confirmed, allergen fractions in common or cross-reacting allergens could be postulated.

Materials, Methods, and Results

The Presence of IgE Antibodies

To confirm the presence of IgE antibodies we performed (in 1982) the Prausnitz-Küstner test using serum of a very highly sensitized patient who showed

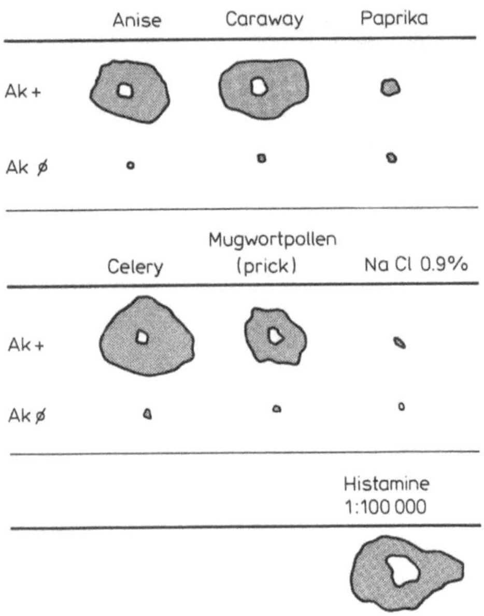

Fig. 2. Results of the Prausnitz-Küstner test with the serum of a patient highly sensitized to mugwort pollen (class 4). The presence of specific antibodies could be proven for anise, caraway, and celery (intradermal) and mugwort pollen (prick)

RAST class 4 with mugwort pollen and positive skin tests with 16 spices and herbs. We were able to demonstrate the presence of antibodies for anise, caraway, and celery (Fig. 2).

Skin Tests and RAST

In recent years we have been performing skin tests routinely both in pollen-allergic patients and also in those suspected of having a food allergy. For these tests we have used commercial extracts (Hollister-Stier, Allergopharma) and extracts from our own laboratory (Frugoni method). We have employed skin prick tests, intradermal tests, and the scratch test method with natural materials (Fig. 3). RAST was performed in cooperation with Kalveram and Forck in a pilot study of ten patients. Good RAST activities, as shown by the skin test results, were found for mugwort pollen (ten patients), wermuth pollen (nine patients), camomile (nine patients), and anise, caraway, and curry (seven patients) [5]. In single cases positive results were found for fennel, basil, paprika, and peppermint.

Figure 4 shows the latest results of skin tests and RAST concerning the frequency of sensitization to spices, herbs, and vegetables in 170 patients with sensitization to mugwort pollen.

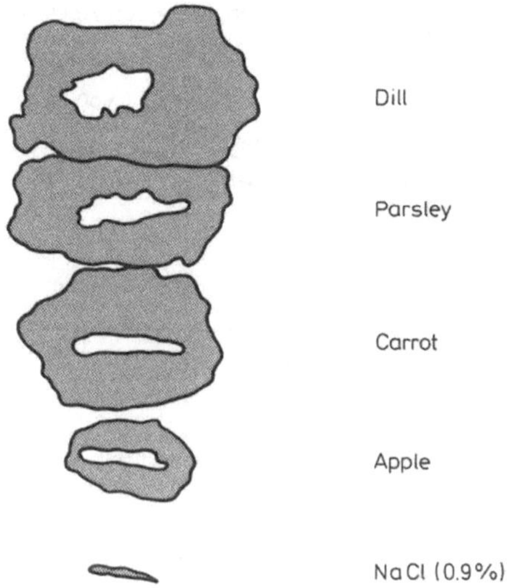

Fig. 3. Scratch test with natural materials

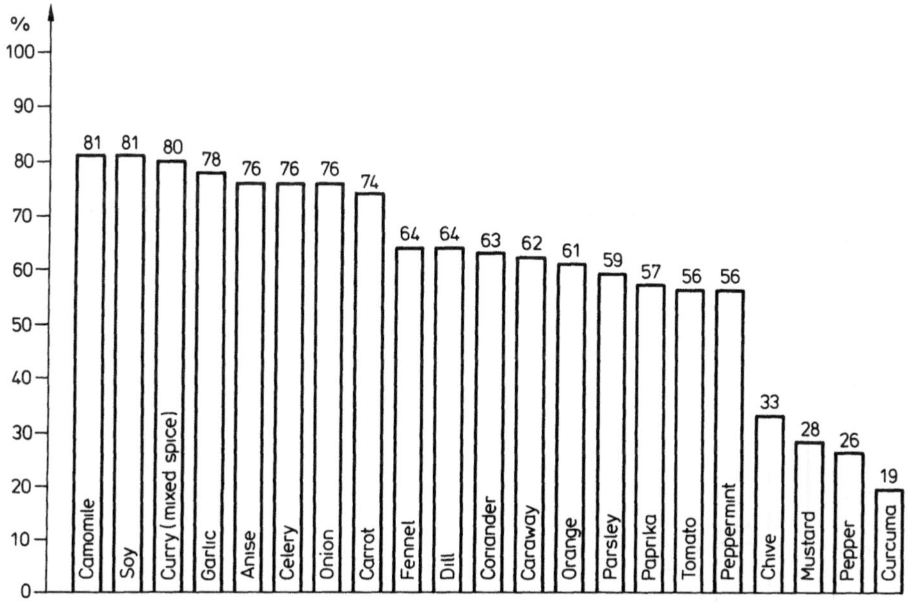

Fig. 4. Analysis of skin test and RAST results with spices, herbs, and vegetables in 170 patients with sensitization to mugwort pollen

RAST Inhibition Tests

In a pilot study RAST inhibition tests were performed in 1983 in cooperation with Kalveram and Forck to investigate the question of possible cross-reacting allergens in mugwort pollen and herb pollen. Figure 5 shows the results, which gave evidence of allergen fractions in common [5].

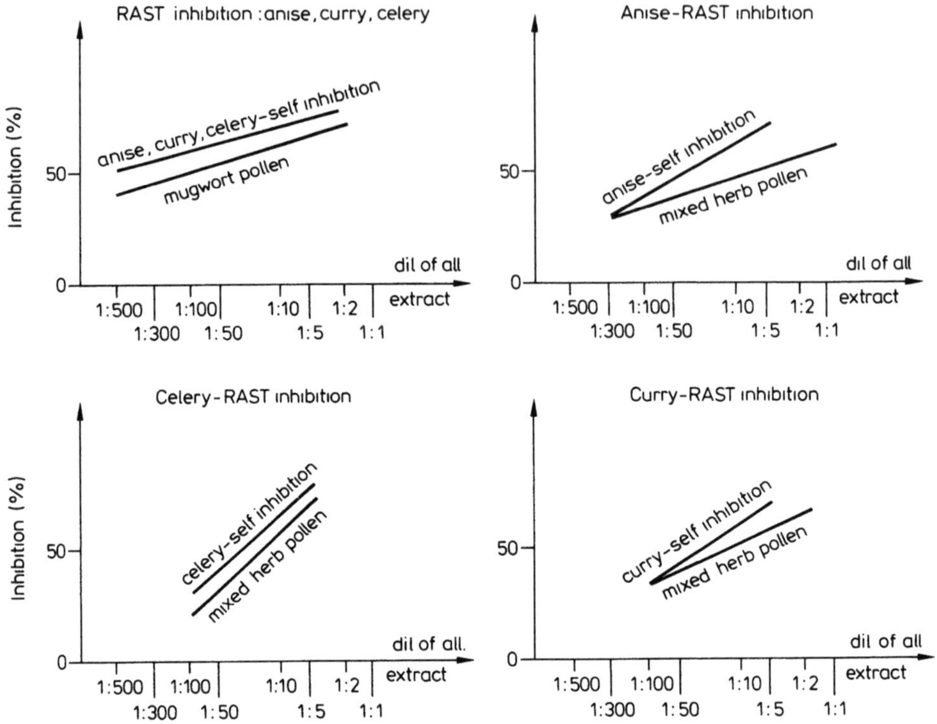

Fig. 5. Results of RAST inhibition and self-inhibition for anise, curry, celery, mugwort pollen, and mixed herb pollen extracts

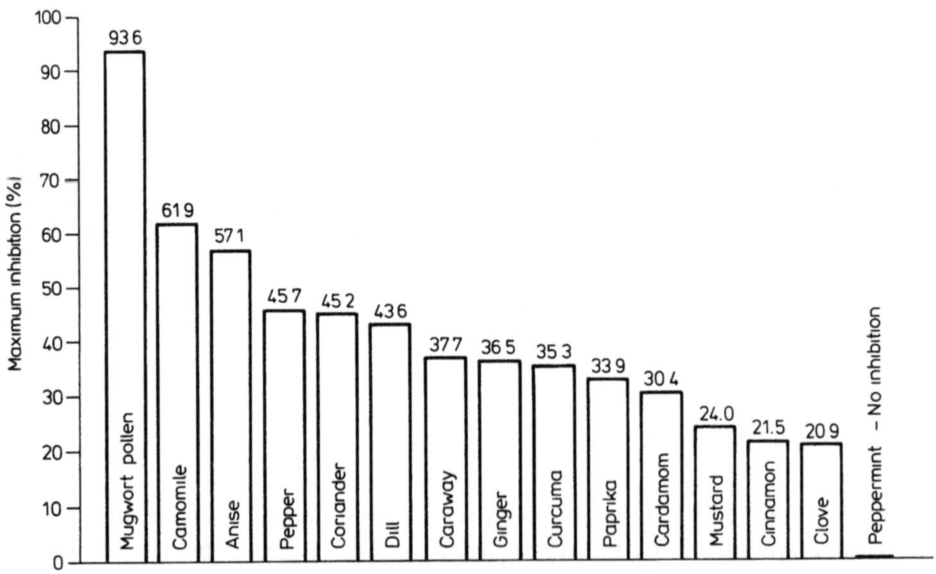

Fig. 6. Results of further RAST inhibition tests for mugwort pollen extract (no 10/116) and a number of herbs and spices

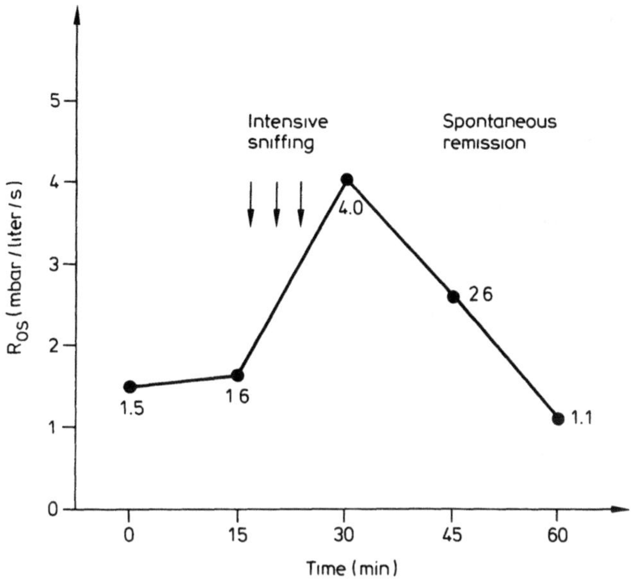

Fig. 7. Increase in nasal resistance and spontaneous remission following a snuff test with sand from bird cages containing anise. Resistance was measured by the oscillation method (Ros)

In 1985 further RAST inhibition tests were performed (Fig. 6) with some other allergens. The highest binding was found (in agreement with skin test results) for camomile and anise (over 50% inhibition). For other allergens we found an inhibition ranging from 45% to 29%. Both camomile and anise, but also pepper, coriander, dill, caraway, celery, and curry, are often used in the German kitchen. Camomile is used in a lot of cosmetics, in brews (beverages), and also for inhalation in cases of bronchitis.

Anise is used in cakes, sweets, bread, alcoholic beverages, and drugs. It is not only oral intake which has to be considered in the case of anise: it is also present in the sand used for bird cages and therefore also acts as an inhalant allergen (it is supposed that more than 50% of the German people have birds in their place of residence). Figure 7 shows the increase in nasal resistance following a snuff test with such sand.

Clinical Disease and Total IgE

Table 2 demonstrates the incidence of clinical symptoms in 121 patients. Total IgE is mostly elevated (above 500 kU/liter), and much higher than in uncomplicated pollen allergy. Allergen restriction by means of diet seems to influence levels of total IgE, if high. Figure 8 demonstrates rises (no diet) and falls (on diet) in some typical patients.

Table 2. Symptoms and total IgE (PRIST) in 121 patients with sensitization to artemisia species, spices, and vegetâbles

Symptoms	%		Total IgE range	Total IgE (mean)
Rhinitis	98.3	76% ($n = 92$)	18–8100 ($n = 87$)	837 kU/Liter
Conjunctivitis	78.5			
Bronchial asthma	61.15			
Urticaria and Quincke's edema	15.7	24% ($n = 29$)	13–1800 ($n = 26$)	569 kU/Liter
Gastrointestinal disorders	13.2			
Life-threatening anaphylaxis	3.3			
No respiratory symptoms	1.6			

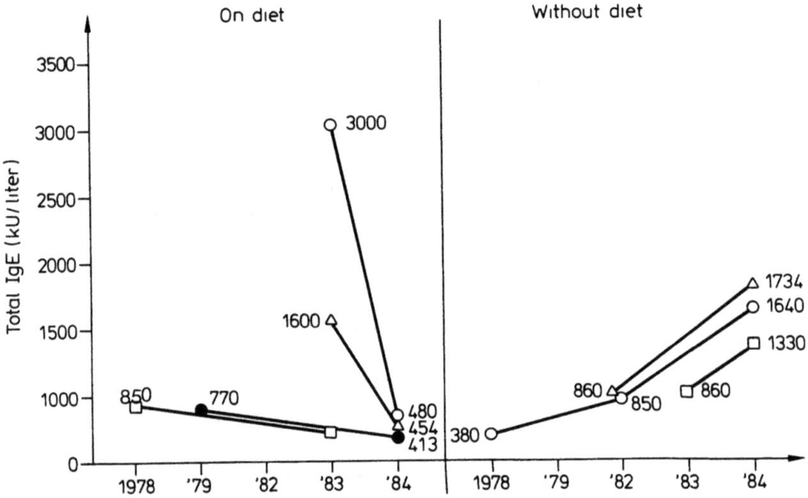

Fig. 8. Rise and fall in total IgE (PRIST) in patients sensitized to spices, herbs, vegetables, and mugwort pollen on a diet or without a diet

Age of Manifestation

Comparing the age of manifestation in 55 patients in 1981 and that in 121 unselected patients in 1984, there seems to be a trend toward younger people (Fig. 9).

Conclusions

There is no longer any doubt that food allergies to spices, herbs, and related vegetables in pollen-allergic individuals are increasing in West Germany, but obviously also in other European countries. Wüthrich and Hofer reported in 1984 [6] a "celery-mugwort-spice syndrome"; through personal communication

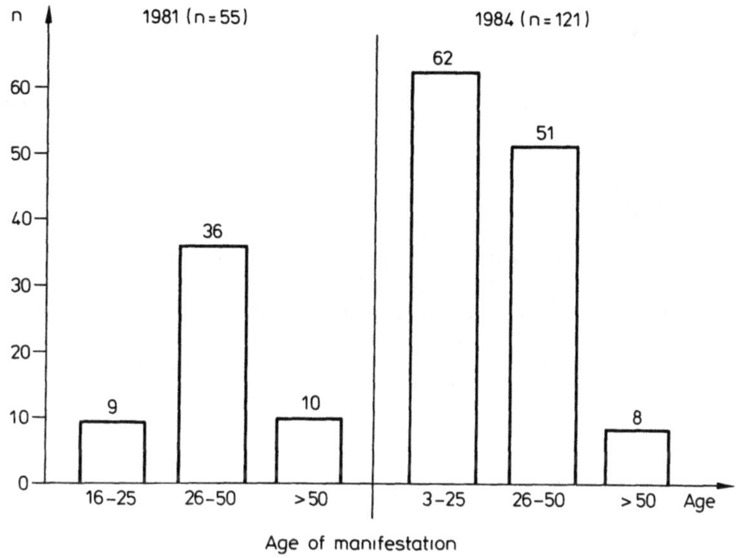

Fig. 9. Age of manifestation of sensitization to spices, herbs, and vegetables in 55 patients in 1981 comared with 121 patients in 1984

we have learned that there may be an increase in this syndrome in Italy and France.

Although the patterns of sensitization to spices, herbs, and vegetables may differ from country to country according to nutritional habits, there may well be a problem of common interest as regards the close relationship between sensitization to allergens of plant origin and pollen allergy.

Since 1980 we have seen more than 500 patients who are more or less sensitive to herbs, spices, and related vegetables and after a follow-up of 5 years we may offer some conclusions.

1. In case of sensitization to herb pollen a high incidence of spice and vegetable allergies can be expected. Mugwort pollen indeed seems a key allergen for detecting these patients. The specificity and presence of IgE antibodies for some allergens in question have been demonstrated by the Prausnitz-Küstner test, skin tests, and RAST.
2. RAST inhibition tests have proven that allergen fractions exist in common for spices, herbs, vegetables, *and* herb pollen.
3. The elimination of mixed and hot spices and industrial products ("ready meals") from the daily diet is usually followed by remission of several symptoms and also sometimes by a decrease in total IgE activity.

The studies are still ongoing, but no longer have the character of a pilot investigation.

The nature of the allergen fractions shared in common by pollen and food still remains unclear and should be investigated. Skin tests have been performed with aqueous extracts and there is no evidence of sensitization to sesquiterpenlactones (described by Hausen in 1979 [2]), which have been found to be responsible for contact allergies.

References

1. Hannuksela M, Lathi A (1977) Immediate reactions to fruits and vegetables. Contact Dermatitis 3:79
2. Hausen BM (1979) Kompositenallergie. Allergologie 4:143–147
3. Moneret DA, Grilliat JP (1980) Allergens alimentaires. In: Charpin J (ed) Allergologie. Flammarion, Paris, p 267
4. Thiel CL, Fuchs E (1981) Über korrelative Beziehungen bei Kräuterpollen- und Gewürzallergenen. 3. Kölner RAST-Symposium. Grosse, Berlin, pp 178–185
5. Thiel CL, Fuchs E, Kalveram KJ, Forck G (1984) Über korrelative Beziehungen bei Kräuterpollen- und Gewürzallergenen. Zweite Mitteilung. 4. Kölner RAST-Symposium 1983. Pharmacia 118–127
6. Wüthrich B, Hofer T (1984) Nahrungsmittelallergie: das Sellerie-Beifuß-Gewürz-Syndrom. Dtsch Med Wochenschr 109:981–986

*Glutamate-Induced Asthmatic Reactions**

D. H. Allen, J. Delohery, and G. Baker
Department of Thoracic Medicine, Royal North Shore Hospital, Sydney, Australia

Abstract

Ingested chemicals are becoming increasingly recognized as provokers of acute severe asthma. Aspirin, tartrazine and the common preservative, metabisulfite, have been recognized for some years. Provocation of asthma by monosodium L-glutamate (MSG), a widely used flavour enhancer, was first reported by our group in 1981. This report describes challenge studies with MSG in 32 asthmatic patients, a number of whom had experienced severe asthma following chinese restaurant meals. The patients received an additive-free diet for 5 days prior to challenge and were challenged in hospital after an overnight fast, with capsules of MSG. They were challenged in a single-blind, placebo-controlled fashion with increasing doses of MSG from 0.5 g to 5 g. Twelve patients reacted and they fell into two groups. Group 1 consisted of 6 patients who developed asthma and symptoms of the Chinese Restaurant Syndrome 1–2 hours after ingestion of MSG. Group 2 patients did not develop symptoms of Chinese Restaurant Syndrome and their asthma was delayed 6–12 hours after ingestion of MSG. These challenge studies confirm that MSG can provoke asthma. The reaction to MSG is dose dependent and may be delayed up to 12 hours, making recognition difficult for both patient and physician.

Introduction

Monosodium glutamate (MSG) is the sodium salt of glutamic acid, a nonessential amino acid that forms 20% of dietary protein. MSG is also present in our diet, most of it being artificially added to enhance the flavour of foods. The average daily intake in western countries is estimated to be 0.3–1 g, but as much as 4–6 g may be ingested in a highly seasoned restaurant meal. Considerable evi-

* A full report of the studies referred to in this review paper has been submitted for publication to the Journal of Allergy and Clinical Immunology

dence exists that MSG, as an additive in food, can indeed cause symptoms [1–3]. In man added MSG is reported to cause epileptic-like shudder attacks in children [4] and the Chinese restaurant syndrome (CRS) [5]. This syndrome, occurring within hours of a Chinese restaurant meal (CRM), is characterized by headache, a burning sensation along the back of the neck, chest tightness, nausea, and sweating.

In its L-isomer form MSG participates in a number of important metabolic and neurologic functions in man and animals [6]. In contrast to its numerous and important endogenous properties, dietary glutamate has only one useful role in man, namely flavour enhancement. In excess of 20000 tons of MSG are manufactured and consumed in the U.S.A. each year. In Australia MSG is regarded as a food ingredient, the addition of which to foods is completely unrestricted, both in the food manufacture and in restaurant industries. In contrast the addition of chemicals regarded as "additives" to foods is closely controlled by laws in all states. MSG was first added to western diets in significant amounts in the 1950s and with the increasing consumption of added MSG there have been a number of reports of adverse effects in humans. However, until our report [7] of asthma provoked by MSG these adverse effects have mainly been in the form of symptoms rather than a measurable effect. It is this lack of any measurable adverse effect that has led the U.S. Food and Drug Administration to classify MSG as "GRAS" or "generally regarded as safe."

The best documented adverse effect of ingested MSG is the Chinese restaurant syndrome, described by Kwok [5] in 1968. Shaumburg et al. [3] showed that the burning sensation was due to a peripheral neuroexcitatory effect by injecting L-glutamic acid into the forearm with the circulation occluded by a cuff. The burning sensation was localized only to the arm until the cuff was removed, when the sensation spread to the upper body and face, which are highly vascular areas.

Ingested chemicals are increasingly recognized as provokers of acute, severe asthma. The asthma-provoking potential of aspirin was first reported more than 60 years ago by Dr. Robert Cooke [8], but it was not until 1959 that an adverse reaction to a food additive was reported by Lockey [9]. He described urticaria in a patient receiving a steroid formulation containing the yellow dye, tartrazine. More recently, the common preservative metabisulfite has been shown to be an important ingested provoker of asthma by ourselves [10] and Stevenson and Simon [11]. Provocation of asthma by MSG was reported by Allen and Baker in 1981 in two patients in a letter to the editor of the New England Journal of Medicine [7]. This report reviews our experience with MSG challenges in asthmatic patients and describes preliminary studies designed to elucidate the mechanism of MSG-induced asthma.

Typical Clinical Histories of CRM-Induced Asthma

Late Reaction

Patient J. W., a 23-year-old registered nurse, with previously documented sensitivities to ingested metabisulfite, tartrazine, benzoic acid, and aspirin, presented to the emergency department at 8 a.m., 11 – 12 h after ingestion of a 15-course Chinese banquet, with Won Ton soup as the first course. On waking the following morning she rapidly developed severe asthma, unresponsive to her usual inhaled bronchodilatators. On arrival at hospital aggressive treatment was begun. Over the next 3 h her asthma increased in severity and a persistent, inappropriate bradycardia was noted. At 11 a.m., 3 h after presentation to the emergency department, she was intubated and mechanical ventilation was instituted. Her bradycardia persisted and blood pressure began to fall despite usual supportive measures. At 12.15 p.m. partial cardiopulmonary bypass was instituted for 5 h until her blood pressure recovered and asthma was improving. She was extubated 24 h later. Six weeks later she had a further small CRM and experienced asthma the following morning.

Patient V. H. was a 42-year-old asthmatic who had unstable asthma but had not observed provocation of her asthma by ingested foods or beverages. Her asthma was difficult to control with corticosteroids and bronchodilators with peak expiratory flow rates (PEFRs) varying between 150 and 300. In order to exclude provocation of her asthma by ingested chemicals or foods, she was placed on a general exclusion diet. Improvement in her PEFRs occurred over a period of 3 – 4 days on the diet. She found the diet very restrictive and broke it one evening to have a CRM. The following morning she had an asthma attack with PEFRs falling to levels similar to those recorded prior to the diet.

Early Reaction

Patient E. G., a 39-year-old female, developed symptoms of CRS shortly after a multicourse Chinese banquet, which included soup. In particular, she recalled a feeling of warmth over the head, together with chest tightness, nausea, and later headache. Shortly after the onset of these symptoms she developed severe asthma, which rapidly progressed to a respiratory arrest requiring resuscitation by paramedics. She was subsequently challenged at her local hospital with each course of the provoking meal on a separate day. When no adverse reaction was observed she was referred for ingested chemical provocation studies.

Challenge Details

Criteria for selection for MSG challenge studies were as follows: (a) a history of asthma occurring within 24 h of a CRM, or (b) unstable asthma usually with sudden, severe, unexplained attacks, or (c) a history suggestive of another ingested chemical sensitivity.

Patients were begun on a general exclusion diet at least 5 days prior to challenge. This diet excludes chemicals known to provoke asthma. Patients were challenged in a single-blind, placebo-controlled dose-response fashion. Capsules containing 1.5 – 2.5 g MSG were shown in a preliminary study to produce similar blood glutamate levels to a CRM containing 5 – 10 g of added MSG. The MSG challenges were randomized with other ingested chemical challenges.

Prior to challenge each subject was allocated to one of four groups; mild, moderate, severe, and very severe. Allocation was determined by two main factors, first the degree of severity of the underlying asthma and second the severity of any previous CRM- or MSG-induced reactions. Patients were allocated in this way in order to determine challenge doses. Challenges were performed with 500 mg capsules of MSG after an overnight fast. Each patient was observed closely and PEFRs recorded hourly for 14 h after each challenge. One dose was administered on each day. A challenge was regarded as positive if there was both a greater than 20% fall in PEFR from baseline of the challenge day and if the lowest recorded PEFR was 20% less than the lowest flow rate recorded on the control day. In view of the possibility of delayed reactions only one dose was administered on each day. Doubtful reactions were confirmed by rechallenge.

Results

Results of the challenge studies of all 32 patients are summarized in Table 1. Of the 32 patients challenged with MSG, 13 had a positive challenge. Eight of these 13 patients gave a history of asthma following CRMs or other similarly spiced meals. In seven subjects asthma developed within a few hours, usually 1 – 2, of ingesting MSG and was accompanied by symptoms of the CRS. In the remaining six patients asthma was delayed many hours, even up to 12, after ingestion of the MSG. Associated symptoms in this group were variable and included nausea and abdominal pain. Two patients (29 and 31) with histories of asthma following CRMs failed to react to MSG.

Figure 1 illustrates typical early asthmatic reactions to MSG challenge of patient E. G. This subject was challenged with 0.5 g, 1.5 g, and 2,5 g on separate days. A clear dose-response effect can be seen.

Table 1. Summary of CRM-induced asthma and results of subsequent MSG challenge in 32 asthmatic patients

	CRM-induced asthma		MSG challenge dose to induce asthma		
	+ CRS	− CRS	0.5 g	1.5 g	2.5 g
Early (< 6 h) reactions to MSG (7 subjects)	3	4		2	5
Late (> 6 h) reactions to MSG (6 subjects)		6			6
Nonreactors to MSG	1	1			0

Abbreviations: + CRS, with Chinese restaurant syndrome; − CRS, without Chinese restaurant syndrome; MSG, Monosodium L-glutamate

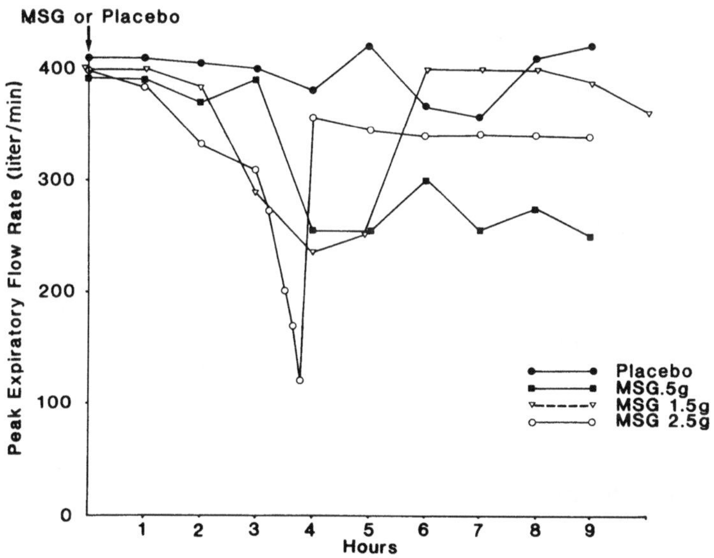

Fig. 1. Typical early asthmatic reactions to challenge with MSG of patient E.G. compared with lactose placebo challenge. The subject was challenged with 0.5, 1.5, and 2.5 g of MSG on separate days

Further Studies of the Mechanism of MSG-Induced Asthma

Inhaled Glutamic Acid Studies

In order to test the hypothesis that early MSG reactions are due to a neuro-hypersensitivity in the lung to circulating L-glutamic acid (L-glu), inhalation challenge studies were performed and compared with a standard histamine reactivity test. Early reactors were as sensitive on a molar basis to inhaled L-glu as they were to histamine, whereas late reactors and non-glutamate-sensitive asthmatics reacted minimally to inhaled glutamic acid.

Blood Level Studies

There is a normal circulating blood glutamic acid level in man and animal. In man the normal range for blood glutamic acid is 5.4–7.6 mg/100 ml. On a normal diet without large boluses of free glutamic acid this plasma or blood level remains fairly constant. Ingestion of capsules containing MSG has shown:

1. Doses of 2.5 g elevate the plasma level to upper normal range.
2. Doses of 5 g produce peak blood levels 2–3 times the upper normal range and occurring 1–2 h after ingestion of capsules of MSG (coinciding with the early asthmatic reaction and the symptoms of CRS).
3. Prolonged elevation of blood glutamate (for up to 12 h) in some subjects after ingestion of capsules containing 5.0 g monosodium glutamate, probably due to saturation of the metabolic pathways by this dose.

Metabolic Studies

Erythrocyte glutamic oxaloacetic transferase (EGOT levels) were measured in sensitive subjects in order to exclude impaired metabolism as a contributing factor. All subjects measured had normal EGOT levels.

Discussion

This study suggests that MSG is an important cause of asthma following CRMs as 11 of the 13 subjects who reported asthma following such a meal reacted to challenge with MSG. The MSG-induced asthmatic reaction was dose dependent and delayed for up to 12 h in some subjects, making recognition difficult for both patient and physician. In addition, the asthmatic reactions were similar in onset and associated symptoms to the CRM-induced reactions.

A number of factors were considered when designing the protocol for MSG challenges, including the form in which MSG was to be administered, the dose, and the timing of each dose. MSG was administered in capsule form in order to blind patients to its very characteristic salty, savory taste. A dosage schedule commencing at 0.5 g, with subsequent doses of 1.5 g, 2.5 g to a maximum of 5 g was employed. Six of our 13 MSG-sensitive patients experienced reactions delayed more than 6 h, and even up to 14 h, after ingestion of MSG; thus a single daily dose of MSG is recommended.

The development of asthma in close association with the onset of symptoms of the CRS suggests a peripheral neuroexcitatory effect e.g., stimulation of irritant receptors in the lung, leading to reflex bronchoconstriction. The inhaled glutamic acid studies indicate that the airways of MSG-sensitive subjects are hyperreactive to inhaled glutamate when compared with nonreactors. The delayed asthmatic reaction observed in several patients was not associated with other neuroexcitatory symptoms. In view of MSG's well known central effects, including the fact that it has recently been shown to be a central nervous system transmitter of baroreceptor afferents [12], a possible explanation for these delayed asthmatic reactions would be a central augmentation of reflex activity to the lung. Further studies will be required to elucidate the mechanism of MSG-induced asthma.

Patients sensitive to MSG need to know not only which foods contain MSG but also the amounts contained in a particular food or meal as it is meals containing 5 – 10 g MSG that are likely to provoke severe asthma. At present it is difficult, if not impossible, for patients to obtain information on the amount of glutamate contained in a particular food because of its unrestricted addition in large amounts to both manufactured and restaurant foods. If our results are confirmed by other groups then there will be an urgent need for the food and drug administration to review monosodium glutamate's "generally regarded as safe" listing. This study suggests that MSG is not safe for some individuals.

Acknowledgments. The writers thank Lyn Scott, Rhonda Williams, and Rae Allen for secretarial and editorial assistance.

References

1. Reif-Lehrer L (1977) Possible significance of adverse reactions to glutamate in humans. Fed Proc 36:1617
2. Kenny RA, Tidball CS (1972) Human susceptibility to oral monosodium L-glutamate. Am J Clin Nutr 25:140
3. Schaumburg HH, Byck R, Gerstl R, Marshman JH (1969) Monosodium L-glutamate: its pharmacology and role in the Chinese-restaurant syndrome. Science 163:826
4. Reif-Lehrer L (1976) A search for children with possible MSG intolerance. Pediatrics 58:771 – 772
5. Kwok RHM (1968) Chinese-restaurant syndrome. N Eng J Med 278:796
6. Olney JW, Ho O (1970) Brain damage in infant mice following oral intake of glutamate, aspartate or cysteine. Nature 227:609 – 610
7. Allen DH, Baker GJ (1981) Chinese-restaurant asthma. N Eng J Med 278:796
8. Cooke RA (1919) Allergy in drug idiosyncrasy. JAMA 73:759
9. Lockey SD (1959) Allergic reactions due to FD and C. Yellow number 5, tartrazine, an aniline dye use as a coloring and identifying agent in various steroids. Ann Allerg 17:719
10. Delohery J, Simmul R, Castle WD, Allen DH (1984) The relationship of ingested metabisulfite reactivity to inhaled SO_2 sensitivity in asthmatic subjects. Am Rev Respir Dis 130:1027 – 1032
11. Stevenson DD, Simon RA (1981) Sensitivity to ingested metabisulfite in asthmatic subjects. J Allergy Clin Immunol 68:26
12. Reis DJ, Granata AR, Perrone MH, Talman WT (1981) Evidence that glutamic acid is the neurotransmitter of baroreceptor afferents terminating in the nucleus tractus sobilarius (NTS). J Autonom Nerv Sys 3:321 – 324

Asthma

Late Phase Reactions

W. Dorsch and J. Ring
Kinderpoliklinik and Dermatologische Klinik der Ludwig-Maximilians-Universität München, 8000 Munich 2, Federal Republic of Germany

Abstract

Late phase reactions (LPR) have been considered generally as Arthus phenomenon (type III allergy according to Coombs and Gell). IgE-antibodies, however, are able to initiate not only immediate (WFR), but also late cutaneous reactions (LCR). Using the skin blister technique we could show LCR to be mediated by inflammatory mediators generated during the preceeding WFR. Histamine, active kallikrein, leukotrienes, thromboxanes and platelet activating property were demonstrable in dual skin reactions. The concentration of these mediators in skin blister fluid was in part related to the time course of skin reactions. LCRs were diminished by eicosatetraynoic acid (not by indomethacin), by dazoxiben (thromboxane synthetase inhibitor) as well as by ethanolic onion extract. Betamimetics as salbutamol and anticholinergics as ipratropium-bromide could reverse late bronchial reactions (LBR), besides disodium cromoglicicum and ethanolic onion extract could prevent LBR. Other authors found prostaglandin D_2 and chemotactic substances during LPRs as well as protective effects of corticosteroids, combined histamine-H_1/H_2 receptor antagonists and tranexamic acid.

Two types of LPR have to be distinguished: type I and type III. The first is initiated by an IgE-dependent mast cell degranulation and maintained by a complex interaction of mediators and cells. It may represent a laboratory model of long lasting asthmatic conditions.

History

Late phase reactions (LPRs) have been observed since the dawn of clinical allergology: In 1873 Blackley [13], who was, like many allergists, himself atopic (he suffered from hay fever), experienced nasal and bronchial discomfort lasting from several hours to 2–4 days after handling pollens. In 1921 Prausnitz and Küstner [104] undertook their famous "studies on hypersensitivity" and discovered the transferability by serum not only of immediate wheal and flare reactions (WFRs), but also of late cutaneous reactions (LCRs). LPRs were also observed by Cooke [23]. In 1952, Herxheimer [63] stressed the clinical importance of late bronchial reactions (LBRs), since this reaction pattern can be observed predominantly in patients with chronic bronchial asthma.

The pathogenesis of LPR was of minor interest until 1968, when Pepys and co-workers [99, 131] observed in patients with bronchopulmonary aspergillosis a close relationship between LCRs and/or LBRs on the one hand and serum precipitins against aspergilli on the other. In skin biopsies they found typical signs of an Arthus reaction: deposits of IgG, IgM, and C_3 as well as infiltrating neutrophil leukocytes. They concluded that LPRs generally represent a type III reaction according to the classification of Gell and Coombs [54]. Doubts regarding this pathogenetic concept arose when Booij-Noord et al. [14] noted in 1971 that there are two types of LBR: LBRs after inhalation of house dust differ distinctly from exogenous allergic alveolitis (= hypersensitivity pneumonitis EAA) by virtue of the lack of fever, leukocytosis, and pulmonary infiltrates. This "late bronchial obstruction" (LBO) was reversed by corticosteroids (similar to EAA) and prevented by disodium cromoglycate (in contrast to EAA).

In the following years (1973–1976), Dolovich et al. [27, 28], Solley et al. [123], de Shazo et al. [117], and Atkins et al. [6] were able to show LCR to be mediated by IgE antibodies. A great number of investigations now focus on the pathogenesis of LPRs and their pharmacological modulation. The central role of mast cell degranulation is generally accepted, while the importance of proinflammatory mediators – including chemotactic factors – and the role of infiltrating cells are subjects of controversy.

Definitions

The term "late phase reaction" describes the time course of an inflammatory response. It lasts longer than the immediate reaction, usually peaks between the 4th and 8th hour after allergen challenge, and subsides within 12–48 h. This definition ("an inflammatory response lasting 2 h to 2 days") abrogates consciously all pathophysiological interpretations because different mechanisms seem to be involved in the pathogenesis of LPR, some acting in combination.

Late Cutaneous Reaction

The intracutaneous injection of an antigen into the skin of sensitive individuals first provokes an immediate reaction: the wheal is sharply distinct from the surrounding flare (which is caused by an axon reflex [21]). Usually this WFR subsides within 90 min. Great wheals (more than 15 mm in diameter) enlarge continually. After 1 h the border of the wheal becomes less distinct and merges with the flare zone. During the next 2–3 h the lesion remains more or less unchanged. Thereafter a second phase of the reaction starts with mild pruritus. Depending on its intensity, the peak of the inflammatory reaction is reached between the 6th and the 12th hour. The fully developed LCR is characterized by edema, erythema, pruritus, tenderness, hyperalgesia, and hyperthermia. The site of the LCR is much more extensive than the preceding WFR, its border less well defined. In some cases a "target lesion" similar to that seen in erythema multiforme may be observed. Thereafter the LCR subsides within hours – first the subjective complaints, then the erythema and edema. In rare cases residual petechiae persist for days [6, 27–29, 39, 57, 104, 117, 118, 123].

Late Nasal Reaction

Late phase reactions of the nose follow a time course similar to LCRs: The immediate reaction is characterized by itching, sneezing, rhinorrhea, and nasal congestion. These symptoms subside within 1 h and peak again 4–12 h later. During late nasal reactions (LNRs) itching and sneezing are less pronounced than nasal congestion. The obstruction of nasal airways can be estimated quantitatively by rhinomanometry [44, 66, 97, 109].

Late Bronchial Reaction

The immediate bronchial reaction peaks 15–20 min after allergen inhalation. After incomplete or complete recovery the airway resistance again increases, reaching a maximum between the 4th and 10th hour. In contrast to the immediate reaction, LBO is manifested predominantly in peripheral areas of the lung. Clinical symptoms and lung function studies make possible easy differentiation of LBO from EAA [14, 34, 110]. LBO must also be distinguished from changes in bronchial tonus due to circadian rhythm [55]. The pathogenesis of LBO will be outlined later; for EAA see reviews from other authors, e.g., Reed [108].

Frequency of Late Phase Reactions

Nearly all common antigens causing immediate reactions in sensitive individuals can initiate dual responses too, i.e., the combination of immediate and late phase reactions. The frequency varies from author to author and from antigen to antigen between 40% and 80%. LBO is ovserved most frequently after house dust or house dust mite inhalation challenges. There is great interindividual variance in the ratio between the intensity of immediate and late bronchial responses [34, 137]. In routine skin (prick) testing LCRs will seldom be observed, probably owing to the low antigen doses used (wheals with 8 mm or less in diameter are seldom follwed by LCRs [27]). Increasing the allergen dose injected leads to wheals greater than 15 mm in diameter and causes LCRs in more than 90% [34, 120, 123]. As in the lung, there is no close relationship between the intensity of immediate and late reactions in the skin [34]. Depending on the sensitivity of the rhinomanometric method used, LNRs are observed in 3% – 50% of positive nasal allergen challenges [45, 109].

Pathogenesis of LCRs

It is generally assumed that bronchial, nasal, and cutaneous LPRs are caused by similar or identical pathomechanisms. This hypothesis has not been proven in all its details. However, it can be stated that studies of LCRs yield valuable insights into the pathogenesis of LBO.

Trigger Mechanisms

Virtually all antigens capable of inducing WFRs can cause LCRs too. In most cases, but not all, the reaction is mediated by IgE antibodies. Besides specific immunological mechanisms there are nonspecific direct mast cell activating pathways for inducing an LPR.

IgE

After the injection of anti-human IgE antibodies ("reverse anaphylaxis") mast cell degranulation occurs in the skin of atopics and nonatopics, followed by WFR and LCR [27]. The Fc part of anti-IgE, which could fix complement and initiate an Arthus-like reaction [64, 65], is not responsible since the same phenomena are observed when only $F(ab)_2$ fragments of anti-IgE are used. Allergen-dependent LCRs as well as WFRs can be passively transferred with the serum of atopics into the skin of nonatopics human beings and primates [32, 95, 104]. Destruction of the heat-labile IgE antibodies by heating the serum (56 °C, 4 h) abolished LCR and WFR in the host. Similarly, extraction of IgE from the graft serum by means of an anti-IgE immunoabsorbent abolishes the host's LCR and WFR after allergen testing. Finally, if the host's IgE receptors are well occupied by myeloma IgE, serum from atopics can no longer sensitize this skin area to WFR or LCR after allergen injection [123].

IgE-Independent Mechanisms

Late cutaneous reactions occur after intracutaneous testing with anti-IgG antibodies, anaphylatoxins, and *Staphylococcus aureus* protein A [126], too. All agents are capable of activating mast cells: anaphylatoxins act directly, protein A and anti-IgG indirectly, e.g., by complement activation and generation of anaphylatoxins [22, 68]. It has to be kept in mind that IgG antibodies can initiate immediate reactions as well [18].

Mast Cell-Derived Mediators

Late cutaneous reactions are often observed after the injection of compound 48/80 [29, 123, 126], a direct mast cell degranulator [96]. In rodents isolated mast cell granules have been shown to induce LCRs [66, 72, 73, 92, 93].

Exudate from Human Skin

Using the skin blister method [12, 39] interstitial fluid from allergen-tested skin was collected at various times after antigen challenge. Reinjection of this fluid caused LCRs similar to those observed after allergen injection (Fig. 1). Possible antigen transfer from one skin site to the other was excluded: as shown in the passive cutaneous anaphylaxis in *Macaca fasciolaris*, there was no detectable antigen contamination of skin blister fluids. These fluids were also free of cellu-

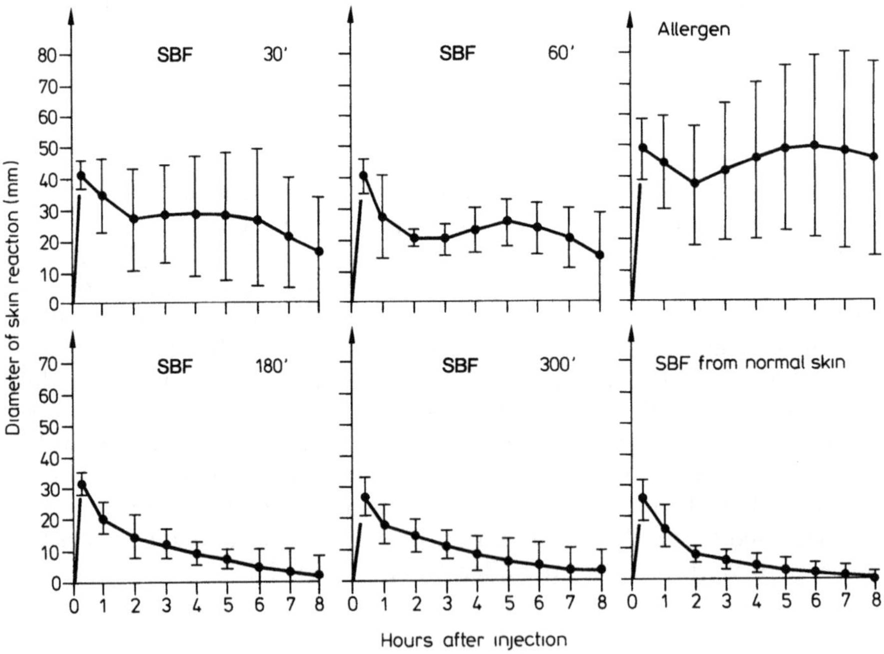

Fig. 1. Induction of late cutaneous reactions by skin blister fluid (SBF). SBF was drawn from allergen-tested skin at different times (30, 60, 180, and 300 min) after antigen injection. 50 µl SBF was reinjected. Diameters of skin reactions were followed up. (Modified from Dorsch and Ring [39])

lar elements. It was concluded that LCRs are caused by soluble mediators generated or released during the early phase of dual skin reactions [39]. When suction blisters were induced over normal skin, higher amounts (250 µl instead of 50 µl after allergen testing) of this skin blister fluid provoked LCRs after intracutaneous injection, too. The intensity and extent of these LCRs, however, were much less pronounced. This observation demonstrates that the exudation of plasma itself – as caused artificially by the generation of skin blisters and naturally during inflammation – generates mediators capable of inducing LCRs [39].

Role of Mediators

Various methods [12, 39, 45, 85, 128] have been used in order to demonstrate the release or generation of inflammatory mediators in the skin during allergic reactions. The suction blister method yields high amounts of mediators, but also causes a slight irritation of the skin [39].

Histamine

Histamine is released from mast cells and circulating basophil leukocytes [8]. In the skin, histamine release was demonstrated during the immediate reaction [45]. Using the skin blister technique [41], a second wave of histamine release from mast cells and/or infiltrating basophil leukocytes during LCR was demonstrable only in a few cases (without correlation to the intensity of the LCR). The skin chamber technique [128] showed histamine release prolonged for up to 4 h in LCR. There was a close interrelationship between the amount of histamine and the intensity of LCR; control studies in isolated WFR, however, were not performed.

The injection of histamine never causes LCRs in normal or atopic persons; however, such reactions have been observed in patients with acute urticaria [65]. Even the combination of allergen and histamine in order to augment WFR to an extent usually follwed by LCR did not alter the frequency of LCR [119]. Antihistamines, both of the histamine H_1- and the histamine H_2-receptor type, did not affect LCR when administered alone; their combination, however, totally abolished it (Fig. 2) [22]. The underlying mechanism is not clear. Interestingly, guinea pigs can be protected against allergen-induced bronchial asthma more effectively by combined H_1-H_2 antagonists than by H_1-blockers alone (see below) [38, 44].

Prostaglandin D_2

Mast cells [75], but not basophil leukocytes, generate prostaglandin D_2 (PGD_2). Maximal concentrations were observed in the skin 2 h after allergen challenge

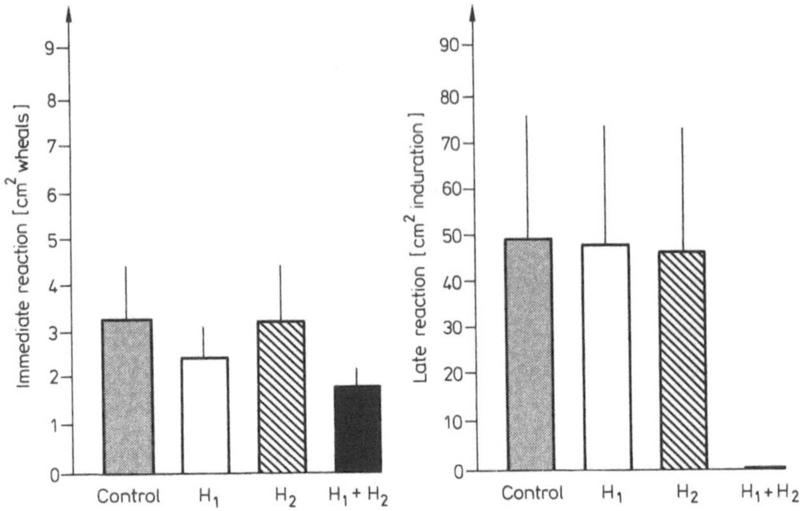

Fig. 2. Antihistamine effects on LCR. Oral pretreatment of eight patients with chlorphenira-mine (H_1-blocker) reduced immediate (WFR) skin reactions ($P < 0.05$) and did not affect LCRs. Cimetidine (an H_2-blocker) influenced neither WFRs nor LCRs. The combination of both (H_1-H_2 blockers) further reduces WFRs ($P < 0.01$) and abolished LCRs (Modified from Smith et al. [122])

in both isolated WFR and dual skin reactions. There was a close relationship between the amount of PGD_2 and the occurrence of LCR (as the authors pointed out, this may be interpreted solely as an epiphenomenon indicating strong mast cell activation [101]). Upon intracutaneous injection PGD_2 (0.5 μg) leads to isolated WFR (peak 30 min after injection). There are synergistic effects with other mediators, such as leukotrienes.

Leukotrienes (LTB_4, LTC_4, LTD_4)

Leukotrienes are formed by several cells types, including mast cells [100, 111, 135]. It seems of special interest that different types of granulocytes seem preferentially to generate different kinds of leukotrienes (e.g., eosinophils especially generate LTC_4 [135]).

The generation of immunoreactive leukotrienes (LTC_4/LTD_4) during the immediate phase of dual skin reactions could be demonstrated by RIA in skin blister fluids: There was a significant increase from 83 ± 13 pg/100 μl (control skin) to 220 ± 23 pg/100 μl (allergen or anti-IgE tested skin) in 13 patients ($P < 0.001$). In this preliminary study neither the intensity of LCR nor that of WFR showed a correlation to the concentration of LTC_4/LTD_4 in the blister fluid. The generation of the leukotactic LTB_4 in LCR has not yet been demonstrated. However, the injection of LTB_4 (0.5 μg) into monkey or human skin is followed within 6 h by infiltration of neutrophil granulocytes accompanied by tenderness and induration. All symptoms are augmented by the simultaneous administration of 0.5 μg PGD_2. LTD_4 (0.5 μg) leads to WFR with maximal intensity after 2 h, followed by erythema lasting 6 h [76]. The pathophysiological role of leukotrienes in LCR is underlined by the fact that neither acetylsalicylic acid [orally, 122] nor indomethacin [topically, 31] prevents LCR, whereas eicosatetraynoic acid does show an inhibitory effect (see below).

Thromboxanes

Thromboxanes (Tx) are not generated by mast cells [100] but by other cell types [114] such as fibroblasts [50] and platelets. In blister fluids from dual skin reactions TxB_2 was detected in progressively increasing concentrations following allergen injection [41]. The biological role of this mediator – which causes long-lasting bronchial asthma in experimental animals [127] – was examined using a selective thromboxane biosynthesis inhibitor [132]: Dazoxiben diminished LCR induced by reverse anaphylaxis in 13 out of 16 patients. However, as an undesired side-effect, this agent increased immediate WFR [42].

Prostaglandins E and $F_{2\alpha}$

These "classical" prostaglandins cause long-lasting erythema when injected into human skin [25]. Their role in LCR is unknown. The relative amount of both PGE_2 and $PGF_{2\alpha}$ generated in the lung during experimental anaphylaxis regulates allergen tachyphylaxis in guinea pigs, i.e., there is a progressive decrease in allergen sensitivity during sequential allergen challenge [37].

Platelet Activation/Coagulation System

Besides thromboxanes other substances can activate platelets, e.g., thrombin or platelet-activating factor (PAF) [10, 26]. PAF is released from several cell types, including mast cells [8, 124]. It has been shown to provoke LCR in human and monkey skin [3]. Thromboxanes are generated by aggregated platelets and thus further promote platelet aggregation. Indeed, in rabbit skin a biphasic accumulation of platelets was demonstrable after injection of compound 48/80 or anti-IgE: a first wave lasting 1 h was followed by a second lasting at least 3 h and exceeding the first by far [70]. IgE-dependent reactions in human lung (and probably also in skin) lead to the activation of Hageman faxtor and thereby the blood clotting system [89]. Fibrin deposits were often seen in LCR [119]. Platelet-activating properties have been found in skin blister fluid from both allergen-tested and normal skin [41].

Kallikrein-Kinin System

Bioassay on the rat uterus demonstrated active kallikrein in skin blister fluid during WFR and LCR [41]. In human skin, kallikrein causes an LCR identical to that seen after compound 48/80 with respect to clinical symptoms and histological pattern [29]. Human leukocytes are known to release kallikrein in vitro by an IgE-dependent mechanism [90].

Conclusion: "a Complex Interaction of Mediators"

At least three mediator systems seem to be involved in the pathogenesis of LCR: arachidonic acid metabolites, kinins, and the coagulation system. It may be that the complement cascade is involved too [9, 11, 61]. It seems of special interest that LCRs are influenced by regulatory mechanisms leading to long-lasting refractory states: the "partial refractory state of LCR" (first described by Umemoto [115, 133]) can last up to 4 weeks. Figure 3 shows the example of a patient with immediate, late, and delayed reactions to *Alternaria tenuis.* One week after the first challenge the skin test was repeated on the same skin area using the same allergen dose. Whereas the WFR was unchanged, the LCR was diminished and the delayed reaction slightly increased. The underlying mecha-

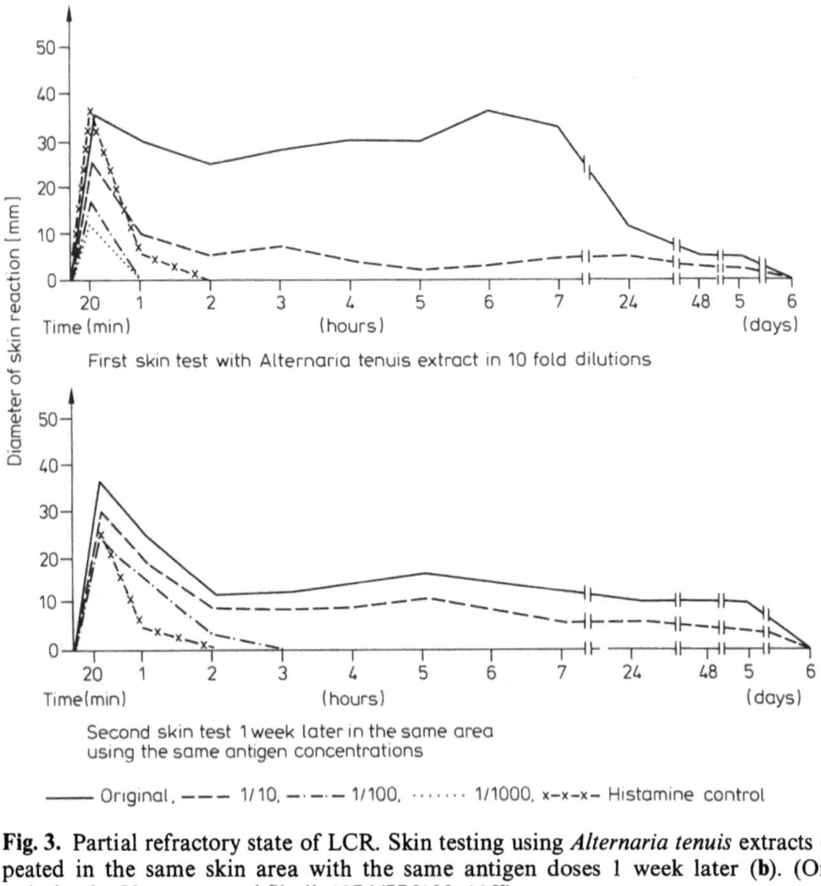

Fig. 3. Partial refractory state of LCR. Skin testing using *Alternaria tenuis* extracts (**a**) was repeated in the same skin area with the same antigen doses 1 week later (**b**). (Original description by Umemoto and Shaik 1976/77 [133, 115])

nism of this refractory state occurring after challenge with allergen, anti-IgE, kallikrein, or compound 48/80 [29] is not known; one might speculate that so-called inflamed tissue factors play some role [121]. An impaired repair mechanism may also be involved in the pathogenesis of LPRs [see 81].

Role of Infiltrating Cells

The chemotactic substances released from mast cells during anaphylaxis involve other cell types in the development of LCRs [57, 117, 118, 123, 140]. Eight hours after allergen injection there are perivascular infiltrates of lymphocytes (35%), monocytes/macrophages (10%), neutrophils (13%), eosinophils (35%), and basophils (3%). The pathogenesic role of these cells is not fully understood as yet, since 6 h [119] or 24 h [109] after allergen injection there is neither a qualitative nor a quantitative difference in cellular infiltrates between isolated WFR and dual skin reactions (in which WFRs of the same extent were followed by LCRs). However, observations in rodents that isolated peritoneal mast cell granules induce LCR [66, 74, 93, 129] support an important role of infiltrating cells in LCR. Neutrophil depletion by immunological [72] or chemical [73] procedures reduces the intensity of LCR. However, species differences have to be kept in mind: LTB_4, which is known to provoke clinical symptoms similar to LCR in human beings (see above), has recently been shown to play no role in LCR in the rat [69]. Basophils also have been considered important in the generation of LCRs [5]. Further arguments for an active role of infiltrating cells in LPRs are the biphasic course of mediator release and leukocyte activation during dual bronchial and nasal reactions (see below).

Pathogenesis of Late Nasal Reactions

Few data are available on this topic. It is most likely that late cutaneous, nasal, and bronchial reactions follow similar pathophysiological pathways. The same antigens which cause LCR by IgE-dependent mechanisms are capable of inducing late nasal reactions. However, passive transfer experiments – analogous to the Prausnitz-Küstner model in skin – were negative in the nasal system [47].

One observation seems to be of special interest: histamine release into nasal secrets was observed throughout the whole immediate and late nasal reaction; by contrast PGD_2 release was seen only during the immediate reaction [87]. Since PGD_2 is generated only by mast cells and not by basophil leukocytes (in contrast to histamine, which is released by both cell types), it was concluded that late nasal reactions are caused by the infiltration of basophil leukocytes.

Pathogenesis of Late Bronchial Obstruction

Trigger Mechanisms

Late bronchial obstruction has been observed after the inhalation of nearly all common allergens known to induce immediate reactions. In most cases LBO is triggered by IgE-dependent mechanisms leading to mast cell degranulation. This may be concluded from indirect evidence: the titer of allergen specific IgE but not IgG antibodies correlates with the frequency of LBO [35, 83]. If the immediate bronchial reaction is prevented by disodium cromoglycate, no LBO will be observed. DNCG given after antigen challenge will affect neither the immediate nor the late bronchial reaction [14].

Exercise-induced immediate asthmatic attacks are often followed by late reactions. The pathogenesis of exercise-induced asthma is not fully understood; according to several authors, however, mast cell degranulation seems to be involved.

Role of Inflammatory Mediators and Cells

During dual bronchial reactions a biphasic increase in neutrophil chemotactic activity was observed in the serum of allergen-challenged patients (Fig. 4) [88]. The same authors recently reported a biphasic increase in immunoreactive leukotrienes (LTB_4, LTC_4, LTD_4) during dual bronchial reactions in the serum of three patients after allergen inhalation [24]. They were also able to demonstrate biphasic activation of leukocytes in allergen-induced dual bronchial responses [46]. The origin of these mediators is not exactly known. They may be released by mast cells activated subsequently or, in analogy to late nasal reactions, by infiltrating cells. The pharmacological action of corticosteroids on LPR favors the latter hypothesis: corticosteroids, while strongly inhibiting LPRs, do not affect immediate reactions (Fig. 5). As shown recently, corticosteroids inhibit the degranulation of basophils, but not that of mast cells [112, 113]. In addition to various other effects (e.g., blockade of phospholipase A_2 [52, 82]) they also depress chemotaxis [120, 136].

Role of Bronchial Hyperreactivity

Bronchial hyperreactivity to nonimmunological stimuli is often seen in patients with chronic asthma. For clinical purposes it is tested by inhalation of acetylcholine or histamine. Bronchial hyperreactivity to these agents is not a prerequisite for the occurrence of LBO [34]. LBOs, however, are followed by bronchial hyperreactivity lasting up to several weeks [20]. This important fact may contribute considerably to the progressive increase in bronchial symptoms after continuous antigen exposure [130].

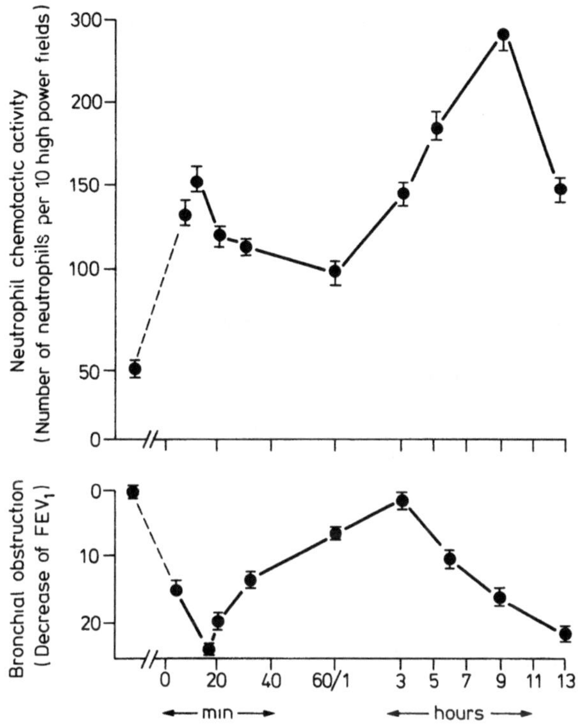

Fig. 4. Biphasic increase of neutrophil chemotactic activity in the serum of nine patients during dual asthmatic reactions after allergen challenge. (Modified from Nagy et al. [88])

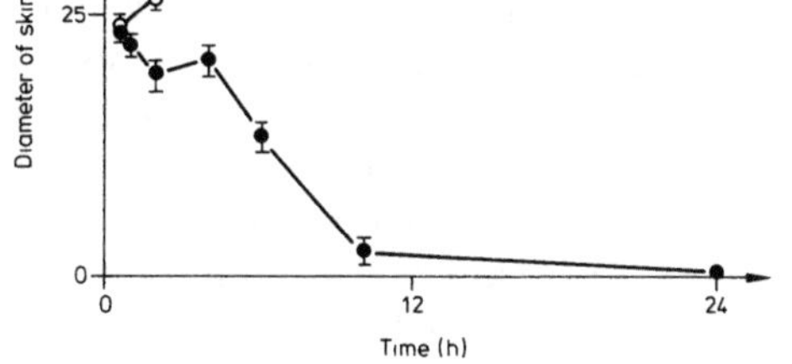

Fig. 5. Inhibitory effect of corticosteroids on LCR after reverse anaphylaxis. 50 μg β-methasone was injected simultaneously with anti-human IgE antibodies. (Modified from Gronneberg et al. [60])

Pharmacological Modulation of Late Phase Reactions

Late phase reactions may be considered as models of chronic asthmatic conditions [39, 57]. They are often ovserved in patients with chronic bronchial asthma [63, 137]; therefore the pharmacological inhibition of LPRs is of great clinical interest [20]. Table 1 summarizes the most important data available.

Table 1. Pharmacologic modulation of late phase reactions in the skin (LCRs) and the bronchial system (LBRs)

Agent	Action on	
	LCRs	LBRs
Corticosteroids	↓	↓
Disodium cromoglycate		↓
β-sympathicomimetics	↓	↓
Anticholinergics		↓
Ketotifen	↓	
Combined H_1-H_2-histamine-receptor antagonists	↓	
Eicosatetraynoic acid (ETYA)	↓	
Acetylsalicylic acid	0	
Indometacin	0 (erythema ↓)	
Dazoxiben (inhibitor of thromboxane biosynthesis)	↓ (immediate reaction ↑)	
Ethanolic onion extract	↓	
Tranexamic acid	↓	

Corticosteroids

Corticosteroids, administered orally or topically, are most efficient in preventing or treating nasal [86, 91, 98], cutaneous [60, 103], and bronchial [14] LPRs. Interestingly, immediate reactions are not affected by these drugs (Fig. 5) [60].

Disodium Cromoglycate

Disodium cromoglycate, (DSCG) can effectively prevent LBO (but not acute hypersensitivity pneumonitis) when it is inhaled prior to allergen (Fig. 6 shows data from 14 of our patients; the original description of this action was made by Booij-Noord [14] in 1971). When it is given after the allergen, DSCG has no effect. The dampening effect of this compound on bronchial hyperreactivity may be explained by its inhibitory effect on LBO [2]. As mentioned above, LBO causes bronchial hyperreactivity lasting up to several weeks. There are, however, also direct effects on bronchial irritant receptors [63].

β-Adrenergic Agents

Late bronchial obstruction can be markedly reduced by the inhalation of β-mimetics such as salbutamol (Fig. 6). This drug also reverses impairments of gas transfer during LBO [33, 48].

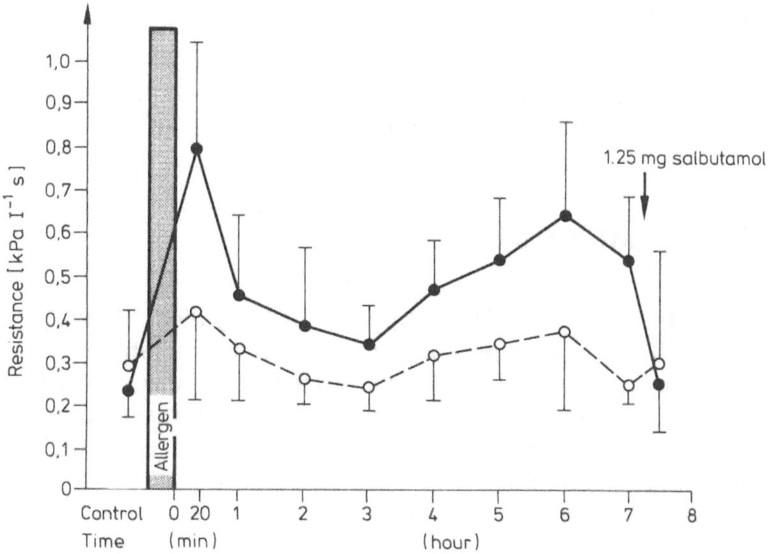

Fig. 6. Protective effect of disodium cromoglycate (DSCG, 40 mg per inhalation) on allergen-induced dual obstructive reactions in 14 patients. The therapeutic effect of β-adrenergic drug (salbutamol, 1.25 mg per inhalation) on allergen-induced LBO is also shown

Anticholinergic Agents

Ipratropium bromide per inhalation has been shown to relieve airway resistance during LBO, thus indicating the involvement of cholinergic mechanisms in LBO [33, see also 52]. The efficacy of this drug, however, is much weaker than that of β-mimetics.

Antihistamines

As mentioned above (Fig. 2), neither histamine H_1- nor histamine H_2-receptor antagonists administered orally affect LCRs when given alone. In combination, however, they abolish LCRs totally [122]. Data on similar experiments on LNRs or LBRs are lacking. H_1-H_2 antagonism has been recommended for preventing pseudo-allergic anaphylactoid [79, 140]. Studium on the effect of combined histamine antagonists on bronchial asthma in human beings will be of great interest [66], since experimental data from animals are promising [37, 38].

Ketotifen

Ketotifen, an orally active agent with mast cell-stabilizing and antihistaminic properties, inhibits both WFRs and LCRs [1].

Eicosatetraynoic acid

Eicosatetraynoic acid (ETYA) applied topically blocks both the cyclooxygenase and the lipoxygenase pathway of arachidonic metabolism. Even high doses (1 mg) do not affect WFRs when injected simultaneously with rabbit anti-human IgE antibodies. The subsequent LCRs, however, are reduced (30% reduction at the 8th hour, $n = 6$, $P < 0.05$; Dorsch et al. to be published). In guinea pigs, inhalation of ETYA shows marked protective effects against allergen-induced bronchial obstruction [43].

Acetylsalicylic Acid and Indomethacin

Neither of these cyclooxygenase inhibitors (oral acetylsalicylic acid, topic indomethacin) altered edema formation or clinical symptoms during LCR [31, 122]. Only the intensity of the erythema was reduced by indomethacin [31], an agent known to diminish erythema in sunburn.

In single cases relief of LBO by cyclooxygenase inhibitors has been reported [49].

Thromboxane Synthetase Inhibitors

Dazoxiben (administered orally) is used in the treatment of vascular diseases [132]. This agent selectively inhibits thromboxane formation in, for example, human platelets while increasing serum levels of prostacyclin and prostaglandins. It depressed edema formation during LCR in 13 out of 16 cases after reverse anaphylaxis and compound 48/80 injection. It showed, however, undesired and potentially serious side-effects by increasing immediate WFR [42].

Onion Extracts

Onion and garlic oils have been shown to inhibit both lipoxygenase and cyclooxygenase pathways of human platelets' arachidonic metabolism in vitro [134]. This biochemical activity may be responsible for the well known antiaggregatory effects of onions. In a double-blind study on 12 volunteers marked suppressive effects of topically applied ethanolic onion extract upon LCR after reverse anaphylaxis were observed [40]. Oral onion treatment effectively protected guinea pigs against allergen-induced bronchial asthma. This observation led to the detection of antiasthmatic properties of mustard oils [30]. In the two patients as yet tested, oral onion treatment (2 × 100 ml extract = 2 × 200 g onions) depressed both immediate and late bronchial obstruction.

Tranexamic Acid

Tranexamic acid is well known as an inhibitor of fibrinolysis. As shown recently, it depresses late cutaneous reactions [29].

Animal Models of LPR

Skin Tests on Monkeys Using Patients' Serum

The skin of primates can be passively sensitized with serum of atopic patients [95]. Intracutaneous injection of the proper antigen causes not only immediate but also late cutaneous reactions [32]. In most of the cases the sensitizing property of patients' serum is heat labile, indicating that IgE antibodies are the active agents. In some cases, however, passive Arthus phenomena can be observed which are mediated by heat-stable antibodies.

Skin Tests on Rats Using Isolated Mast Cell Granules

The injection of anti-IgE or compound 48/80 into the skin of rats is followed by increased vascular permeability and perivascular cell infiltration. Polymorphonuclear leukocytes present 1–2 h later are gradually replaced by mononuclear cells (predominantly macrophages) at 24 h. The same symptoms occur after injection of mast cell granules isolated from rat peritoneal mast cells [67, 74, 129]. From these membrane-free granules a so-called inflammatory factor of anaphylaxis (IFA) was isolated [93] and characterized in part as a polypeptide containing 12 amino acids (molecular weight 1400). IFA caused both early polymorphonuclear and late mononuclear cell infiltrations.

Immunologically or chemically induced neutropenia diminished LCRs in this animal model [72, 73]. Both corticosteroids and combined histamine H_1-H_2 receptor antagonists are inhibitory, as in human LCRs [71, 92].

Bronchial Provocation Test in Rabbits

If neonatal rabbits are immunized with *Alternaria tenuis* they produce only IgE antibodies to this antigen. By the age of 1 week they synthesize precipitating antibodies of various isotypes. IgE-sensitive animals react to inhalative allergen challenges with immediate and late bronchial obstruction. This biphasic pulmonary response can be passively transferred with IgE serum to nonimmunized animals. Transfusion of IgG serum to IgE animals diminishes their biphasic pulmonary response after *Alternaria* aerosol challenge. Especially the latter observation may be important for the understanding of the beneficial effects of specific hyposensitization [116].

Clinical Consequences

In the past, patients with LPRs were excluded from hyposensitization because these reactions were generally considered to be the Arthus phenomenon. In our opinion, IgE-dependent LPRs certainly are not a contraindication to hyposensitization. Recent studies have even shown that hyposensitization will ameliorate IgE-dependent LPR rather than the corresponding immediate reaction [78, 102]. In clinical practice, however, demonstration of the IgE dependency of a certain LPR may be difficult. When there is doubt, bronchial provocation tests should be performed. LBO can be differentiated from hypersensitivity pneumonitis by clinical symptoms (lack of crepitations, chills, fever, marked leukocytosis), lung function tests (bronchial obstruction instead of impaired gas transfer), and its response to drugs such as DSCG and β-mimetics. Measurements of complement factors in the serum are not useful [9]. During hyposensitization, allergen-specific IgG antibodies occur. They may cause adverse reactions, but hyposensitization can be continued if certain precautions are taken [19, see also 78, 116].

Summary and Conclusion

Late phase reactions have generally been considered as the Arthus phenomenon (type III allergy according to Coombs and Gell). IgE antibodies, however, are able to initiate not only immediate (WFR), but also late cutaneous reactions. Using the skin blister technique we could show LCRs to be mediated by inflammatory mediators generated during the preceding WFR. Histamine, active kallikrein, leukotrienes, thromboxanes, and platelet-activating properties were demonstrable in dual skin reactions. The concentration of these mediators in skin blister fluid was in part related to the time course of skin reactions. LCRs were diminished by ETEA (but not by indomethacin), by dazoxiben (thromboxane synthetase inhibitor), and by ethanolic onion extract. β-Mimetics such as salbutamol and anticholinergics such as ipratropium bromide were able to reverse LBRs, whereas disodium cromoglycate and ethanolic onion extract were able to prevent LBR. Other authors have found PGD_2 and chemotactic substances during LPRs, as well as protective effects of corticosteroids, combined histamine H_1-H_2 receptor antagonists, and tranexamic acid.

Two types of LPR have to be distinguished: type I and type III. Late phase reactions are caused by IgE antibodies in most of the cases. They are initiated by mast cell degranulation and maintained by a complex interaction of inflammatory mediators and cells. LPRs represent models of chronic asthmatic conditions. Studies on their pharamcological modulation may yield new insights in the pathophysiology and therapy of bronchial asthma.

References

1. Aas K (1979) Effects of ketotifen and clemastine on passive transfer of reaginic reaction. Allergy 34:121–124
2. Altounyan REG (1980) Review of clinical activity and mode of action of sodium cromoglycate. Clin Allergy [Suppl] 10:481–489
3. Archer CB (1983) Early and late inflammatory effects of PAF-Acether in the skin of experimental animals and man. J Invest Dermatol 80:346 (Abstract)
4. Arroyave GM, Stevenson DD, Vaughan JH, Tah EH (1977) Plasma complement changes during bronchospasm provoked in asthmatic patients. Clin Allergy 7:173–182
5. Askenase PW (1977) Role of basophils, mast cells and vasoamines in hypersensitivity reactions with a delayed time course. Prog Allergy 3:211–215
6. Atkins PC, Green GR, Zweiman B (1973) Histologic studies of human skin test responses to ragweed, compound 48/80 and histamine. J Allergy Clin Immunol 51:263–273
7. Atkins PC, Norman M, Weiner H, Zweiman B (1976) Release of neutrophil chemotactic activity during immediate hypersensitivity reactions in humans. Ann Intern Med 86:415–418
8. Austen KF, Orange RP (1975) Bronchial asthma: The possible role of the chemical mediators of immediate hypersensitivity in the pathogenesis of subacute disease. Am Rev Respir Dis 112:423–451
9. Baur X, Dorsch W, Becker T (1980) Levens of complement factors in human serum during immediate and late asthmatic reactions and during acute hypersensitivity pneumonitis. Allergy 35:383–390
10. Benveniste J, le Couedie JP, Polansky J, Tence M (1977) Structural analysis of purified platelet-activating factor by lipases. Nature 269:170–171
11. Berrens L, van Rijswijk-Verbeck J (1973) Inactivation of complement (C3) in human serum by atopic allergens. Int Arch Allergy 45:30–39
12. Black AK, Greaves MW, Hensby CN, Plummer NA (1976) A new method of obtaining human skin inflammatory exudate for pharmacological analysis. Br J Pharmacol 58:317 (Abstract)
13. Blackley CH (1873) Experimental researches in the causes and nature of catarrhus aestivus (hayfever or hay asthma). Bailliere, Tindall and Cox, reprinted by Dawson's of Pail Mall, London, 1959, pp 77–81
14. Booij-Nord II, Orie NGM, de Vries K (1971) Immediate and late bronchial obstructive reactions to inhalation of house dust and protective effects of disodium cromoglycate and prednisolone. J Allergy Clin Immunol 43:344–354

15. Brady R, Glovsky M, Hugli T (1978) Complement (C) activation by house dust extract; Implications in immediate hypersensitivity. J Allergy Clin Immunol 61:187–188
16. Brocklehurst WE (1971) Role of kinins and prostaglandins in inflammation. Proc R Soc Med 64:4–6
17. Brostoff J, Roitt IM (1969) Cell mediated (delayed) hypersensitivity in patients with summer hayfever. Lancet 2:1269–1272
18. Bryant DH, Burns MW, Lazarus L (1975) New type of allergic asthma due to IgG "reaginic" antibody. Br Med J 4:580 (Abstract)
19. Busse WW, Storms WW, Flaherty DK, Crandall M, Reed CE (1976) Alternaria IgG precipitating an adverse reaction. J Allergy Clin Immunol 57:367–372
20. Cartier A, Thomson NC, Frith PA, Roberts R, Tech M, Hargreave FE (1982) Allergen-induced increase in bronchial responsiveness to histamine: relationship to the late asthmatic response and change in airway caliber. J Allergy Clin Immunol 70:170–177
21. Chapman LF (1977) Mechanism of the flare reactions in human skin. J Invest Dermatol 69:88–97
22. Cochrane CG, Dixon FJ (1976) Antigen-antibody complex induced disease. In: Miescher PA, Müller-Eberhard HJ (eds) Textbook of immunopathology. Grune & Stratton, New York, pp 137–156
23. Cooke RA (1922) Studies in specific hypersensitiveness IX. On the phenomenon of hyposensitization (the clinically lessened sensitiveness of allergy). J Immunol 7:219–227
24. Cromwell O, Shaw RJ, Durham SR, Kay AB (1984) Plasma LTB_4 concentrations during early and late phase antigen-induced asthmatic reactions. J Allergy Clin Immunol 73:147 (Abstract)
25. Crunkhorn P, Willis AL (1971) Cutaneous reactions to intradermal prostaglandins. Br J Pharmacol 41:49–56
26. Demopoulos CA, Pinckard RN, Hanahan DJ (1976) Platelet activating factor. J Biol Chem 254:9355–9358
27. Dolovich J, Hargreave FE, Chalmers R, Shier KJ, Gauldie Bienenstock J (1973) Late cutaneous allergic responses in isolated IgE dependent reactions. J Allergy Clin Immunol 52:38–46
28. Dolovich J, Little DC (1972) Correlates of skin test reactions to *Bacillus subtilis* enzyme preparations. J Allergy Clin Immunol 49:43–53
29. Dor PJ, Vervloet D, Sapene M, Andrac L, Bonerandi JJ, Charpin J (1983) Induction of late cutaneous reaction by kallikrein injection: comparison with allergic-like late response to compound 48/80. J Allergy Clin Immunol 4:363–370
30. Dorsch W, Adam O, Weber J, Ziegeltrum T (1985) Antiasthmatic effects of onion extracts – detection of benzyl- and other isothiocyanates (mustard oils) as antiasthmatic compounds of plant origin. Eur J Pediatr 141:264 (Abstract) Eur J Pharmacol 107:17–24
31. Dorsch W, Baur X (1980) Effect of topical indomethacin on allergen-induced dual skin reaction. Allergy 35:503–508
32. Dorsch W, Baur X, Becker TH (1979) Zur Pathogenese verzögerter Immunreaktionen beim Asthma bronchiale. Atemwegs Lungenerkrankungen 5:294–297
33. Dorsch W, Baur X, Emslander HP, Fruhmann G (1980) Zur Pathogenese und Therapie der verzögerten Bronchialobstruktion. Prax Pneumonol 34:461–468
34. Dorsch W, Baur X, Polke H (1980) Quantitative Beziehungen zwischen Hauttestreaktionen, allergenspezifischem Serum-IgE-Spiegel und bronchialer Reagibilität bei Patienten mit exogen allergischem Asthma bronchiale. Allergologie 3:12–16
35. Dorsch W, Baur X, Vogelmeier C (1979) IgE- und IgG-RAST bei Asthma-Patienten mit verzögerten Testreaktionen. Ein Beitrag zur Pathogenese der verzögerten Immunantwort in der cutanen und bronchopulmonalen Allergiediagnostik. II. RAST-Symposium Köln, Berichtsband. Grosse, Berlin (1981), pp 138–143
36. Dorsch W, Hintschich C, Neuhauser J, Weber J (1985) Sequential histamine inhalations cause increased bronchial histamine reactivity in guinea pigs: Role of platelets, thromboxanes and prostacyclin. Naunyn-Schmiedebergs Arch Pharmacol 327:148–155
37. Dorsch W, Frey L, Müller W (1984) In vitro allergen tachyphylaxis of guinea pig lung is mediated by endogenous prostaglandin E biosynthesis. Naunyn-Schmiedebergs Arch Pharmacol 325:275–282

38. Dorsch W, Reimann HJ, Neuhauser J (1982) Histamine$_1$-histamine$_2$-antagonism: effect of combined clemastine and cimetidine pretreatment on allergen and histamine induced reactions of the guinea pig lung in vivo and in vitro. Agents Actions 12:113–118
39. Dorsch W, Ring J (1981) Induction of late cutaneous reactions by skin blister fluid from allergen tested and normal skin. J Allergy Clin Immunol 67:117–123
40. Dorsch W, Ring J (1984) Suppression of immediate and late anti-IgE-induced skin reactions by topically applied alcohol/onion extract. Allergy 39:43–49
41. Dorsch W, Ring J, Reimann H, Geiger R (1982) Mediator studies in skin blister fluid from patients with dual skin reactions. J Allergy Clin Immunol 70:236–244
41a. Dorsch W, Ring J, Strasser T, Weber PC (1985) Detection of immunoreactive leukotrienes (LTC_4/LTD_4) in skin blister fluid after allergen testing in patients with late cutaneous reactions. Arch Dermatol Res 277:400–401
42. Dorsch W, Ring J, Melzer H (1983) A selective inhibitor of thromboxane biosynthesis enhances immediate and reduces late cutaneous allergic reactions in man. J Allergy Clin Immunol 72:168–173
43. Dorsch W, Waldherr U, Rosmanith J (1981) Continuous recording of intrapulmonary "compressed air" as a sensitive noninvasive method of measuring bronchial obstruction in guinea pigs. Pflügers Arch 391:236–241
44. Dvoracek JE, Yunginger JW, Kern EB, Hyatt RE, Gleich GJ (1984) Induction of nasal late-phase reactions by insufflation of ragweed-pollen extract. J Allergy Clin Immunol 73:363–368
45. Dunsky EH, Zweiman B (1978) The direct demonstration of histamine release in allergic reactions in the skin using a skin chamber technique. J Allergy Clin Immunol 62:127–130
46. Durham SR, Carrol M, Walsh G, Boghossian S, Kay AB (1984) Leucocyte activation during antigen-induced early and late-phase asthmatic reactions. J Allergy Clin Immunol 73:146 (Abstract)
47. Edwards JH, Baker JR, Davies BH (1974) Precipitin test negative farmer's lung-activation of the alternative pathway of complement by mouldy hay dusts. Clin Allergy 4:379–388
48. Emslander HP, Dorsch W, Baur X (1979) Airway resistance and $C^{18}O$-gas transfer in the late reaction following inhalant challenge by allergen. International congress on respiratory diseases, Basel, Switzerland, p 79
49. Fairfax AJ (1982) Inhibition of the late asthmatic response to house dust mite by non-steroidal anti-inflammatory drugs. Prostaglandins Leukotrienes Med 8:239–248
50. Feinmark SJ, Bailey JM (1982) Lipid metabolism in cultured cells: activation of endogenous thromboxane A_2 synthesis in cultured lung fibroblasts. J Biol Chem 257:2816–2821
51. Flower R (1978) Steroidal antiinflammatory drugs as inhibitors of phospholipase A_2. Adv Prostaglandin Thromboxane Leukotriene Res 3:103–107
52. Folco G, Omini C, Rossini G, Vigan'o T, Berti F (1982) Anticholinergic agents prevent guinea-pig airway constriction induced by histamine, bradykinine and leukotriene C_4: relationship to circulating TXA_2. Eur J Pharmacol 78:159–165
53. Geiger R (1985) The kallikrein-kinin systems. In: Türk VLJ (ed) Proteinases and their inhibitors. Mladinska Knjian – Pergamon, Ljubljana Oxford, pp 353–376
54. Gell PGH, Coombs RRA (1968) Clinical aspects of immunology, vol 3. Blackwell, Oxford, p 3
55. Gervais R, Reinberg A, Gervais C, Smolensky M, de France O (1977) Twenty-four-hour rhythm in the bronchial hyperreactivity to house dust in asthmatics. J Allergy Clin Immunol 59:207–213
56. Gigli I (1976) Immunochemistry and immunobiology of the complement system. J Invest Dermatol 67:346–350
57. Gleich GJ (1982) The late phase of the immunoglobulin E-mediated reaction – a link between anaphylaxis and common allergic disease? J Allergy Clin Immunol 70:160–169
58. Gleich GJ, Muller SA (1980) Atopic dermatitis: a review with emphasis on pathogenesis. Clin Immunol 43:1316–1335
59. Goetzl EJ (1980) Occasional notes: mediators of immediate hypersensitivity derived from arachidonic acid. N Engl J Med 303:822–824

60. Gronneberg WE, Strandberg K, Stalenheim G, Zetterstrom O (1981) Effect in man of anti-allergic drugs on the immediate and late cutaneous allergic reaction induced by anti-IgE. Allergy 36:201–208
61. Grönneberg R (1984) Inhibition of the late phase reaction to antihuman IgE in man by oral tranexamic acid. Allergy 39:115–118
62. Harris MG (1981) Bronchial irritant receptors and a possible new action for cromolyn sodium. Ann Allergy 46:156–158
63. Herxheimer H (1952) The late bronchial reaction in induced asthma. Int Arch Allergy Appl Immunol 3:189–207
64. Ishizaka TCM, Sian K, Ishizaka K (1972) Complement fixation by aggregated IgE through alternate pathway. J Immunol 108:848–851
65. Juhlin L, Michaelsson G (1969) Cutaneous reactions to kallikrein, bradykinin and histamine in healthy subjects and in patients with urticaria. Acta Derm Venerol 49:26–36
66. Kaliner M (1984) Hypotheses on the contribution of late phase allergic responses to the understanding and treatment of allergic diseases. J Allergy Clin Immunol 73:311–315
67. Kaliner M, Lemanske RF (1985) Inflammatory responses to mast cell granules. Fed Proc (in press)
68. Keller R (1968) On the role of secondary mast-cell damage and histamine-release in the course of immune reactions. In: Dusten K, Becker EL (eds) Biochemistry of acute allergic reactions. Blackwell, Oxford, pp 253–265
69. Kopp D, Esser B, Goetzl E, Lemanske R, Madison WI (1984) The role of leucotriene B_4 in rat cutaneous late phase reactions. J Allergy Clin Immunol 73:158 (Abstract)
70. Kravis TC, Henson PM (1977) Accumulation of platelets at sites of antigen-antibody-mediated injury: a possible role for IgE antibodies and mast cells. J Immunol 118:1559–1573
71. Lemanske RF, Barr L, Guthman DA, Kaliner M (1983) The biologic activity of mast cell granules. V. The effect of antihistamine treatment on rat cutaneous early late phase allergic reactions. J Allergy Clin Immunol 72:94–99
72. Lemanske RF, Guthman DA, Kaliner M (1983) The biologic activity of mast cell granules. VII. The effect of antineutrophil antibody induced neutropenia on rat cutaneous late phase reactions. J Immunol 131:929–933
73. Lemanske RF, Guthman DA, Oertel H, Barr L, Kaliner M (1983) The biologic activity of mast cell granules. The effect of vinblastine-induced neutropenia on rat cutaneous late phase reactions. J Immunol 6:2837–2842
74. Lemanske RF, Kaliner M (1982) Mast cell dependent late phase reactions. Clin Immunol Rev 1:547–580
75. Lewis RA, Holgate ST, Roberts LJ, Oates JA, Austen KF (1971) Preferential generation of prostaglandin D_2 by rat and human mast cells. In: Becker EL, Simon AJ, Austen KF (eds) Biochemistry of the acute allergic reaction. Blackwell, Oxford, pp 239–254
76. Lewis RA, Soter YA, Corey EJ, Austen KF (1981) Local effects of synthetic leukotrienes on monkey and human skin. Clin Res 29:492 (Abstract)
77. Lichtenstein LA, Gillespie E (1973) Inhibition of histamine release by histamine controlled by H_2 receptors. Nature 244:287–288
78. Lichtenstein LM, Valentine MD, Norman PS (1984) A reevaluation of immunotherapy for asthma. Am Rev Respir Dis 129:657–659
79. Lorenz W, Doenicke A, Schoening B, Mamorski J, Weber D, Hinterlang E, Schwarz B, Neugebauer E (1980) H_1-H_2-receptor antagonists for premedication in anaesthesia and surgery. Agents and Actions 10:114–124
80. Lotner GZ, Lynch JM, Betz SJ, Henson PM (1980) Human neutrophil-derived platelet activating factor. J Immunol 124:676–684
81. Mayno G (1964) Mechanism of abnormal vascular permeability in acute inflammation. In: Thomas L, Uhr J, Grant L (eds) Injury inflammation and immunity. Williams and Wilkins, Baltimore, pp 58–93
82. Marone G, Kagey-Sobotka A, Lichtenstein LM (1981) Possible role of phospholipase A_2 in triggering histamine secretion from human basophils in vitro. Clin Immunbiol Immunopathol 20:231–239

83. Metzger WJ, Dorminey HC, Robbins D, Richerson HB (1981) Late asthmatic responses during allergen bronchoprovocation. Correlation with specific IgE and symptoms. J Allergy Clin Immunol 67:11 (Abstract)
84. Metzger WJ, Richerson HB, Kregel K, Barfknecht C, Moore K (1982) Late phase obstructive airways responses (LPR) in a rabbit model: physiology and anatomic findings. Am Rev Dis 125:62 (Abstract)
85. Michel B, Russell TH, Winkelmann RK, Gleich GJ (1970) Release of kinins from site of wheal- and flare allergic skin reactions. Int Arch Allergy 39:616–624
86. Mygind N, Johnson NJ, Thonsen J (1977) Intranasal allergen challenge during corticosteroid treatment. Clin Allergy 7:69–74
87. Naclerio R, Togias A, Proud D, Adkinson NF, Kagey-Sobotka A, Plaut M, Norman PS, Lichtenstein LM (1984) Inflammatory mediators in nasal secretions during early and late reactions. J Allerg Clin Immunol 73:148 (Abstract)
88. Nagy L, Lee Th, Kay AB (1982) Neutrophil chemotactic activity in antigen-induced late asthmatic reactions. N Engl J Med 306:497–501
89. Newball HH, Meier HL, Kaplan AP, Revak SD, Cochrane CG, Lichtenstein LM (1981) Activation of the Hageman factor dependent systems during IgE mediated reactions of the human lung. Int Arch Allergy Appl Immunol 66:165 (Abstract)
90. Newball HH, Talamo RC, Lichtenstein LM (1975) Release of leucocyte kallikrein mediated by IgE. Nature 254:635–636
91. Norman PS (1983) Review of nasal therapy: update: J Allergy Clin Immunol 72:421–429
92. Oertel H, Kaliner M (1981) The biologic activity of mast cell granules in rat skin. II The effects of adrenocorticosteroids upon late phase inflammatory responses induced by mast cell granules. J Allergy Clin Immunol 68:238–245
93. Oertel H, Kaliner M (1981) The biologic activity of mast cell granules. III Purification of inflammatory factors of anaphylaxis (IF-A) responsible for causing late phase reactions. J Immunol 1127:1398–1402
94. Parish PE (1970) Short-term anaphylactic IgG antibodies in human sera. Lancet 2:591–592
95. Patterson R, Fink JN, Nishimura ET (1965) The passive transfer of immediate type hypersensitivity from man to other primates. J Clin Invest 44:140–148
96. Paton WDM (1951) Compound 48/80: A potent histamine liberator. Br J Pharmacol Chemother 6:499–508
97. Pelikan Z (1978) Late and delayed responses of the nasal mucosa to allergen challenge. Ann Allergy 41:37–47
98. Pelikan Z, Pelikan-Filipek M (1982) The effects of disodium cromoglycate and beclomethasone diproprionate on the immediate response of the nasal mucosa to allergen challenge. Ann Allergy 49:238–292
99. Pepys J, Turner-Warwick M, Dawson PL, Hinson KFW (1968) Arthus (type III) skin test reactions in man. Clinical and immunopathological features. In Excerpta Medica International Congress Series, Allergology, Proceedings of the Sixth Congress of the International Association of Allergology 162:221–235
100. Peters SP, MacGlashan DW, Schulman ES, Schleimer RP, Hayes EC, Rokach J, Adkinson NF, Lichtenstein LM (1984) Arachidonic acid metabolism in purified human mast cells. J Immunol 4:1972–1979
101. Pienkowski M, Adkinson NF, Norman PS, Lichtenstein LM (1984) Mediators during cutaneous allergic immediate and late-phase reactions. J Allergy Clin Immunol 73:147 (Abstract)
102. Pienkowski M, Norman PS, Lichtenstein LM (in press) Suppression of late phase skin reaction in patients on immunotherapy with ragweed. Ann Allergy (Abstract)
103. Poothullil J, Umemoto L, Dolovich J, Hargreave FE, Day RP (1976) Inhibition by prednisone of late cutaneous allergic responses induced by antiserum to human IgE. J Allergy Clin Immunol 57:164–167
104. Prausnitz C, Küstner H (1921) Studien über die Überempfindlichkeit. Zentralbl Bakteriol 86:160–169
105. Price JF, Hey EN, Soothill JF (1982) Antigen provocation to the skin, nose and lung in

children with asthma; immediate and dual hypersensitivity reactions. Clin Exp Immunol 47:587–594

106. Radermecker M, Maldague MP (1981) Depression of neutrophil chemotaxis in atopic individuals: an H_2 histamine receptor response. Int Arch Allergy Appl Immunol 65:144–152
107. Ratnoff OD (1971) A tanglet web: the interdependence of mechanism of blood clotting fibrinolysis, immunity and inflammation. Thromb Diath Haemorrh [Suppl] 45:109–129
108. Reed CHE (1974) Allergic mechanisms in extrinsic allergic alveolitis. In: Brent L, Holborow S (eds) Progress in immunology, vol 4, part 2. North Holland, Amsterdem, pp 271–281
109. Richerson HB, Rajtora DW, Penik GD, Dick FR, Yoo TJ (1979) Cutaneous and nasal allergic responses in ragweed hay fever: lack of clinical and histopathologic correlations with late phase reactions. J Allergy Clin Immunol 64:67–77
110. Ring J, Rothenberger KH, Clauß W (1985) Prevention of anaphylactoid reactions after radiographic contrast media infusion by combined histamine H_1- and H_2-receptor antagonists: results of a prospective controlled trial. Int Archs Allergy appl Immun 78:9–14
111. Robertson DG, Kerigan AT, Hargreave FE, Chalmers K, Dolovich J (1974) Late asthmatic responses induced by ragweed pollen allergen. J Allergy Clin Immunol 54:244–254
112. Samuelsson B (1982) The leukotrienes: an introduction. In: Samuelsson B, Paoletti R (eds) Leukotrienes and other lipoxygenase products. Raven, New York, pp 1–17
113. Schleimer RP, MacGlashan DW, Gillespie E, Lichtenstein LM (1982) Inhibition of basophil histamine release by antiinflammatory steroids. II. Studies on the mechanism of action. J Immunol 129:1632–1635
114. Schleimer RP, Schulman ES, MacGlashan DW (1983) Effects of dexamethasone on mediator release from human lung fragments and purified human lung mast cells. J Clin Invest 71:1830–1835
115. Schulman ES, Newball HH, Demers LM, Fitzpatrick FA, Adkinson NF (1981) Anaphylactic release of thromboxane A_2, prostaglandin D_2 and prostacyclin from human lung parenchyma. Am Rev Resp Dis 124:402–406
116. Shaikh W, Umemoto L, Poothullil J, Hargreave FE, Dolovich J (1977) Relative refractory state for late cutaneous allergic response. J Allergy Clin Immunol 60:242–246
117. Shampain MP, Behrens BL, Larsen GL, Henson PM (1982) An animal model of late pulmonary responses to *Alternaria* challenge. Am Rev Respir Dis 126:493–498
118. Shazo De RD, Dvorak H, Davis R, Evans R (1978) The late phase skin reaction. J Allergy Clin Immunol 61:186–202
119. Shazo de RD, Boehm TM, Kuman D (1982) Dermal hypersensitivity reactions to insulin: correlations of three patterns to their histopathology. J Allergy Clin Immunol 69:229–237
120. Shazo de RD, Levinson AI, Dvorak HF, Davis RW (1979) The late phase skin reaction: evidence for activation of the coagulation system in an IgE-dependent reaction in man. J Immunol 122:692–698
121. Shea C, Morse ED (1978) Inhibition of human neutrophil chemotaxis by corticosteroids. Ann Clin Lab Sci 8:30–33
122. Smith MHJ, Ford-Hutchinson AW (1979) Inflamed tissue factors. In: Vane JR, Ferreira SH (eds) Antiinflammatory drugs. Springer, Berlin Heidelberg New York, pp 675–677 (Handbook of experimental pharmacology, vol 50, part 2)
123. Smith JA, Mansfield LE, Shazo de RD, Nelson HS (1980) An evaluation of the pharmacologic inhibition of the immediate and late cutaneous reactions to allergen. J Allergy Clin Immunol 65:185–222
124. Solley GO, Gleich GJ, Jordon RE, Schroeter AL (1976) The late phase of immediate wheal and flare skin reactions. J Clin Invest 58:408–420
125. Soter NA, Austen KF (1976) The diversity of mast cell-derived mediators: implication for acute, subacute and chronic cutaneous inflammatory disorders. J Invest Dermatol 67:313–319
126. Staszewska-Barezak J, Vane JR (1975) The role of prostaglandins in the local control of circulation. Clin Exp Pharmacol Physiol 2:71–78

127. Stalenheim G, Zetterström O (1979) Late cutaneous reactions without the participation of IgE. Monogr Allergy 14:264–267
128. Svensson J, Strandberg K, Turemo T, Hamberg M (1977) Thromboxane A_2: Effects on airway and vascular smooth muscle. Prostaglandins 14:425–436
129. Talbot S, Atkins P, Zweiman B (1984) Prolonged histamine release in cutaneous allergic reactions. J Allergy Clin Immunol 73:147 (Abstract)
130. Tannenbaum S, Oertel H, Henderson W, Kaliner M (1980) The biologic activity of mast cell granules. I Elicitation of inflammatory responses in rat skin, J Immunol 125:325–335
131. Tiffeneau R (1960) Über nicht kontinuierliche (Pollen) und kontinuierliche (Hausstaub) Allergeneffekte und deren Einfluß auf die bronchomotorische Erregbarkeit der Asthmatikers. Allergie Asthma 6:10–15
132. Turner-Warwick M (1978) Immunology of the lung. Edward Arnold, London, p 165
133. Tyler HM, Saxton CATD, Parry JM (1981) Administration to man of UK-37, 248-01, a selective inhibitor of thromboxane synthetase. Lancet:629–632
134. Umemoto L, Poothullil J, Dolovich KE, Hargreave AP, Day RP (1976) Factors which influence the late cutaneous allergic response (LCAR). J Allergy Clin Immunol 58:60
135. Vanderhoek JY, Makheja AN, Bailey JM (1980) Inhibition of fatty acid oxygenases by onion and garlic oils. Evidence for the mechanism by which these oils inhibit platelet aggregation. Biochem Pharmacol 29:3169–3173
136. Verhagen J, Bruynzeel PLB, Koedam JA, Wassink GA, de Boer M, Terpstra GK, Kreukniet J, Veldink GA, Vliegenthart JFG (1984) Specific leukotriene formation by purified human eosinophils and neutrophils. FEBS Lett 168:23–28
137. Ward PA (1966) The chemosuppression of chemotaxis. J Exp Med 124–209
138. Warner JA (1976) Significance of late reactions after bronchial challenge with house dust mite. Arch Dis Child 51:905–911
139. Williams TJ, Morley J (1973) Prostaglandins as potentiators of increased vascular permeability in inflammation. Nature 246:215–217
140. Zetterström O (1978) Dual skin test reactions and serum antibodies to subtilisin and *Aspergillus fumigatus* extracts. Clin Allergy 8:77–91

Aspirin-Induced and Intrinsic Asthma

D. A. Mathison, R. A. Simon, and D. D. Stevenson

Division of Allergy & Immunology and Department of Basic & Clinical Research, Scripps Clinic & Research Foundation, 10666 North Torrey Pines Road, La Jolla, CA 92037, USA

Abstract

Asthma is a syndrome characterized by increased responsiveness of the trachea and bronchi to various stimuli and manifested by widespread hyperreactivity of the airways that changes in severity either spontaneously or as a result of therapy. The increased responsiveness can be documented and the diagnosis confirmed by spirometric measurements of bronchodilatation following inhalations of beta-adrenergic drugs or broncho-constriction following inhalations of methacholine or histamine or exercise. When the asthmatic patient has attacks precipitated by exposures to aeroallergens to which he has IgE antibodies, the asthma is turned "allergic", "atopic" or "extrinsic"; however, most of such patients also have the bronchospasticity "intrinsic" to the disease.

One subset of asthmatic patients has a syndrome of chronic hyperplastic and eosinophilic rhinosinusitis with polyp formation and acute and severe rhinitic and asthmatic reaction to ingestion of ordinary doses of aspirin and aspirin-like non-steroidal antiinflammatory drugs (NSAID). Even though these patients avoid NSAID, their disease is progressive and frequently requires corticosteroid treatment for control. Cautious challenges in a hospital setting, beginning with 3 mg of aspirin and increasing doses at 2–3 hour intervals while monitoring spirometric function, may be undertaken to confirm sensitivity and repetitively to desensitize a patient who has need to take NSAID. Desensitization followed by continued daily NSAID treatment reduces the respiratory disease in some patients but not of sufficient degree to ordinarily warrant such treatment.

The mechanism of the sensitivity reaction to NSAID is not completely understood. IgE or an immunologic reaction has not been found; mast cell mediators (histamine, neutrophil chemotactic factor) and complement activation are not consistently associated with the reaction. There may be a genetic predisposition/marker, involvement of platelet, contact-kinin or arachidonate metabolite mediator or other mechanism; none has yet been confirmed.

The "intrinsic" abnormalities underlying asthma are likely multiple with one or more operative in an individual patient. Possibilities include:

1. immunologic dysfunction such as IgE mediated immediate and late reaction to aeroallergens or microbes (*Aspergillus fumigatus,* for example);

2. mast cell dysfunction with 'easy releasability' as to osmotic, chemical or mechanical stimuli;
3. enzyme dysfunction – metabolic error;
4. autonomic imbalance – afferent, central synaptic, efferent, receptor, secretory or contractile responses;
5. psychophysiologic reactions.

Asthma – The Syndrome

To the lay person, asthma means labored breathing accompanied by wheezing, by a sense of chest constriction, and often by attacks of coughing or gasping caused by conditions that interfere with the normal inflow and outflow of air in the lungs (according to Webster's Third New International Dictionary). In the scientific sense, asthma has been defined as a disease (more correctly, a syndrome – a commonly occurring collection of symptoms and signs) characterized by an increased responsiveness of the trachea and bronchi to various stimuli and manifested by a widespread narrowing of the airways that changes in severity either spontaneously or as a result of therapy (American Thoracic Society [2]). Several subsequent attempts to update the scientific definition of asthma have not yielded consensus.

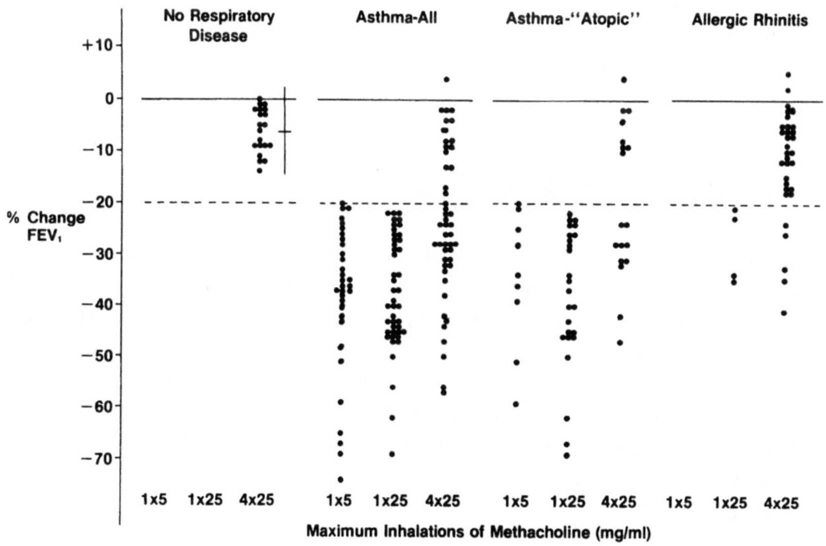

Fig. 1. Percent change in 1-s forced expiratory volume (FEV_1) after successive inhalations of methacholine in 20 adult subjects without a history of respiratory disease; 124 patients with a history of cardinal symptoms of asthma of all varieties but without spirometric evidence of airways obstruction at the time of study; 52 of the asthmatics had "atopic" asthma associated with specific IgE antibodies to aeroallergens; and 36 subjects with rhinitis associated with specific IgE antibodies but without history of spirometric evidence of asthma

The increased responsiveness of the bronchi can be documented and the diagnosis confirmed by spirometric measurements of bronchodilitation following inhalations of β-adrenergic drug or bronchoconstriction following inhalations of methacholine or histamine or, though less universally, exercise [28]. When the asthmatic patient has attacks precipitated by exposures to aeroallergens to which he has IgE antibodies, the asthma may be termed "allergic," "atopic," or "extrinsic"; however, most such patients also have the bronchospasticity "intrinsic" to the disease (Fig. 1) [19].

Initiating, Aggravating, and Perpetuating Factors

In the evaluation and management of the individual asthmatic patient, it is important for the physician to recognize and treat or alter the initiating, aggravating, and perpetuating factors that contribute to the asthma [20]. These may include immediate and late hypersensitivity (IgE-mediated) reactions, aeroirritant exposures, exercise, respiratory infection, sensitivity to aspirin or other chemicals, meteorologic changes, psychological factors, occupational exposures and associated disorders such as chronic bronchitis, emphysema, heart failure, gastroesophageal reflux, or hyperthyroidism.

To the investigator, each of these factors offers a challenge to unfold the precise cells, mediators, and mechanisms which lead to the airways' obstruction. Some combination of inflammatory cell (especially mast cell and eosinophil) activation, autonomic-psychological dysfunction and/or mucous accumulation are present in all asthmatic patients.

Aspirin Sensitivity in Asthma

Aspirin has been used for over 80 years as an anti-inflammatory, antipyretic, and analgesic agent, and more recently as a platelet-inhibiting agent to prevent thrombotic and embolic disease. The average per capita consumption is more than 60 5-grain tablets per year. Asthmatic reaction to aspirin was first reported in 1911; the intervening history of observations on idiosyncratic reactions to aspirin is summarized by VanArsdel [38]. Idiosyncratic reaction to aspirin may be manifested by either flare of respiratory disease or urticaria-angioedema; only very few individuals have been reported to have both respiratory and cutaneous response to aspirin.

The Typical Aspirin-Sensitive Respiratory Syndrome

The typical aspirin-sensitive syndrome [21] primarily affects adults, though onset may be in childhood. The disease evolves over decades and ordinarily begins with a perennial vasomotor-irritant aggravated type of rhinitis, though a third of these patients also have IgE-mediated cutaneous reactions to aeroallergen extracts. Next an eosinophilic hyperplastic rhinosinusitis with nasal polyps ensues, and, not infrequently, this is complicated by boüts of purulent bacterial sinusitis. Intrinsic asthma then appears and progresses to require treatment with systemic steroids. The earmark of aspirin sensitivity is the appearance of facial or generalized flush, ocular and nasal congestion, and acute, often severe, asthmatic attack within one-half to several hours after ingesting an ordinary dose of aspirin or aspirin-like drug. Even though the patient soon learns to avoid aspirin and similar drugs, the underlying respiratory disease continues.

Prevalence

The prevalence of aspirin sensitivity in patients with asthma varies according to the population studied and the methods used to detect the sensitivity. Giraldo et al. [10] found that 3%–5% of hospitalized asthmatic patients had a history of reaction to aspirin. At Scripps Clinic, a secondary and tertiary medical center, we found that about 10% of our asthmatic population were aspirin sensitive [22]. At the National Jewish Hospital, where an even more highly selected group of severely asthmatic patients were studied, 19% were found by oral challenges to have idiosyncratic reaction to aspirin [29]. Among asthmatic patients with pansinusitis and nasal polyps, 30%–40% are aspirin sensitive [32].

Cross-Sensitivity with Aspirin-Like Drugs

The Nobel Prize in Medicine in 1982 was awarded to Dr. John Vane, Dr. Bengt Samuelsson, and Dr. Sune Bergstrom for their studies of metabolites of arachidonic acid (Fig. 2). Dr. Vane identified a mechanism of action of aspirin to be the inhibition of prostaglandin synthesis from the cyclooxygenase pathway of arachidonate metabolism. Other nonsteroidal anti-inflammatory drugs which inhibit this pathway also can provoke a respiratory reaction in aspirin-sensitive asthmatic subjects. As shown in Table 1, cross-sensitivity correlated with the effectiveness of cyclooxygenase inhibition.

Variability in Expression

When we studied 50 consecutive asthmatic patients who had a history of aspirin sensitivity by cautious oral challenges with aspirin, we found a spectrum of reactions [25]. The majority of these patients experienced a typical ocular, nasal, and asthmatic response; however, 12% had a nasal-ocular response with-

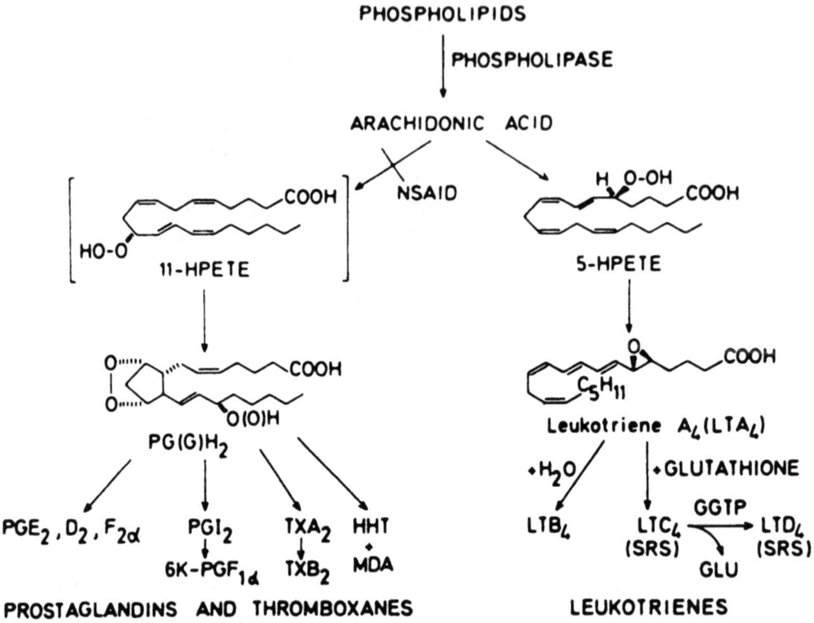

Fig. 2. Phospholipid-arachidonate metabolic pathways of presumed relevance to aspirin sensitivity in asthma; nonsteroidal anti-inflammatory drugs (NSAIDs) block cyclo-oxygenase pathways

Table 1. Cross-sensitivity between aspirin and other nonsteroidal anti-inflammatory drugs

Cyclooxygenase inhibition	Prevalence of cross-sensitivity with aspirin
Inhibitors	
Indomethacin (Indocin)	High – 90%
Fenoprofen (Nalfon)	
Naproxen (Anaprox, Naprosyn)	
Ibuprofen (Advil, Motrin, Rufen)	
Mefenamic acid (Ponstel)	
Sulindac (Clinoril)	
Meclofenamate (Meclomen)	
Tolmetin (Tolectin)	
Piroxicam (Feldene)	
Partial inhibitors	
Aminopyrine (Pyramidon)	Occasional
Oxphenbutazone (Oxalid, Tandearil)	
Phenylbutazone (Butazolidin)	
Non-inhibitors	
Sodium salicylate	Isolated case reports
Choline salicylate	
Salicylamide	
Propoxyphene	
Acetaminophen	

out definite asthmatic reaction, and 16% had no adverse reaction whatsoever. Further, in several patients in whom we repeated the aspirin challenges, there was variation of an individual's response, including one patient challenged on four occasions over a 9-year interval who had typical ocular, nasal, and asthmatic reactions following the first two challenges, no reaction following the third, and only a nasal response following the fourth.

Avoidance

As aspirin sensitivity may occur in up to 15% of asthmatic patients, but appears only after years of progression of the respiratory disorder and varies in its expression, and since the vast majority of asthmatic patients can avoid aspirin and aspirin-like drugs, the prudent approach to all asthmatic patients is to advise them to avoid these drugs by substituting acetaminophen. For the occasional patient with aspirin-sensitive respiratory disease who also has vascular disease requiring an inhibitor of platelet aggregation/embolization or musculorheumatic disease that is inadequately responsive to non-aspirin-like drugs, desensitization with oral challenges with incremental doses of aspirin or aspirin-like drugs, followed by at least daily administration of the drug, can be accomplished [24].

Challenges – Desensitization with Aspirin

Challenges/desensitizations must be performed using a number of safety practices. At Scripps Clinic, we perform challenges within the hospital, where emergency resuscitative equipment, an intensive care unit, and trained personnel are readily available. Challenges are always started in the morning so that optimal time and treatment are available to ensure ease of recovery from reaction. Patients are challenged at a time when their asthma is in remission; if need be, we administer additional corticosteroid for several days prior to challenge to ensure that there is full remission. In addition, to proceed with the challenge, the patient must have a 1-s forced expiratory volume (FEV_1) greater than 70% of predicted or his best previously recorded, and, in absolute numbers, this must be greater than 1.5 liters. We observe our patients not only for asthmatic but also for ocular and nasal responses.

Asthmatic patients who have a history of severe reaction to aspirin are challenged/desensitized over at least a 2-day interval with aspirin given at 3-h intervals, beginning with a dose of 3 mg followed by 30, 60, and 100 mg, and then, on the 2nd day, 150, 325, and 650 mg of aspirin. For patients who do not have a history of aspirin sensitivity, but also have not taken aspirin in recent months, a 1-day challenge with doses of 30, 60, 100, 325, and 650 mg at 2-h intervals can be initiated. If there is a fall in FEV_1 greater than 25% from baseline, the challenge is always suspended and inhalations of sympathomimetic and additional doses of corticosteroid and aminophylline administered. The challenge is resumed the following morning (if criteria are met), beginning with the dose which provoked reaction on the previous day. Up to ten or more provoked asthmatic attacks may be required before a desensitized state is achieved.

Sensitization may recur from 1 to 5 days after interruption of therapy; for this reason it is imperative that the patient continue taking the aspirin or aspirin-like drug on a daily basis if continuous desensitization is the objective.

We followed up two patients who had undergone aspirin desensitization and continued taking daily aspirin treatment and found them to have improvement in their respiratory disease and less need for steroid treatment [33]. We subsequently studied the efficacy of treatment with aspirin in 25 aspirin-sensitive asthmatic patients in a 7-month, randomized, placebo-controlled, double-blind, cross-over trial [34]. A significant improvement in rhinosinusitis occurred in about two-thirds of the patients during aspirin maintenance compared with the placebo, and a majority of the patients had improvement in their asthma, though not reaching statistical significance. A few of the patients had even greater respiratory symptoms while taking aspirin compared with the placebo. We are continuing investigative studies aimed at better identifying those subsets of aspirin-sensitive patients who might benefit from this treatment; we do not ordinarily recommend this treatment for aspirin-sensitive patients seen at the Clinic.

Mechanisms

The mechanism(s) underlying sensitivity to aspirin has not been identified. There is a preliminary report suggesting DRQ/HLA genetic association [36]. Thus far, there have been mostly negative results from tests of hypotheses for aspirin sensitivity. IgE antibodies or an other immunologic response to aspirin have not been identified. There does not appear to be an imbalance of the bronchodilating PGE_2 or bronchoconstricting PGF_2 following aspirin ingestion. Benoxaprofen, a nonsteroidal anti-inflammatory drug which may inhibit the lipoxygenase pathway of arachidonate metabolism, does not block the aspirin reaction. Mast cell mediators (histamine, neutrophil chemotactic factor, PGD_2), activation of complement, and release of platelet factor 4 have not consistently been measured in association with the aspirin-sensitive response [12, 26]. Evidence for abnormal platelet activation by aspirin has been reported by one group of investigators [1]. There may be activation of the contact-kinin system as evidenced by reduced in vitro bradykinin-releasable high molecular weight kininogen, endogenous heparin release, and enhanced in vitro stimulated appearance of kallikrein [17]. Whatever the mechanism, its identification offers promise of greater understanding of intrinsic asthma.

New Trends in Asthma

Mortality

Mortality rates for asthma in the United Kingdom have remained constant [30] and those in the United States appear to have risen during the 1980s [27]. Severe sudden attacks account for a significant proportion of the deaths and occur in individuals who have previously had such attacks. Psychological factors were prominent in a group of children who died of asthma [35]. Mortality from asthma persists despite or conceivably because of intensified applications of modern pharmaceuticals.

Etiology

The etiology of the bronchial hyperreactivity, the sine qua non of asthma remains uncertain in the sense of a single mechanistic pathway common to all with the clinical syndrome. Several associations have been noted.

Fresh bronchial biopsies taken from asthmatic patients at carinal, lobar, and lobular levels and studied by electron microscopy showed epithelial destruction, especially of ciliated cells, prominent enough to expose mast cells and epithelial nerves to immunologic and irritant stimuli [16].

About one-fourth of "hay fever" patients show bronchial reactivity to methacholine, even in the absence of clinical asthma (Fig. 1) [19]. Bronchial hyperreactivity increases transiently during the pollenating season or following allergen inhalation challenge in aeroallergen-sensitive asthmatic patients [8] and for years in people with occupational asthma due to western red cedar [7]. Reduction of bronchial hyperreactivity has been noted during prolonged avoidance of dust mites in asthmatic patients allergic to mites [23].

The hypothesis that IgE-mediated immediate and especially late asthmatic responses to allergen with generation of neutrophilic and eosinophilic inflammation produces or at least compounds bronchial hyperreactivity derives from these and other observations [3, 8, 15].

Viral infection, especially respiratory syncytial virus bronchiolitis, and even viral immunization have been associated with asthma and bronchial hyperreactivity [6, 39, 40], as has ozone exposure in healthy subjects [5].

These various associations need not prove mutually exclusive nor commonly linked to ultimately account for the bronchial hyperreactivity of asthma.

Exercise-Provoked Bronchospasm

It is likely that exercise-provoked bronchospasm is dependent upon an intrabronchial hyperosmotic state brought on by hyperventilation – heat exchange-facilitated water loss, resultant epithelial injury, and/or mast cell mediator release and the hyperresponsive asthmatic state [9, 11].

Sulfur Dioxide

Sulfur dioxide (SO_2) is a common fossil fuel air pollutant; at a concentration of 0.5 parts per million, within the range commonly experienced in air pollution episodes, SO_2 facilitates bronchoconstriction in asthmatic subjects during exercise [4]. SO_2 and a variety of sulfiting agents, including potassium metabisulfite ($K_2S_2O_5$), have been used for centuries as preservatives, selective inhibitors of microorganisms in the fermenting of beverages, and inhibitors of discoloration during the preparation, distribution, and storage of foods. The estimated consumption of sulfites in U.S. diets is 2–3 mg per day in the home, 5–10 mg/30 ml of beer or wine consumed, and 25–100 mg per restaurant meal. Foods and beverages commonly preserved with SO_2 and/or sulfites are listed in Table 2.

Table 2. Foods and beverages commonly preserved with sulfur dioxide and/or sulfites

Dried and packaged fruits and beverages
Beers, wines, and other fermented beverages
Salads including all ingredients (salad bars)
Avocado – guacamole and other dips
Potatoes – chips, fries, dehydrated
Cider and wine vinegars, pickled vegetables
Shrimp and other seafoods
Processed, preserved, "ready to eat" foods and beverages

There are several reports in recent years of acute severe choking within minutes of ingesting as little as 5 mg of $K_2S_2O_5$ [31], inhalation of bronchodilator, and intravenous injection of metachlopramide preserved with sulfite [37].

Sulfites are in equilibrium with SO_2 so that at the acid pH of saliva or gastric juice, ingested sulfites generate SO_2 gas which probably acts as an irritant to the hyperresponsive airway. Sulfites are ordinarily oxidized to sulfites, a reaction catalyzed by the enzyme sulfite oxidase; heterozygous deficiency of this enzyme may account for the exquisite sensitivity to ingested sulfites found in a few asthmatic patients [13].

Psychological Factors

Psychological factors affect asthma in some patients, especially those with chronic severe disease as measured by intensity of prescribed medications, length of hospitalizations [14], and death [35]. Patients with severe disease are more frequently characterized by response styles involving disregard of breathing difficulties and/or helplessness in coping with distress, and histrionic and somatization dynamics [18]. Self-monitoring of pulmonary function and medication usage, an aerobic conditioning program, and/or behaviorally oriented psychotherapy in addition to conventional antiasthma treatments may benefit these patients.

References

1. Ameisen JC, Joseph M, Tonnel AB et al. (1985) Specific abnormal platelet activation in aspirin sensitive asthma. J Allergy Clin Immunol 75:123
2. American Thoracic Society (1965) Chronic bronchitis, asthma and pulmonary emphysema: a statement by the committee on diagnostic standards for nontuberculous respiratory diseases. Am Rev Resp Dis 85:762–8
3. Atkins PC, Zweiman B (1985) Bronchial asthma – what are those inflammatory cells doing there anyway? J Allergy Clin Immunol 75:239–41
4. Bethel RA, Epstein J, Sheppard D et al. (1983) Sulfur dioxide induced bronchosensitization in free breathing, exercising, asthmatic subjects. Am Rev Resp Dis 128:987–90
5. Boushey HA, Holtzman MJ (1985) Experimental airway inflammation and hyperreactivity. Searching for cells and mediators. Am Rev Resp Dis 131:312–3
6. Busse WW (1985) The precipitation of asthma by upper respiratory infections. Chest 87:44S–8S
7. Chan Yeung M (1982) Immunologic and non-immunologic mechanisms in asthma due to western red cedar (*Thuja plicata*). J Allergy Clin Immunol 70:32–7
8. Cockroft DW, Ruffin RE, Dolovich J, Hargreave FE (1977) Allergen-induced increases in non-allergic bronchial reactivity. Clin Allergy 7:503–13
9. Eggleston PA, Kagey-Sobotka A, Schleimer RP, Lichtenstein LM (1984) Interaction between hyperosmolar and IgE mediated histamine release from basophils and mast cells. Am Rev Resp Dis 130:86–91
10. Giraldo B, Blumenthal MN, Spink WN (1969) Aspirin intolerance and asthma. Ann Intern Med 71:479–96
11. Hahn A, Anderson SD, Moton AR et al. (1984) A reinterpretation of the effect of temperature and water content on the inspired air in exercise-induced asthma. Am Rev Resp Dis 130:575–9
12. Hollingsworth HM, Center DM (1985) Neutrophil chemotactic factor in aspirin induced bronchospasm. Chest 87:1675–85
13. Jacobsen DW, Simon RA, Singth MA (1984) Sulfite oxidase deficiency and cobalamin protection in sulfite-sensitive asthmatics. J Allergy Clin Immunol 73:135
14. Jones NF, Kinsman RA, Dirkes JF et al. (1979) Psychological contributions to chronicity in asthma: patient response styles influencing medical treatment and its outcome. Med Care 17:1103–18
15. Kaliner MM (1984) Hypotheses on the contribution of late-phase allergic responses to the understanding and treatment of allergic diseases. J Allergy Clin Immunol 73:312–5
16. Laitinen LA, Heino M, Laitinen A et al. (1985) Damage of the airway epithelial and bronchial reactivity in patients with asthma. Am Rev Resp Dis 131:599–606
17. Lasser EC, Lang JH, Curd JG et al. (1983) The plasma contact system in asthma. J Allergy Clin Immunol 72:83–8
18. Mathison DA, Jacobsen LD (1985) Psychomaintenance of asthma: Scripps Clinic experiences. International congress of allergology and clinical immunology (abstract). Ann Allergy 55:339
19. Mathison DA, Stevenson DD, Tan EM, Vaughan JH (1973a) Methacholine challenge and the diagnosis of bronchial asthma. J Allergy Clin Immunol 51:94

20. Mathison DA, Stevenson DD, Tan EM, Vaughan JH (1973b) Clinical profiles of bronchial asthma. JAMA 224:1134–9
21. Mathison DA, Stevenson DD, Simon RA (1984) Precipitating factors in asthma: aspirin, sulfites and other drugs and chemicals. Chest 87:50S–4S
22. McDonald JR, Mathison DA, Stevenson DD (1972) Aspirin intolerance in asthma. J Allergy Clin Immunol 50:198–209
23. Platts-Mills TA, Mitchell EB, Noch P et al. (1982) Reduction of bronchial hyperreactivity during prolonged allergen avoidance. Lancet 1:675–9
24. Pleskow WW, Stevenson DD, Mathison DA et al. (1982) Aspirin desensitization in aspirin-sensitive asthmatic patients. J Allergy Clin Immunol 69:11–9
25. Pleskow WW, Stevenson DD, Mathison DA et al. (1983) Aspirin sensitive rhinosinusitis/asthma: spectrum of adverse reactions to aspirin. J Allergy Clin Immunol 73:574–9
26. Simon R, Pleskow W, Kaliner M et al. (1983) Plasma mediator studies in aspirin sensitive asthma. J Allergy Clin Immunol 71:146
27. Sly RM (1984) Increases in death from asthma. Ann Allergy 53:20–5
28. Spector S (1983) Provocative challenge procedures: bronchial, oral, nasal and exercise. CRC Press, Boca Raton, Florida
29. Spector SL, Wangaard CH, Farr RS (1979) Aspirin and concomitant sensitivities in adult asthmatic patients. J Allergy Clin Immunol 64:500–6
30. Stableforth D (1983) Death from asthma. Thorax 38:801–5
31. Stevenson DD, Simon RA (1981) Sensitivity to metabisulfites in asthmatic subjects. J Allergy Clin Immunol 68:28–32
32. Stevenson DD, Mathison DA, Tan EM, Vaughan JH (1976) Provoking factors in bronchial asthma. Arch Intern Med 135:77–83
33. Stevenson DD, Simon RA, Mathison DA (1980) Aspirin sensitive asthma: tolerance to aspirin after oral aspirin challenges. J Allergy Clin Immunol 66:82–8
34. Stevenson DD, Pleskow WW, Simon RA, Mathison DA et al. (1984) Aspirin sensitive rhinosinusitis-asthma: a double-blind crossover study of treatment with aspirin. J Allergy Clin Immunol 73:500–7
35. Strunk RC, Mrazek DA, Wolfson F et al. (1985) Physiologic and psychological characteristics associated with deaths due to asthma in childhood. JAMA 254:1193–1198
36. Thomas PS, Mullarkey MF, Webb DR et al. (1985) Genetic markers in aspirin-sensitive asthma. J Allergy Clin Immunol 75:156
37. Twarog FJ, Laung DYM (1982) Anaphylaxis to a component of isoetharine (sodium bisulfite). JAMA 248:2030–2
38. VanArsdel PP (1984) Aspirin idiosyncracy and tolerance. J Allergy Clin Immunol 72:431–4
39. Weiss ST, Tager IB, Munoz A, Speizer FE (1985) The relationship of respiratory infections in early childhood to the occurrence of increased levels of bronchial responsiveness and atopy. Am Rev Resp Dis 131:573–8
40. Welliver RC, Wong DT, Sun M et al. (1981) The development of respiratory syncytial virus-specific IgE and the release of histamine in nasopharyngeal secretions after infection. N Engl J Med 305:841–6

Isocyanate-Induced Asthma

X. Baur

Pneumologische Abteilung der I. Medizinischen Klinik, Klinikum Grosshadern, Ludwig-Maximilians-Universität München, 8000 Munich 70, Federal Republic of Germany

Abstract

Diisocyanates with the general formula $R(-N=C=O)_2$ play an important role in modern industry and are used for production of a great variety of polyurethane materials. It is thought that 5% of the 1 million workers being regularly exposed to isocyanate vapors and aerosols develop acute or chronic respiratory diseases. The underlying mechanisms depend on the concentrations and consist of:

a) toxic effects at high air concentrations,
b) IgE-mediated hypersensitivity,
c) pharmacologic reactions.

Toxic lesions on the mucosa of the respiratory tree are known from animal exposure tests at isocyanate concentrations of $\geq$ 1 ppm. Corresponding diseases can be observed in humans who have been involved in accidents, e.g. spilling of isocyanates.

According to immunologic investigations of our group, 14% of symptomatic isocyanate workers (35/247) possess IgE antibodies to isocyanate compounds. Intracutaneous skin tests with isocyanate-albumin conjugates produced typical immediate wheal and flare reactions in RAST-positive workers. RAST-inhibition studies demonstrated various degrees of cross-reactivity between aromatic and aliphatic isocyanates. In addition, there is evidence for formation of new antigenic determinants upon reaction of inhaled isocyanates with human proteins.

By means of in-vitro assays we were able to demonstrate potent inhibition of human erythrocyte cholinesterase by industrially used diisocyanates. This inhibition is a very fast and long-lasting process. We believe that inhibition of cholinesterase and the consequent increase of the bronchoconstrictor acetylcholine are implicated in the pathogenesis of asthmatic disease following exposure to higher concentrations of isocyanates.

In conclusion, there is evidence which indicates that isocyanates induce obstructive pulmonary disease due to different pathophysiologic mechanisms. Isocyanate air concentrations at workplaces should be maintained at low levels, which is possible by means of modern processing and effective ventilation systems. Workers with preexisting bronchial asthma or in whom pulmonary symptoms are observed should be protected from exposure to isocyanates in order to prevent chronic illness.

Introduction

Isocyanates are nowadays the most important low molecular weight chemicals associated with occupational asthma. Their characteristic residue is composed of one nitrogen atom, one carbon atom, and one oxygen atom, connected by two double bonds. Due to these double bonds, isocyanates behave as highly reactive substances and will react immediately upon contact with active hydrogen atoms as found in hydroxy, sulfhydryl, or amino groups.

Diisocyanates and their prepolymers are extensively used in modern industry and trade handicraft. Upon reaction with diols or polyols, a large variety of polyurethanes with different properties can be obtained, e.g., smooth or rigid foams with more or less elasticity.

Production and processing of isocyanates is associated with a certain degree of uptake through inhalation; this is especially the case with the widely used aromatic TDI, because of the relatively high steam pressure. Therefore, in several countries TDI has now been replaced in foam production by another aromatic diisocyanate, MDI, which has a much lower steam pressure. However, what is not recognized by most authorities is that this compound forms a considerable amount of aerosol which is inadequately monitored by routine isocyanate procedures.

The aliphatic diisocyanate HDI is predominantly used for varnishes, e.g., in the automobile and aircraft industries. Methyl isocyanate, which caused the great disaster in Bhopal, India, is an important precursor of insecticides (Fig. 1).

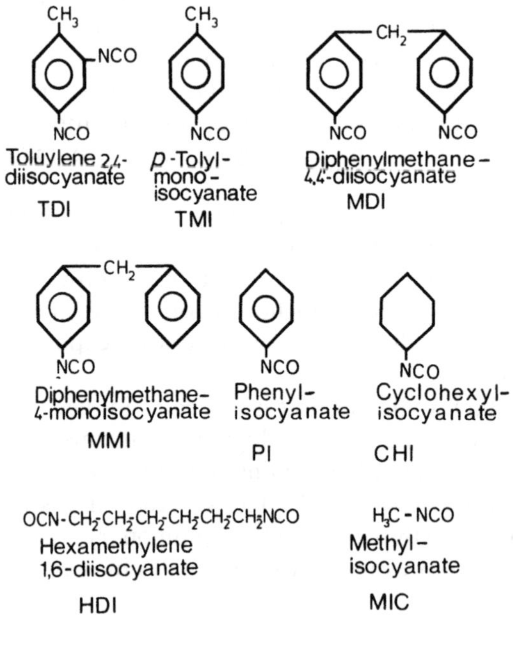

Fig. 1. Chemical formulas of some isocyanates and their derivatives

Shortly after the commencement of industrial production of isocyanates in the late 1930s, it became evident that some of the exposed workers developed asthmatic diseases. Investigations by others as well as by our group have shown the incidence of symptoms to vary greatly between different firms, depending predominantly on the air concentrations at workplaces. On average, approximately 5% of the workers are affected.

For many years the underlying pathogenetic mechanisms remained unknown. In 1978 Karol et al. [1] were the first to detect isocyanate-specific IgE antibodies. In the following years, a great controversy arose concerning the incidence and clinical role of such antibodies.

Results of Clinical and Immunological Studies

We have investigated more than 750 isocyanate workers using lung function tests, skin tests, measurement of specific IgE antibodies by RAST, and inhalation challenges. As can be seen from Table 1, 247 persons were symptomatic. Predominant clinical diagnoses were bronchial asthma, chronic obstructive pulmonary disease, nonobstructive bronchitis, rhinitis, and conjunctivitis. However, immediate-type skin responses, eczema, fever, and symptoms coincident with hypersensitivity pneumonitis could also be observed.

The patterns of the asthmatic responses included immediate and late reactions. In addition, dual as well as prolonged asthmatic reactions could be observed. In one case, inhalation challenge by MDI showed a rare combination of an immediate asthmatic response as indicated by decreases in FEV_1 and specific airway conductance, followed by typical signs of hypersensitivity pneumonitis such as decreases in diffusing capacity and vital capacity, increases of blood leukocytes up to $19\,000/mm^3$, and a rise in temperature up to 39° C; this man was engaged in spraying a mixture of an isocyanate (MDI) and polyol to produce a polyurethane foam for use as a packing material.

RAST studies were performed with a panel of different isocyanates bound to human serum albumin, HSA, in our laboratory. These investigations showed that 15% of the symptomatic group, but only 0.3% of the asymptomatic group, had specific IgE antibodies. Most of the RAST-positive symptomatic workers

Table 1. Frequencies of clinical diagnoses in 247 symptomatic isocyanate workers

Bronchial asthma	153 (62%)
COPD	26 (11%)
Nonobstructive bronchitis	43 (17%)
Rhinitis	42 (17%)
Conjunctivitis	26 (11%)
Urticaria, erythema, eczema	12 (5%)
Fever	7 (2%)
Hypersensitivity pneumonitis	4 (2%)

showed reactivity with several of the isocyanate compounds. Some workers even had antibodies against all investigated isocyanate conjugates.

In our studies, the results of RAST were found to depend on several characteristics of the isocyanate carrier conjugate used: for instance, we found that the molar ratio of isocyanates to carrier may be of great importance. We have used different methods for preparation of TDI-HSA and found that conjugates containing 20–25 mol isocyanate/mole protein are superior to those containing greater amounts of the hapten (40–50 mol/mole). Therefore, in our opinion it is always necessary to indicate the chemical composition of the RAST antigens used. In addition, nearly all RAST-positive persons exhibit immediate-type skin test responses to the same compounds, whereas RAST-negative workers as well as control persons have negative skin tests [2].

Further evidence for immunological sensitization is the induction of rhinitis and asthmatic reactions following inhalation of a low amount of albumin-bound isocyanates [2]. In addition, inhalation challenges by native isocyanates exhibit low bronchial threshold concentrations in persons with positive skin test and RAST results; that means threshold concentrations far below the threshold limit value of 0.01 ppm.

Immunological Cross-reactivity Between Different Isocyanate Compounds and Evidence for New Antigenic Determinants

One interesting aspect of the IgE responses to isocyanates is the high degree of immunological cross-reactivity between different isocyanate compounds, even among aliphatic and aromatic ones [3]. In RAST inhibition experiments, sera of sensitized patients were preincubated with different isocyanate conjugates. Afterwards, the sera were tested for their reactivity with TDI-HSA. The reduction in the RAST value due to preincubation of the sera correlated with the degree of reactivity of IgE antibodies both with the inhibitor used for preincubation and with the solid phase antigen. Figure 2a demonstrates a dose-dependent inhibition of IgE binding to TDI-HSA by various isocyanate conjugates; this took place at low concentrations, as is typical for immunological cross-reactivity. There was no inhibition by the carrier molecule HSA or isocyanates bound to nonhuman proteins, such as ovalbumin in this case.

It should be mentioned, however, that the degree of individual cross-reactivity differs from one patient to another. As an example, only weak cross-reactivity between some isocyanate compounds, indicated by weaker inhibition, was observed in worker no. 2 (Fig. 2b). Another interesting aspect in this case was the rare finding of a certain degree of antigenicity of TDI bound to a nonhuman protein, ovalbumin. Recent studies by our group demonstrate that immunological cross-reactivity also exists between albumin-bound methyl isocyanate, the chemical which caused the tragedy of Bhopal, and the diisocyanate HDI, as can be seen in Figs. 2c, d.

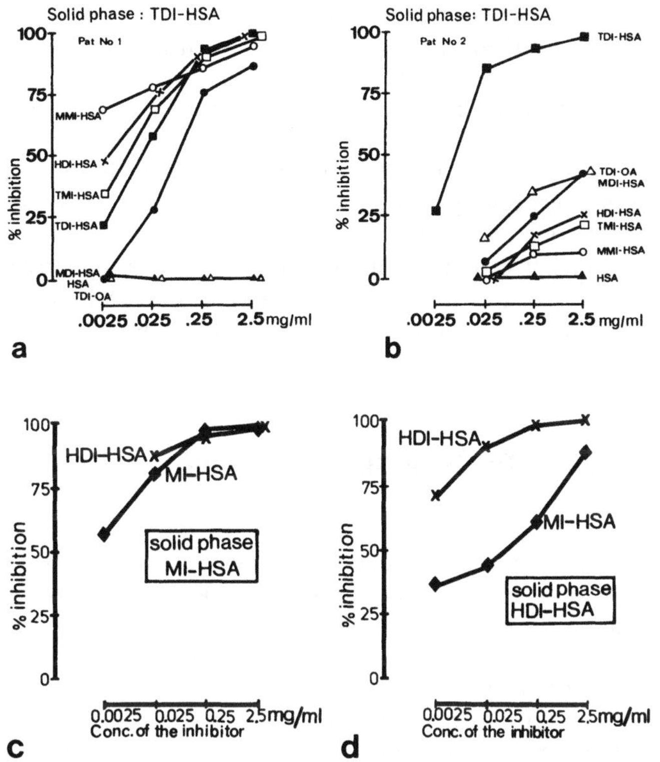

Fig. 2a–d. RAST inhibition experiments using different isocyanate-albumin conjugates

Our results suggest the involvement of various new antigenic determinants, which include parts of the isocyanate molecules, altered human protein structures, and especially the bond regions between the two moieties. At least some isocyanates are too small to form complete antigenic determinants. However, when bound to a carrier molecule, for example to albumin molecules which are available in the bronchial fluid, new antigenic determinants may arise. These can be composed mainly of:

1. The binding region of the two molecules. This is indicated by immunological cross-reactivity between HSA-bound isocyanates with different residues.
2. Parts of the isocyanates on the one hand and auxiliary groups, that means free side chains of the protein carrier, on the other, including or not including the binding region.
3. Altered structures of the carrier molecule.

The results of our RAST studies and RAST inhibition experiments provide evidence for antibodies with different specificities which may react with various antigenic determinants in one or in different individuals. For example, antibodies directed against the binding region of the two molecules are thought to be responsible for cross-reactivity between compounds containing different isocyanates or different carriers. As opposed to this, in other cases immunological cross-reactivity occurs only between isocyanate conjugates with different carriers, not between those with different isocyanate residues, because the latter are involved in antibody binding. Such antibodies may be the reason for the absence or weakness of immunological cross-reactivity in some patients.

Isocyanates may also react with components in surface membranes or parenchymal cells and behave as haptens or as parts of antigenic determinants or as new antigenic determinants similar to those mentioned. Binding of antibodies, especially of the IgG class, can induce activation of the complement system, thus inducing cytotoxic lesions.

Further evidence for immunological cross-reactivity between different isocyanates comes from clinical studies showing hypersensitivity reactions upon exposure to various of these compounds in many symptomatic workers.

Evidence for Nonimmunological Responses to Isocyanates

Evidence for nonimmunological responses comes from provocation tests performed on 13 previously nonexposed asthmatics. We were able to demonstrate that exposure to 0.02 ppm of TDI for up to 30 min resulted in an increase in airway resistance of at least 50% in 8 of these 13 workers, and an increase of at least 100% in 3 workers.

In addition to induction of asthmatic reactions in previously nonexposed asthmatics, nonimmediate reactions such as late onset asthma or prolonged bronchial obstruction in symptomatic isocyanate workers indicate the importance of nonimmunological mechanisms by isocyanate vapors.

Possible Biochemical/Pharmacological Effects of Isocyanates

Isocyanates may evoke biochemical/pharmacological effects. We have also studied in some detail the in vitro effects of three industrially used diisocyanates on human erythrocyte acetylcholinesterase. The inhibition potency was found to be in the order HDI, TDI, MDI. This inhibition is a very fast process which runs to completion in less than 1 min. Furthermore, the final spontaneous reactivation percentages of HDI-, MDI-, and TDI-inhibited enzyme were only in the ranges of 30%, 40%, and 90% respectively.

This persisting inhibition of acetylcholinesterase and its subsequent limited spontaneous reactivation may be implicated in the acute and chronic effects of isocyanate vapors and aerosols on lung function, due to local accumulation of the bronchoconstrictor acetylcholine. The daily delivery of isocyanates into the lungs may be faster than the rate of spontaneous reactivation. This interpretation seems to be supported by the clinical observation that in many cases several days' exposure to isocyanates is necessary for the appearance of complaints. On the other hand, in the case of immunological sensitization, onset of respiratory symptoms should take place immediately upon reexposure.

In vitro studies on possible further physiological mechanisms of isocyanates were carried out by some other investigators. McKay et al. [4] demonstrated no effect of isocyanates on tracheal smooth muscles in response to isoproterenol, which indicates no specific influence on β-adrenergic receptors as suggested by some other authors. On the other hand, cholinergic effects could be established, insofar as tracheal smooth muscle strips from TDI-exposed animals were significantly more responsive to carbachol than were those from control animals.

Concluding Remarks

There is no doubt that isocyanates induce asthmatic diseases via IgE-mediated sensitization in a subgroup of exposed workers. However, nonspecific toxic and irritative effects as well as biochemical/pharmacological reactions have to be taken into consideration, especially when air concentrations are high.

Our present conclusions relating to the effects of different isocyanate air concentrations on the bronchopulmonary system are as follows:

- Immunological responses occur at all concentrations.
- Biochemical/pharmacological effects begin at higher concentrations and can be expected to be related in some degree to inhaled amounts.
- Toxic effects are observed at very high concentrations, markedly above the threshold limit values, and show a dose-related response.

The predominant type of reaction may depend on the nature of the chemical, the concentration to which the patient is exposed, and host-specific factors; e.g., high air concentrations of isocyanates are known to cause irritative effects in the majority of exposed people. Host-specific factors are especially important for immunological response, which can be observed only in a small proportion of the workers after a latent period and usually at extremely low levels of the causative agents. Until now, no correlation between atopy and susceptibility to these substances could be found.

References

1. Karol MH, Ioset MH, Alarie YC (1978) Tolyl-specific IgE antibodies in workers with hypersensitivity to toluene diisocyanate. Am Ind Hyg Assoc J 39:454
2. Baur X, Dewair M, Fruhmann G (1984) Detection of immunologically sensitized isocyanate workers by RAST and intracutaneous skin tests. J Allergy Clin Immunol 73:610–618
3. Baur X (1983) Immunologic cross-reactivity between different albumin-bound isocyanates. J Allergy Clin Immunol 71:197–205
4. McKay R, Brooks S, Johnson C (1981) Mechanism to explain isocyanate-induced asthma: abnormality of beta-adrenergic receptors. Chest 80 [Suppl]:61

Contact Allergy

Molecular Recognition in Allergic Contact Dermatitis

C. Benezra

Laboratoire de Dermatochimie, Associé au CNRS, Université Louis Pasteur, Clinique Dermatologique, CHU, F-67091 Strasbourg, France

Abstract

Most of contact sensitizers are *electrophiles,* i.e. they are electron-deficient and able to accept electrons from skin protein *nucleophilic* (electron-rich) groups such as NH_2, SH etc., thus forming a strong *covalent* bond. In order to understand the mechanism of Allergic Contact Dermatitis (ACD), we have synthesized *models* of plant allergens and studied their sensitizing power in guinea-pigs. These molecules included α-methylene-γ-butyrolactones (models of natural sesquiterpene lactones, and of tulipalins A and B), with and without a β-hydroxy substituents, allyldisulfides (from garlic), long chains pyrocatechols and 1,2-cyclohexanediols (models of poison ivy and poison oak allergens), etc. ...

The majority of these model haptens were skin sensitizers. In particular, β-hydroxy-α-methylene-γ-butyrolactones, once claimed to be nonsensitizers, are actually able to induce ACD. Long-chain pyrocatechols and 1,2-cyclohexanediols seem to operate via a mechanism different from the electrophile-nucleophile scheme, probably via insertion into cell membranes (Langerhans cells?).

The importance of the nature of the bond in inducing either sensitization or tolerance will also be discussed.

Introduction

What makes a compound a skin sensitizer? A critical look at the structures of known contact allergens convinces one that, in order to induce contact sensitivity, a substance must have well-defined chemical properties. These include as a first prerequisite *electrophilic* properties, that is the capacity to form strong, covalent bonds with cutaneous (essentially epidermal) protein *nucleophilic* groups (such as $-NH_2$, $-SH$, and imidazole). Electrophiles are electron-poor and nucleophiles electron-rich entities [3, 7]. The cutaneous protein formely recognized as *self* by the organism, is therefore modified by the electrophilic hapten, becoming nonself, i.e., antigenic:

Protein-Nu +	E	→	Protein-Nu-E
nucleophile	electrophile (hapten)		antigen Œ

Some cutaneous sensitizers are not initially electrophiles. They must undergo in vivo reactions (oxidations, reductions, hydrolysis, etc.) in order to become electrophilic. These sensitizers are called *prohaptens* [3, 7]. An example is paraphenylenediamine, which is probably oxidized into quinonimine and eventually hydrolyzed into benzoquinone, a remarkable nucleophile acceptor.

Such strong covalent bonds can also be formed through photosensitization: under the action of light, some bond breaking with radical formation takes place (for instance tetrabromosalicylanilide can lose a bromine atom, Br). As some protein groups can also undergo oxidation into radicals (e.g., $-SH \rightarrow -S + H$), the combination of the two radicals (protein + hapten) leads to the formation of a new bond:

Protein + Hapten → Protein−hapten
antigen

Finally, some well-known contact allergens (such as those present in poison ivy or poison oak) are long straight-chain pyrocatechols. Through these hydrophobic chains, these haptens could (and do, as shown by in vitro studies) insert into the double layer lipidic cell membranes [4]. Another mechanism might be operating here and will be exemplified later.

Two topics will be discussed: the nature of protein-hapten bonds and the specificity of cross-reactivity.

Nature of the Protein-hapten Bond

Among the nucleophilic groups present in proteins, the most likely candidates for bond formation with hapten are amino groups, NH_2 (such as the $-NH_2$ group of lysine), and thiol groups, SH (such as in cysteine). Recent results from three different research groups seem to show that in the induction of contact sensitivity thiols and amines are not equivalent.

Castagnoli and Byers' group in San Francisco have shown [8] that the attack of $R-NH_2$ exclusively occurs at position 5 in 3-heptadecyl orthoquinone (the oxidation product of heptadecylcatechol), while thiols add at position 6 (Fig. 1).

Compounds with blocked 5-position (5-methylpentadecyl-catechols) did not induce sensitization but rather produced tolerance, while blocking position 6 did not prevent contact sensitivity in the mouse [6] and the guinea pig [15].

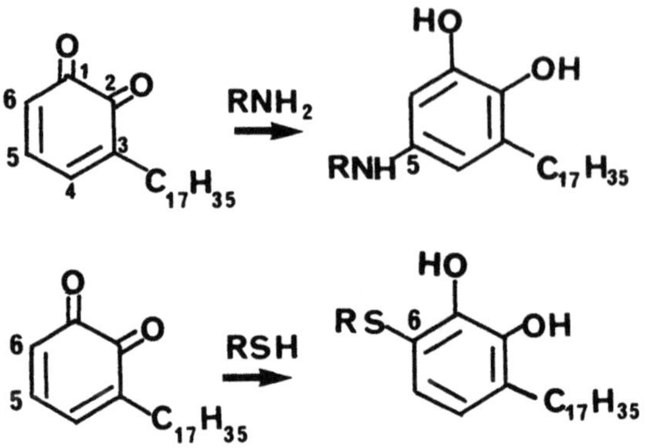

Fig. 1. Bond formation with heptadecylquinones

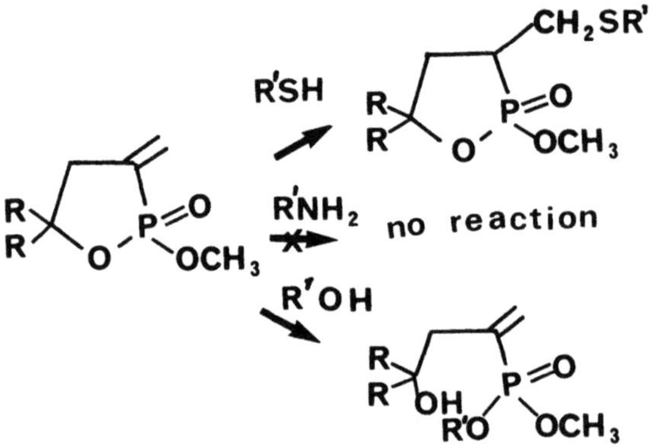

Fig. 2. Reactions of α-methylene-γ-phostones with thiols (R'SH), amines (R'NH), and alcohols (R'OH)

Parker and Turk's group in London have compared the bond-making reaction of DNCB (2,4-dinitrochlorobenzene) and DNTB (2,4-dinitrothiocyanobenzene) with several nucleophiles from proteins. They concluded that thiols preferentially attack DNTB (a known tolerogen when applied epicutaneously) while amino groups react with DNCB (a strong sensitizer). Can it be gathered as a preliminary conclusion from the above results that a nitrogen-protein bond is necessary to induce sensitization while a sulfur-protein bond rather provokes tolerance? Interpretation is not so simple, as recent results from the same group in London on acrylate derivatives did not give clear-cut results (Parker and Turk 1984, personal communication).

Finally in Strasbourg, we have prepared [5] phosphorus analogs of α-methylene-γ-lactones, e.g., α-methylene-γ-phostones which were unable to induce contact sensitivity when there was no substituent (R=R'=H) or a methyl group (R=R'=CH_3) in the γ-positions. Model studies with amines, thiols, and alcohols showed that (a) thiol groups attack the methylene group exclusively; (b) there is *no reaction with amines* $R''NH_2$, and (c) alcohols and water attack the phosphorus atom (Fig. 2). Again, when no nitrogen-protein bond can be formed, no sensitization seems to occur. The trend is reversed when a long chain substituent (R=H, R'=$C_{10}H_{21}$ or R=H, R'=$C_{15}H_{31}$) is present, enabling the phostone to insert into cell membranes (Collard and Benezra 1984, unpublished results).

If one could in some way or another direct protein-hapten formation to form sulfur-protein bonds only, one might hope to produce new tolerogens.

Is Cross-sensitivity Specific?

We have gone a long way from "group sensitization" as viewed in the 1950s (sensitivity to the "para group," aromatic amines, phenols, nitro derivatives etc.) to modern molecular recognition. Not everything is understood in cross-sensitivity reactions but one thing is certain: it does not suffice, for instance, for two haptens to share a common group (such as the α-methylene-γ-butyrolactone group) to observe cross-sensitivity reactions. Thus, people sensitive to some Compositae sesquiterpene lactones do not necessarily react to all Compositae or other families of plants containing sesquiterpene lactones (such as Lauraceae, Frullaniaceae, and Magnoliaceae).

How specific is cross-reactivity? It is a well-known fact that natural products usually exist in only one *enantiomeric* form (enantiomers are nonsuperimposable mirror-image compounds). There are some exceptions: for instance, usnic acid exists in nature in the (−)-form, the (−)-form, as well as the (+/−) or racemate form. Also well known is the *enantiospecific* activity of one enantiomer in pharmacology (only *one* enantiomer is biologically active).

What about allergic contact dermatitis (ACD)? In 1969, Mitchell and Shibata [9] reported that lumberjacks in British Columbia suffering from ACD to lichens only reacted to the *d*- (or +) form of usnic acid. No reaction to *l*- (or −) usnic acid was observed even when multiplying 50-fold (!) the test concentration. It was concluded that only *d*-usnic acid was a sensitizer. In fact, it turned out that *l*-usnic acid was also a contact allergen, as shown by Salo et al. [13] in Finland in lichen pickers (Fig. 3).

We undertook to verify the *enantiospecificity* of ACD by making mirror-images of γ-methyl-α-methylene-γ-butyrolactones, sensitizing guinea pigs to each mirror image, and exposing them to each enantiomer. The results were quite disappointing: no enantiospecificity was observed, i.e., (+)-lactone-sensitized guinea pigs recognized the (−)-lactone and conversely (−)-lactone-sensitized guinea pigs recognized the (+)-lactone [1]. We interpreted these results by assuming that, due to its small size, γ-methyl-α-methylene-γ-butyrolactone was "buried" into the protein carrier in such a way that a (+)-lactone-protein

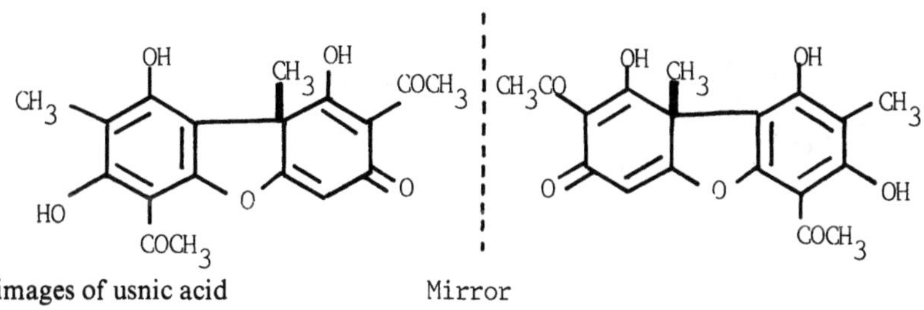

Fig. 3. Mirror images of usnic acid

antigen could not be differentiated from a (−)-lactone-protein antigen. We then turned to a larger hapten, frullanolide, a sesquiterpene lactone extracted from *Frullania.* Remarkably, the main two species of liverworts this compound is extracted from contain nonsuperimposable mirror-image derivatives: *F. dilatata* (L.) Dum. produces (−)-frullanolide while *F. tamarisci* yields (+)-frullanolide, its enantiomer (Fig. 4). Two groups of guinea pigs were sensitized to each of the lactones and almost total enantiospecificity was observed: all (+)-frullanolide-sensititized animals reacted to (+)-frullanolide (the primary sensitizer), with an average + 2 intensity reaction, while only a small fraction of animals (two of six) showed a weak (0.2 + average) reaction to the (−)-enantiomer; (−)-frullanolide-sensitized animals did not react to (+)-frullanolide [2].

We extended the study of enantiospecific ACD to "pseudo-enantiomers" [14], i.e., compounds with opposite configuration (= three-dimensional arrangement of atoms in space) and differing by one substituent. Polygodial, a dialdehyde present in *Polygonum hydropiper* L., a spice used to flavor the

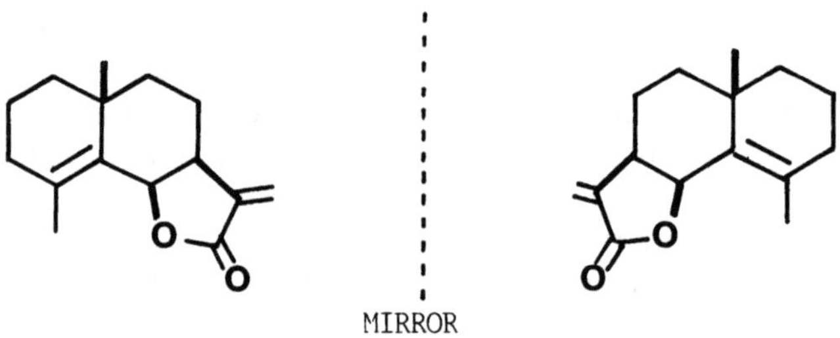

Fig. 4. (−)- and (+)-frullanolides

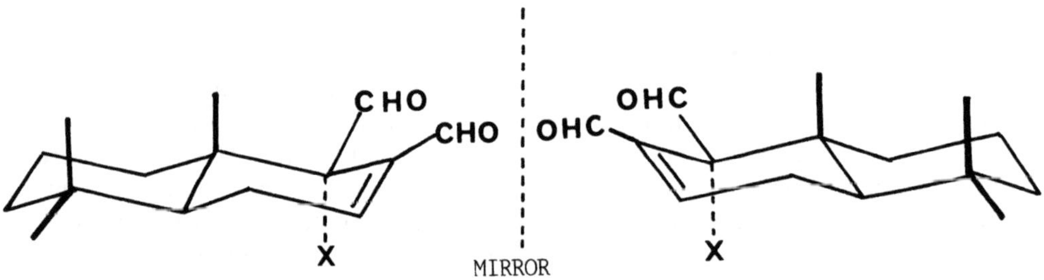

Fig. 5. Polygodial (X=H) and (−)- and (+)-warburganals (X=OH)

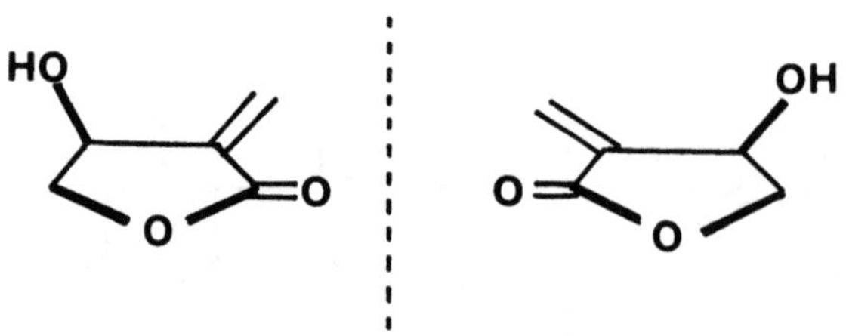

Fig. 6. (−)- and (+)-tulipalins B

Japanese raw fish, sashimi, was used to sensitize guinea pigs (giving an average + 2 reaction). These animals were then tested with (−)-warburganal, a hydroxy substituted polygodial derivative, with a configuration identical to that of polygodial. The average test reaction was + 1 (down from the stronger reaction to polygodial). However, with a *racemic* mixture of (+)- and (−)-warburganals (i.e., a mixture containing 50% of each enantiomer) (Fig. 5), the average skin test reaction was 0.4 +, i.e., what would be expected if the pseudo-enantiomer, (+)-warburganal, was nonreactive and only the compound with identical 3-D arrangement of atoms in space, (−)-warburganal, elicited a cross-reaction. Again, this is a case of true enantiospecific ACD.

Finally, we were recently able to synthesize both (−)-tulipalin B, the natural enantiomer present in tulip bulbs, and its nonnatural enantiomer, (+)-tulipalin B (Fig. 6) [10]. Again, two groups of guinea pigs were sensitized. *Complete enantiospecificity* was observed: (+)-tulipalin B-sensitized animals reacted to (+)-tulipalin B only and not at all to (−)-tulipalin B, and the reverse was true for (−)-tulipalin B-sensitized animals (Papageorgiou and Benezra 1985, unpublished results). In this case the *chiral* center (OH-bearing carbon atom) is close to the probable site of attack by the nucleophilic protein, enabling specificity to take place.

Conclusion

The last few years have seen quite important development in the understanding of the molecular properties of skin sensitizers. An attempt to relate sensitizing power to electrophilic and lipopholic properties of cutaneous allergens was made recently in the U.K. [12]. The nature of the carrier protein-hapten bond as well as structural factors seems to be of major importance. The aims of such studies are multiple: (a) to try and understand what makes a compound a contact sensitizer (structure-activity relationships), (b) to establish how specific the cell-mediated response is [it is quite remarkable that T-lymphocytes able to recognize either the (+)- or its nonsuperimposable mirror image (−)- derivatives can be induced], and (c) to try and develop compounds capable of inducing tolerance and, hopefully, desensitization.

In conclusion, the joint efforts of dermatologists, immunologists, chemists, and biochemists have been extremely productive and should help us to understand in the near future what the mechanisms of ACD are and possibly to try and control them.

References

1. Barbier P, Benezra C (1982a) Allergenic α-methylene-γ-butyrolactones. Stereospecific syntheses of (+)- and (−)-γ-methyl-α-methylene-γ-butyrolactones. A study of the specificity of (+)- and (−)- enantiomers in inducing allergic contact dermatitis. J Med Chem 25:943–946

2. Barbier P, Benezra C (1982b) Stereospecificity of allergic contact dermatitis induced by two natural enantiomers, (+)- and (−)-frullanolides in guinea pigs. Naturwissenschaften 69:296–297
3. Benezra C, Dupuis G (1983) L'allergie de contact. La Recherche 14:1062–1072
4. Byers VS, Epstein WL, Castagnoli N, Baer H (1979) In vitro studies of poison oak immunity. I. In vitro reactions of human lymphocytes to urushiols. J Clin Invest 64:1437–1448
5. Collard JN, Benezra C (1982) α-Methylene-γ-phostones. Tetrahedron Lett:3725–3728
6. Dunn IS, Liberato DJ, Castagnoli N Jr, Byers VS (1982) Contact sensitivity to urushiol: role of covalent bond formation. Cell Immunol 74:220–233
7. Dupuis G, Benezra C (1982) Allergic contact dermatitis to simple chemicals: a molecular approach. Dekker, New York
8. Liberato DJ, Byers VS, Dennick RG, Castagnoli N Jr (1981) Region-specific attack of nitrogen and sulfur on quinones derived from poison oak/poison ivy catechols (urushiols) and analogs as models of urushiol-protein conjugate formation. J Med Chem 24:28–33
9. Mitchell JC, Shibata S (1969) Immunological activity of some substances derived from lichenized fungi. J Invest Dermatol 52:517–320
10. Papageorgiou C, Benezra C (1985) Use of enzymatic hydrolysis of dimethyl malates for a short synthesis of tulipalin B and of its enantiomer. J Organic Chem 50:1145–1147
11. Parker D, Long PV, Turk JL (1983) A comparison of the conjugation of DNTB and other dinitrobenzenes with free protein radicals and their ability to sensitize or tolerize. J Invest Dermatol 81:198–201
12. Roberts DW, Williams DL (1982) The derivation of quantitative correlations between skin sensitization and physicochemical parameters for alkylating agents and their application to experimental data for sulfones. J Theor Biol 99:807–825
13. Salo H, Hannuksela M, Hausen B (1981) Lichen pickers' dermatitis *Cladonia alpestris* (L.) (Rab.). Contact Dermatitis 7:9–13
14. Stampf JL, Benezra C, Asakawa Y (1982) Stereospecificity of allergic contact dermatitis to enantiomers. III. Experimentally induced ACD to a natural sesquiterpene dialdehyde, polygodial, in guinea pigs. Arch Dermatol Res 274:277–281
15. Stampf JL, Byers VS, Benezra C, Castagnoli N Jr (1986) Induction of tolerance to poison ivy urushiol by epicutaneous application of the structural analog 5-methyl-3-pentadecylcatechol. J Invest Dermatol 86:535–538

Regulation of Contact Allergy by Interferon

J. Knop

Department of Dermatology, University of Münster, 4400 Münster, Federal Republic of Germany

Abstract

Interferon (α, β and γ) has multiple effects on the immune system and it seems most likely that it is an important immune regulatory molecule. Original observations using experimental contact allergy models have shown that high doses of interferon α, β can suppress or enhance contact sensitivity in vivo, depending on the time of administration in relation to the sensitizing application of the contact sensitizer. We have observed that interferon released by C. parvum treatment of BALB/c mice enhanced contact sensitivity to 2,4-dinitrofluorobenzene (DNFB) and further analysis of this phenomenon showed that interferon α, β and γ in very low doses blocked the T suppressor pathway of this delayed type hypersensitivity reaction. We further tried to analyze the mechanism of this interferon-mediated blockade of the T suppressor pathway, using an in vitro model of contact sensitivity. From the observation obtained in this model we concluded that interferon blocked the T suppressor lymphocyte directly and not via antigen-presenting macrophages. It was further shown that antigen-presenting macrophages particularly able to activate T suppressor cells produced much less interferon than those able to activate T effector lymphocytes. Adding antiinterferon globulin to cultures containing macrophages able to induce T effector cells but unable to activate T suppressor cells resulted in an activation of T suppressor lymphocytes; this indicates that the ability of macrophage populations to produce interferon could be related to the ability to activate T effector or T suppressor lymphocytes.

Introduction

Less than a quarter of a century ago, interferon was a rather mysterious and elusive entity recognized only on the basis of its antiviral activity. Today interferons are known to form a system of many different and well-defined molecules exerting a wide variety of biological effects. Many activities of cells that make up the immune system can be influenced by interferon α, β and interferon

γ and it has been proposed that the interferons are very important immune regulatory molecules [1]. Which role does interferon play in the activation and maintenance of the contact sensitivity reaction? Contact sensitivity is a type of T cell-mediated delayed-type hypersensitivity reaction and there are many experimental data which show that this type of reaction can be significantly influenced by interferon. De Maeyer and co-workers were the first to describe that interferon α, β can influence contact sensitivity in animals, whereby these reactions could be suppressed by relatively high amounts of interferon, but also be enhanced depending on the time schedule of application (for review see [2]). We became interested in interferon as an immune regulatory factor in contact sensitivity by the initial finding that an interferon inducer *Propionibacterium acnes* (*P. acnes,* identical with *Corynebacterium parvum*) enhanced the contact sensitivity response in animals in which this response was reduced due to the action of T suppressor cells [3]. In the following we describe some of the results we obtained with interferon in contact sensitivity and propose a role of interferon in the induction process of contact sensitivity.

Experimental Design

Contact sensitivity was induced in BALB/c mice using 2,4-dinitrofluorobenzene (DNFB) which was painted twice onto the abdomen. After 4 days contact sensitivity was elicited by applying a lower concentration of DNFB onto the right ear of the animals, measuring the inflammatory response (ear thickness in 10^{-2} mm) after 24 h [4]. T effector cells of delayed-type hypersensitivity (T_{DH}) and T suppressor (T_s) cells which were induced in these animals either by intravenous injection of the contact sensitizer or by applying an antigen overload onto the skin of the animals were demonstrated by transferring spleen and lymph node cells to recipient animals which were ear challenged shortly after cell transfer (assay for T_{DH} cells) or sensitized twice and ear challenged 4 days later (assay for T_s cells).

For in vitro induction of T_{DH} and T_s cells bone marrow-derived macrophages (BM-Ma) were used as antigen-presenting cells. These macrophages were grown from bone marrow stem cells in conditioned medium, harvested, and then further cultured in culture dishes using Dulbecco's MEM. This method provides a very pure population of macrophages. The macrophages were labeled with the contact sensitizer 2,4-dinitrobenzene sulfonic acid ($DNBSO_3$) and washed carefully. Lymphocytes from nonsensitized animals were added to these cells and cocultured for 3 days. The lymphocytes were harvested after this culture period and injected intravenously into naive BALB/c mice which were then either ear challenged immediately afterwards (T_{DH} assay) or sensitized and ear challenged (T_s assay) [5].

Interferon α, β was obtained from Dr. De Maeyer, Paris; purification, purity, and activity have been described [6].

Results and Discussion

As mentioned above, injection of the contact sensitizer DNFB intravenously or application of a high dose onto the skin did not result in an induction of T_s-lymphocytes in animals treated before with *P. acnes*. Furthermore, pretreatment of the animals with serum obtained from *P. acnes*-treated animals also inhibited the T_s response (Table 1). Since *P. acnes* is a strong interferon inducer we added anti-interferon α, β to this serum before injecting it into the donor animals of T_s-lymphocytes [7]. We found that anti-interferon α, β completely blocked the T_s inhibitory factor in this serum. We concluded that interferon may be the T suppressor-inhibitory factor. Pretreatment of the animals, therefore, with interferon α, β or γ [8; Taborsky et al. 1985, submitted for publication] also blocked the T_s pathway (Table 1). It should be mentioned that the T_{DH} cell was not inhibited by interferon or the other treatments described above. We therefore concluded that interferon α, β possibly produced by the accessory macrophage or other cells may preferentially block the T_s cell pathway, allowing the T_{DH} cell to become activated. Interferon γ, which is produced by activated T-lymphocytes after contact with the corresponding antigen, may maintain the contact sensitivity response by further blocking the T_s pathway. How do the interferons act on the T_s pathway? Interferon may directly block the T-lymphocytes, suggested by some of the in vivo experiments, or it may act via the antigen-presenting macrophages.

In order to study these questions we developed an in vitro sensitization method which is briefly described in the Experimental Design section. In this system T effector or T_{DH} and T_s lymphocytes were induced separately by different antigen-presenting bone marrow-derived macrophages (BM-Ma). Cocultivation of lymphocytes from nonsensitized animals with young, 5-day-old BM-Ma activated T_{DH} but no T_s cells, as demonstrated by transfer of these cells to naive recipients. On the other hand, older, 10- to 14-day-old BM-Ma preferentially induced T_s-lymphocytes (Lyt 2^+ afferent acting T_s cells) without inducing Lyt 1^+ T_{DH} cells. Using this model we either treated the lymphocytes

Table 1. Inhibition of the T_s cell circuit by interferon (IFN) in vivo

Treatment before T_s-induction[a] with	T_s-induction/ function[b] inhibited
Saline/buffer	No
P. acnes	Yes
P. acnes serum	Yes
P. acnes serum + anti-IFN α, β	No
IFN α, β or γ	Yes

[a] By intravenous or epicutaneous (antigen overload) application of the contact sensitizer

[b] Determined by spleen and lymph node cell transfer followed by sensitization

Table 2. Inhibition of the T_s cell response by interferon (IFN) in vitro

Treatment of		T_s induction[c] inhibited
BM-Ma[a]	Lymphocytes[b]	
–	Buffer	No
–	IFN α, β	Yes
Buffer	–	No
IFN α, β	–	No
IFN γ	–	Yes

[a] Day 14 bone marrow-derived macrophages (BM-Ma) incubated for 24 h with IFN before DNP labeling and cocultivation with lymphocytes
[b] Treated for 2 h with IFN before cocultivation with antigen-labeled BM-Ma
[c] Assayed by i.v. injection of in vitro educated lymphocytes followed by sensitization with DNFB

with interferon α, β before cocultivation with antigen-presenting BM-Ma or in a second set of experiments pretreated the antigen-presenting BM-Ma with interferon α, β or γ before adding the lymphocytes. The results are summarized in Table 2. Pretreatment of the lymphocytes with interferon α, β prevented the induction of T_s cells but had no effect on the induction of T_{DH} cells. This confirmed our recent finding in vivo. Pretreatment of the macrophages with interferon α, β had no effect on the induction of T_s lymphocytes. However, pretreatment of the macrophages with interferon γ prevented the induction of T_s cells. We do not know yet whether interferon γ changed the macrophage phenotype in such a way that they would now induce T_{DH} cells. Experiments to solve this question are in progress.

We then asked the following question: Why do young, 5-day-old BM-Ma not activate T_s cells? One answer to this question could be that this accessory cell population is particularly able to produce interferon during the culture period which would then prevent the development of T_s cells, in contrast to the older accessory cell population which would not produce sufficient interferon. Supernatants taken from cultures of young and old macrophages without any further stimulation did not contain any detectable amounts of interferon. This, of course, could be due to the insensitivity of our assay system. However, there are two lines of evidence which would support the notion that interferon produced during the culture period may directly influence the development of T_s cells. In cooperation with Dr. Sorg's department we could show that young, 5- to 7-day-old BM-Ma produce significant amounts of interferon upon stimulation with lipopolysaccharide. Ten- to 14-day-old BM-Ma, on the other hand, do not produce any or very little interferon. Direct evidence for the participation of interferon in the activation process of T_s cells in this system was derived from experiments in which we added a highly specific anti-interferon α, β globulin to cultures with 5-day-old antigen-presenting bone marrow macrophages and lymphocytes. While no T_s cells were induced in the normal serum control in the presence of anti-interferon α, β,T_s cells were clearly activated.

There are still many questions to be answered, such as why do macrophages treated with interferon γ not induce T_s cells and what are the changes in this population of cells. Which role does Ia expression play in this system and many more. Considering all these data, we would propose that in the absence of interferon the immune response in contact sensitivity would be shifted toward suppression by activation of the T_s circuit. However, in the presence of interferon during the sensitization process (the interferon might be derived from keratinocytes or Langerhans cells induced by interferon-activating contact sensitizers or by bacterial or viral infections) the activation of T_{DH} cells would be facilitated by blocking the T_s pathway. Interferon α, β acts directly on the T_s cells while interferon γ will in addition change the phenotype of the antigen-presenting accessory cells in such a way that it will not allow the induction of T_s cells.

References

1. De Maeyer E (1984) The interferon system and the immune system. In: Vilcek J, De Maeyer E (eds) Interferons and the immune system. Interferon 2:1–6
2. De Maeyer-Guignard J (1984) Effects of interferon on cell-mediated immunity as manifested by delayed hypersensitivity and allograft rejection. Vilcek J, De Maeyer E (eds) Interferons and the immune system. Interferon 2:133–145
3. Knop J, Riechmann R, Macher E (1981) Modulation of suppressor mechanisms in allergic contact dermatitis II. Inhibition of suppressor-T-lymphocytes by *C. parvum.* J Invest Dermatol 76:396–399
4. Knop J, Riechmann R, Macher E (1981) Modulation of suppressor mechanisms in allergic contact dermatitis I. Effect of *C. parvum* on the induction phase of contact allergy. J Invest Dermatol 76:193–196
5. Knop J, Malorny U, Macher E (1984) Induction of T effector and T suppressor lymphocytes in vitro by haptenized bone marrow-derived macrophages. Cell Immunol 88:411–420
6. De Maeyer-Guignard J, Tovey MG, Gresser I, De Maeyer E (1978) Purification of mouse IFN by sequential affinity chromatography on poly (U-) and antibody-agarose columns. Nature 271:622–623
7. Knop J, Riechmann R, Macher E (1981) Modulation of suppressor mechanisms in allergic contact dermatitis IV. Selective inhibition of suppressor-T-cells by serum derived from *C. parvum* treated mice. J Invest Dermatol 77:469–473
8. Knop J, Stremmer R, Neumann C, De Maeyer E, Macher E (1982) Interferon inhibits the suppressor T cell response of delayed-type hypersensitivity. Nature 296:775–776

Contact-Allergy Time

G. Burg, B. Przybilla, and J. Bogner
Dermatologische Klinik und Poliklinik, Ludwig-Maximilians-Universität München, 8000 Munich 2, Federal Republic of Germany

Abstract

The most commonly used techniques for the in vivo evaluation of the cellular immune response include intracutaneous testing with microbial recall antigens or sensitization with neoantigens. The reliability of these tests for the individual patient usually is low due to the lack of standardization and quantification. Moreover only the efferent branch of the immune response can be judged.

The dinitrochlorobenzene-contact allergy time (DNCB-CAT) is a quantitative approach for the assessment of the cellular immune response. 2% DNCB-ointment is applied on the upper arm in a 1 cm^2 area. On the following days patch-testing with 0.05% DNCB-ointment is done on the homolateral forearm in alternating localizations till an allergic contact dermatitis reaction appears.

As assessed in patients with malignant melanoma (MM, $n = 115$) and with lymphoproliferative disorders (LD, $n = 25$), the DNCB-CAT correlates with the age of the patients and can be expressed by a formula given by the age (years) × factor (MM = 0.16; LD = 0.17) + constant figure (MM = 5.5; LD = 4.3). There was no significant difference between the two groups or subgroups investigated.

By DNCB-CAT quantitative analysis of the cellular immune response in vivo is possible. It is an appropriate model for further investigations of the cellular immunity under different clinical, histological, prognostic, and therapeutic aspects.

Introduction

Immune status is an ill defined term, reflecting the capacity of the organism to exhibit immunologic defense mechanisms following antigenic stimulation. Evaluation of the immune status may be of interest in various disciplines, such as oncology, hematology, and transplantation medicine. In dermatology alteration of the immune status has been described in sarcoidosis, leprosy, atopic eczema, collagenosis, chronic infectious diseases, AIDS, malignant neoplasms (including squamous and basal cell carcinoma, malignant melanoma and lymphoma), and several other conditions [1, 5].

Reports in the literature are controversial. For example in malignant melanoma, cell-mediated immunity assessed by recall antigens or by neoantigens has been claimed to be normal [22], impaired [19], and even increased [20]. The reasons for the contradictory results are manifold. They may be due to the method applied, to the patient and his disease, or to the test material or antigens used: Firstly the various in vitro and in vivo tests for the assessment of immune status can scarcely be compared since they reflect different functional capacities of the immune system. Secondly the contradictory results may be related to the patient and his disease in that factors claimed to modulate the immune response, like atopy [15, 16], clinical stage of tumoral diseases [14], sex [11, 17], or surgical stress [3], have been neglected in many of the reports on the immune status of patients tested. Thirdly the in vivo methods used are not standardized with respect to either the test procedure and the number and type of antigens tested or the evaluation of the test reaction [12]. Comparison of six recall antigens provided by two different manufacturers tested simultaneously in each of 20 patients revealed different test reactions in 10% for tuberculin, in 20% for trichophytin, in 30% for diphtheria, in 35% for streptococci or candidin, and in more than 50% for tetanus antigen (Table 1). In the same group of patients there was complete anergy in one patient tested with seven recall antigens from manufacturer M and in another patient tested with antigens from manufacturer B. The mean numbers of positive reactions in the two groups were 40% and 25% respectively (Table 2).

One step towards standardization and quantification of delayed type hypersensitivity tests for the evaluation of immune status is the multitest. The application of seven recall antigens and the control is standardized; the result is

Table 1. Comparison of six recall antigens from two different manufacturers tested in each of 20 patients

Recall antigen	% discordance
Tuberculin	10%
Trichophytin	20%
Diphtheria	30%
Streptococci	35%
Candidin	35%
Tetanus	55%

Table 2. Comparison of DTH reactions of recall antigens from two different manufacturers (M and B) ($n = 20$)

Manufacturer	M	B
Number of recall antigens	7	11
Complete anergy	5% (1)	5% (1)
Mean number of positive reactions	40% (3/7)	25% (3/11)

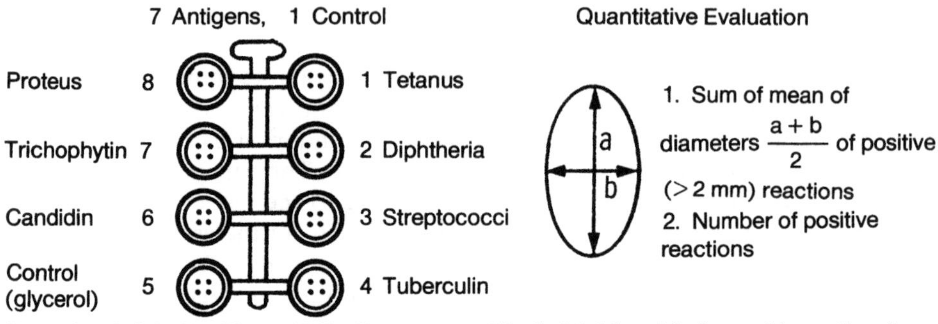

Fig. 1. Multitest Merieux with recall antigens

given in a score calculated from the number and the sum of diameters of positive test reactions (Fig. 1). The disadvantage, as with all tests using recall antigens, is that the multitest depends partly on regional vaccination programs, on geographic and epidemic factors, and on the sex of the patient without correlation to age [13]. Therefore testing with neoantigens like DNCB would seem more reliable [7].

Potential hazards of therapeutic use of dinitrochlorobenzene (DNCB), like mutagenicity or cross-reaction with other substances, can be ignored when it is used as a test allergen [2, 6, 8, 21]. The common procedure for DNCB testing consists in the application of a toxic 2% concentration of DNCB on the arm and a threshold challenge test with DNCB in various concentrations 2–4 weeks later. This neglects two important factors:

1. Only some of the patients will be sensitized at the time of the challenge test.
2. If the challenge test is performed when more time has elapsed since the first contact, the degree of sensitization will be slowly fading, so that determination of the threshold dose will not quantitatively reflect the immune status of the patient [10].

The disadvantage of all classical in vivo tests of the immune status – intracutaneous with recall antigens or epicutaneous with neoantigens – is the fact that only the efferent limb of the immune reaction process is measured, not the afferent limb, which is more complex, more important, and affords greater insight into the integrity or disturbance of the immune system [9].

Method and Patient Material

We tried to evaluate the complete process of development of hypersensitivity, as expressed by the time needed by the patient to build up an immunological reaction to DNCB, including both the afferent and the efferent limb (Fig. 2). A patch with 2% DNCB was applied on day 0 on a 1 cm^2 area of the upper arm. Subsequently 0.05% DNCB was applied daily on the forearm in alternating locations. The day when an allergic reaction appeared was registered. One week later a challenge test was performed in order to determine the threshold dose, using various concentrations of DNCB, from 0.001% to 0.05%.

Table 3. DNCB-CAT test results in 115 patients with malignant melanoma

		Patients		DNCB-CAT (days)		
		No.	Mean age	Mean	Shortest	Longest
Type	SSM	54	54	14	6	58
	NM	48	48	15	6	62
	LMM	3	59	23	10	49
	ALM	4	51	10	8	12
Stage	I	103	51	14	6	62
	II	8	47	14	9	25
	III	4	51	13	10	16
Level	II	10	56	14	8	30
	III	40	52	17	8	62
	IV	46	51	13	6	31
	V	5	51	12	10	14
Prognostic index (18)	0–1	29	51	14	8	62
	1.1–13	46	48	15	6	58
	>13	21	56	14	9	31

Abbreviations: SSM, superficial spreading melanoma; NM, nodular melanoma; LMM, lentigo maligna melanoma; ALM, acrolentiginous melanoma

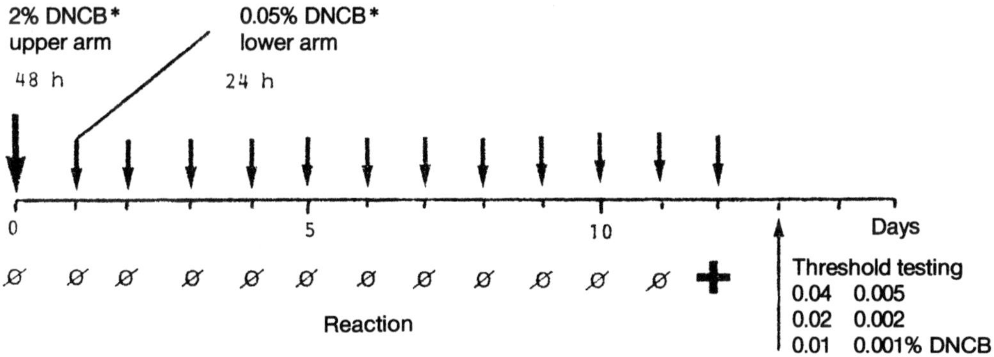

Fig. 2. DNCB-CAT for testing the immune status. * in Eucerin anhydricum

The test was applied to 115 patients with malignant melanoma (46 men, 69 women, age range 19–79 years, mean 51 years). Further information on their clinical features, stage, level, and prognostic index (PI [18]) is given in Table 3.

Results

The figures given in Table 3 illustrate the DNCB contact-allergy time (DNCB-CAT) in various subgroups of malignant melanoma patients. The shortest time measured (6 days) was found in one patient with superficial spreading melanoma (SSM) and in another with nodular melanoma (NM). Eleven patients showed a DCNB-CAT of longer than 20 days; the longest, 62 days, occurred in a patient with stage I, level III, low risk (prognostic index below 1) NM.

No significant correlation could be detected between the DNCB-CAT in various clinical types of malignant melanoma (SSM, NM, lentigo maligna melanoma, acrolentiginous melanoma) and stage (I–III), level (II–V), or prognostic index score (< 1, 1.1–13, > 13).

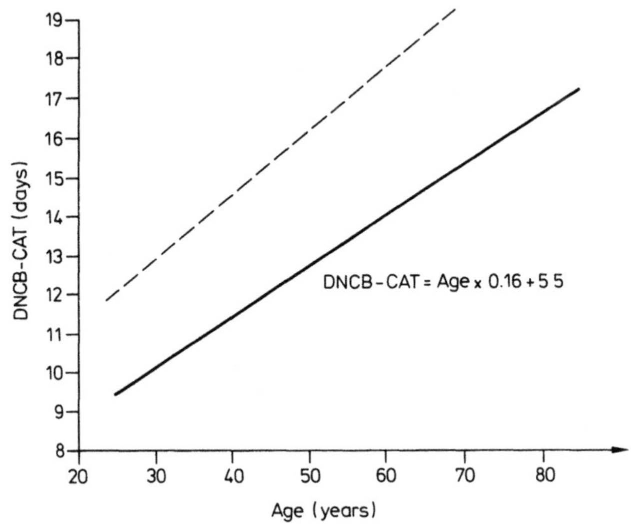

Fig. 3. Age-dependent regression curve of DNCB-CAT in malignant melanoma and 125% percentile (– –)

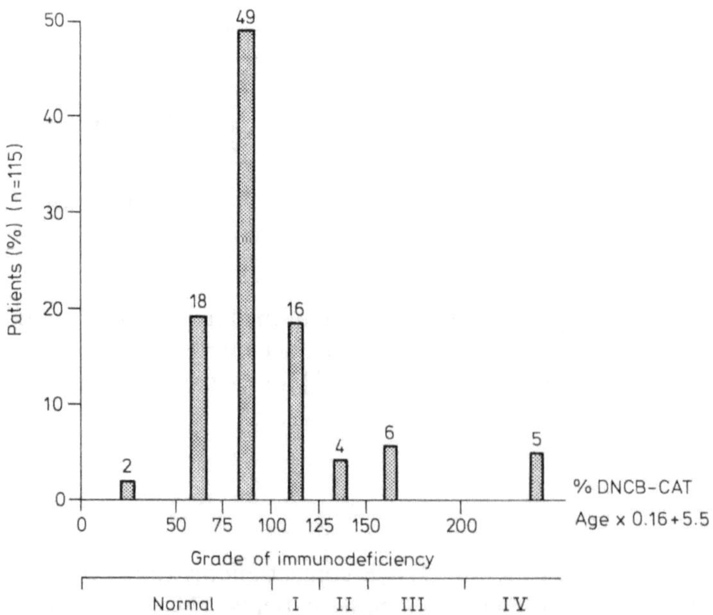

Fig. 4. DNCB-CAT exceeding the age-dependent calculated average: grades I–IV of immune deficiency

The most important finding was a strong correlation between DNCB-CAT and age of the patient. The expected DNCB-CAT was found to equal the age of the patient multiplied by a constant factor (0.16) plus a constant figure (5.5). Thus the DNCB-CAT in a 20-year-old patient is on average about half that expected in an 80-year-old patient (Fig. 3). Of the 115 patients, 69% ($n = 79$) exhibited a DNCB-CAT below the expected value as calculated by the above means. On the other hand 16% ($n = 18$) exceeded the expected figure by more than 25%, 11% by more than 50%, and 5% by more than 100% (Table 4, Fig. 4).

Table 4. Grading of immune deficiency by DNCB-CAT

Grade	% exceeding normal value (age × 0.16 + 5.5)	No. of patients	%
0 (normal)	0	79	69
I	≦ 25%	18	16
II	≦ 50%	5	4
III	≦ 100%	7	6
IV	> 100%	6	5

Table 5. Details of melanoma patients (n = 18) exhibiting an increased DNCB-CAT

Immuno-deficiency grade	% DNCB-CAT calcu-lated	Age (years)	MM (type)	Stage[a]	Level	Depth of in-vasion (mm)	PI[b]	Fol-lowup (years)	Stage[c]
II	136	42	SSM	II	–	–	–	3.5	0
125%–150%	140	41	SSM	I	II	0.27	< 1	1	0
	140	41	SSM	I	II	0.85	3	3	0
	142	43	SSM	I	II	0.27	< 1	2	0
	146	45	SSM	II	IV	–	33	4.5	+
III	152	42	SSM	I	IV	1.1	5	2	0
151%–200%	152	74	NM	I	IV	1.1	5	3	+
	156	21	NM	II	V	–	–	0.2	+
	166	50	SSM	I	III	0.45	< 1	3	0
	168	46	NM	I	III	0.48	2	3.5	0
	177	52	NM	II	IV	5.1	82	1.5	0
	184	68	NM	I	IV	–	32	3	II/0
IV	203	56	SSM	I	II	0.68	< 1	2	0
> 200%	208	42	ALM	I	IV	3.3	3	2	+
	248	54	SSM	I	III	1.37	5	2.5	0
	295	67	LMM	I	III	1.2	13	4	0
	365	69	NM	I	III	0.43	< 1	3	0
	433	47	SSM	I	III	–	9	3	0

[a] At time of diagnosis
[b] Prognostic index [18]
[c] At end of follow-up

Table 6. DNCB-CAT and multitest results in 15 patients with malignant melanoma

DNCB-CAT \ Multitest	Normal	Pathologic
Normal	9 (60%)[a]	3 (20%)[b]
Pathologic	2 (13%)[b]	1 (7%)[a]

[a] Concordance between tests = 67%
[b] Discordance between tests = 33%

Table 7. Correlation between DNCB-CAT and DNCB threshold concentration in 13 melanoma patients

DNCB-CAT[a]	Degree of hypersensitivity	
	High[b]	Low[c]
+	2 (15%)[d]	8 (62%)[e]
–	1 (8%)[e]	2 (15%)[d]

[a] + = normal or below; – = > 25% above normal
[b] 0.005%, 0.002%, or 0.001% DNCB
[c] 0.04%, 0.02%, or 0.01% DNCB
[d] Concordance = 30%
[e] Discordance = 70%

If the patients whose DCNB-CATs were higher than expected were categorized into four immunodeficiency groups (I = 101% – 125% of normal age-related DNCB-CAT; II = 126% – 150%; III = 151% – 200%; IV > 200%) and the patients of groups II – IV were listed in order of their DNCB-CAT (Table 5), no correlation was seen either with the type of melanoma or with stage, level, prognostic indices, or survival within the different categories.

In 15 patients we compared the result of the Merieux multitest with the DNCB-CAT test. A multitest score below 5 in women and below 10 in men and a DNCB-CAT exceeding the expected value by more than 25% were considered pathologic. Concordance between the multitest and the DCNB-CAT test was found in about two-thirds of the patients tested (Table 6).

Correlation between the DNCB-CAT and the degree of sensitization expressed by the threshold concentration of DNCB was found in only about one-third of the 13 patients tested (Table 7).

Discussion

Abnormalities of the cell-mediated immune status have been reported in a variety of dermatoses, including inflammatory and proliferating disorders [5]. It has been speculated that tumor induction and tumor growth are controlled by specific immune reactions against tumor cells, including enhancing and blocking mechanisms. However, there is little evidence that, for example, PHA stimulation of peripheral lymphocytes, the type and degree of the peritumoral infiltrate [4], or reactivity against recall antigens or neoantigens provide any reliable information as to the induction and growth of solid tumors. Nevertheless, in advanced stages of tumoral diseases with widespread metastases the immune system may be severely affected and a single test may elucidate dysfunctioning delayed type sensitivity provided the procedure is standardized and individual factors (e.g., age) are considered. Moreover it is important that the afferent and efferent limbs of the delayed type reactivity are measured. Therefore neoantigens are preferable to recall antigens.

The DNCB-CAT test is recommended as a standardized test for the assessment of immune status since it is simple, covers the complete process of building up delayed type hypersensitivity, and considers the most important individual factor, namely age. When using the DNCB-CAT test, grades (I–IV) of immunodeficiency can be differentiated in accordance with the percentage by which the actual DNCB-CAT exceeds the average-figure calculated for the individual age group.

Summary

The DNCB-CAT test is a quantitative approach for the assessment of the cellular immune response. 2% DNCB ointment is applied on the upper arm over a 1 cm^2 area. On subsequent days patch testing with 0.05% DNCB ointment is done on the homolateral forearm until an allergic contact dermatitis reaction appears. By this the afferent and the efferent limb of the delayed hypersensitivity reaction is measured.

In a group of 115 patients with solid tumors (malignant melanomas) DNCB-CAT correlated with the age of the patient and could be expressed by the following equation:

$$[\text{DNCB-CAT} = \text{Age (years)} \times 0.16] + 5.5$$

Deviations from the calculated agedependent regression curve were categorized into grades I–IV of immunodeficiency.

DNCB-CAT is an appropriate model for quantitative age-related analysis of cellular immune responsiveness in relation to various clinical, histologic, prognostic, and therapeutic factors.

References

1. Ahmed AR, Blose DA (1983) Delayed-type hypersensitivity skin testing. Arch Dermatol 119:934–945
2. Black HS, Castrow FF, Gerguis J (1985) The mutagenicity of dinitrochlorobenzene. Arch Dermatol 121:348–349

3. Bröcker EB, Macher E (1981) Der Einfluß von Narkose und Operation auf das Immunsystem. Klin Wochenschr 59:1291–1301
4. Burg G, Kohdam M, Kaudewitz D, Detmar U, Mason DY (1984) Plasma cells accumulating around epidermal neoplasms. Immunoenzymatic staining of paraffin sections. MacDonald D (ed) Immunodermatology. Butterworth, London, pp 167–171
5. Burg G, Rehle R (1981) Immunological work up. In: Ring J, Burg G (eds) New trends in allergy. Springer, Berlin Heidelberg New York, pp 115–128
6. Djawari D, Körner E, Haneke E (1980) Kreuzallergien nach Sensibilisierung mit Dinitrochlorbenzol (DNCB) Hautarzt 31:F198–202
7. Friedmann PS, Moss C, Shuster S, Simpson JM (1983) Quantitation of sensitization and responsiveness to dinitrochlorobenze in normal subjects. Br J Dermatol 109 [Suppl]:86–88
8. Happle R (1985) The potential hazards of dinitrochlorobenzene. Arch Dermatol 121:330–331
9. Knop J (1984) Immunologische Grundlagen des allergischen Kontaktekzems. Hautarzt 35:617–622
10. Magnusson B, Kligman AM (1970) Allergic contact dermatitis in the guinea pig. Thomas, Springfield
11. Marcano NB, Rivas A, Figarella EV, Blanca I, Penchaszadeh GK, Pérez-Rojas G, Bianco NE (1982) Cell-mediated effector mechanisms in aging humans. Int Archs Allergy Appl Immunol 69:7–11
12. Mayenburg JV, Heymer B, Düngemann H, Schleifer KH, Seidl HP, Galle J, Neiß A, Borelli S (1980) Hautreaktionen gegen isolierte bakterielle Zellwandkomponenten insbesondere bakterielle Peptidoglycane. Z Hautkr 55:710–733
13. Multitest Mérieux (1984) Institut Mérieux, Norderstedt
14. Pritchard DI, Ritts RE, Taylor WF, Miller GC (1978) A prospective study of immune responsiveness in human melanoma. Cancer 41:2165–2173
15. Rajka G (1968) Delayed dermal and epidermal reactivity in atopic dermatitis (prurigo Besnier). Acta Dermatol Venereol 48:186–191
16. Rajka G, Barlinn C (1979) On the significance of the trichophytin reactivity in atopic dermatitis. Acta Dermatol Venereol 59:45–47
17. Rosenthal M, Steinmann A (1978) Lebensalter und Immunität. Dtsch Med Wochenschr 103:409–412
18. Schmoeckel C, Kaviani Nejad K, Braun-Falco O (1980) Der prognostische Index beim malignen Melanom. Pathologie 1:71–78
19. Seigler HF, Stringleton WW, Metzger RS, Buckley CE, Bergoc PM, Miller DS, Fetter BF, Phaup MB (1972) Non-specific and specific immunotherapy in patients with melanoma. Surgery 72:162–174
20. Stenger D, Delbrück H, Krumrey K, Zaun H (1983) Standardisierte Recall-Antigentestung bei Patienten mit malignem Melanom, endogenen Ekzematikern und Gesunden. Z Hautkr 58:293–304
21. Strick RA (1983) Lack of cross-reaction between DNCB and chloramphenicol. Contact Dermatitis 9:484–487
22. Ziegler JL, Lewis MG, Luyombya J Lus, Kiryaboire JWM (1969) Immunologic studies in patients with malignant melanoma in Uganda. Br J Cancer 23:729–734

Drug Reactions

Histopathological Patterns of Drug Eruptions

H. H. Wolff and M. Winzer
Klinik für Dermatologie und Venerologie, Medizinische Universität zu Lübeck, 2400 Lübeck, Federal Republic of Germany

Abstract

"Drug eruption" is a term used for a broad spectrum of pathomechanisms and clinical pictures. It is not restricted to allergic reactions alone but comprises pharmacodynamical, toxic, phototoxic effects and reactions of still unknown origin.

The clinical appearance of drug eruptions includes wheals, macules, nodules, blisters and purpura among many others. A similar variety of histopathological alterations appears in the skin specimen. All well-known histological patterns of inflammatory dermatoses may be recognized, e.g. spongiotic, superficial and deep dermatitis, vasculitis, folliculitis and panniculitis.

An additional diagnostic clue is the composition of the cellular infiltrate, which may be further characterized using monoclonal antibodies.

Introduction

The use and abuse of drugs has resulted in an enormously increasing incidence of adverse drug reactions, especially skin eruptions. Inflammatory skin diseases may be attributed to drugs in about 5% of our dermatological patient population [15].

In this symposium on allergy, it must be mentioned, however, that by no means all "drug eruptions" are due to "allergic" mechanisms [4]. Any of the classical types of allergic reaction may be responsible for drug eruptions; nevertheless, there are many other possible mechanisms of drug-induced inflammation of the skin (Table 1).

Both the clinician and the dermatohistologist encounter two major problems: First, it is almost impossible to differentiate a drug eruption from identically looking dermatoses; it is well known that drug eruptions may mimic a broad spectrum of well defined skin diseases [9] like viral rashes, lichen planus [12], lupus erythematosus [3, 14], and psoriasis [2]. Second, if an eruption is definitely caused by a pharmaceutical agent, it cannot be concluded whether the pathogenesis is immunological or nonimmunological from pure morphology.

Table 1. Pathomechanisms of drug eruptions

Allergic
– IgE dependent
– Cytotoxic
– Immune complex dependent
– Cell mediated
Nonallergic
– Nonspecific effector activation
– Pharmacodynamic ("side") effects
– Overdosage
– Cumulation
– Drug interactions
– Ecological disturbances

Table 2. Histological patterns of drug eruptions (according to Kind and Ackerman)

1. Superficial perivascular dermatitis
2. Superficial and deep perivascular dermatitis
3. Vasculitis
4. Nodular and diffuse dermatitis
5. Intraepidermal vesicular and pustular dermatitis
6. Subepidermal vesicular dermatitis
7. Folliculitis and perifolliculitis
8. Fibrosing dermatitis
9. Panniculitis

Table 3. Histological patterns of drug eruptions

Architecture	Cytology
Epidermis	Lymphocytes
Epidermodermal interface	Histiocytes
Superficial plexus	Eosinophils
Deep plexus	Neutrophils
Subcutis	Plasma cells

Dermatopathologists can recognize neither a single histological finding nor a typical constellation of histological features specific or even typical of a drug reaction. Kind and Ackerman recently pointed out (unpublished work, 1985) that each of the nine basic histological patterns of inflammatory skin diseases can be induced by drugs (Table 2). As Fig. 1 illustrates, combinations may even occur in the same patient: desquamation, pustulation, and hemorrhagic vasculitis (in this case after intake of ampicillin). Nevertheless, certain constellations are more frequent, as shown in the examples below. Each histological pattern (Table 3) is recognized by:

– The general architecture, i.e., the type of pathological changes (necrosis, edema, etc.), their distribution and
– the cytological characterization of the inflammatory infiltrate.

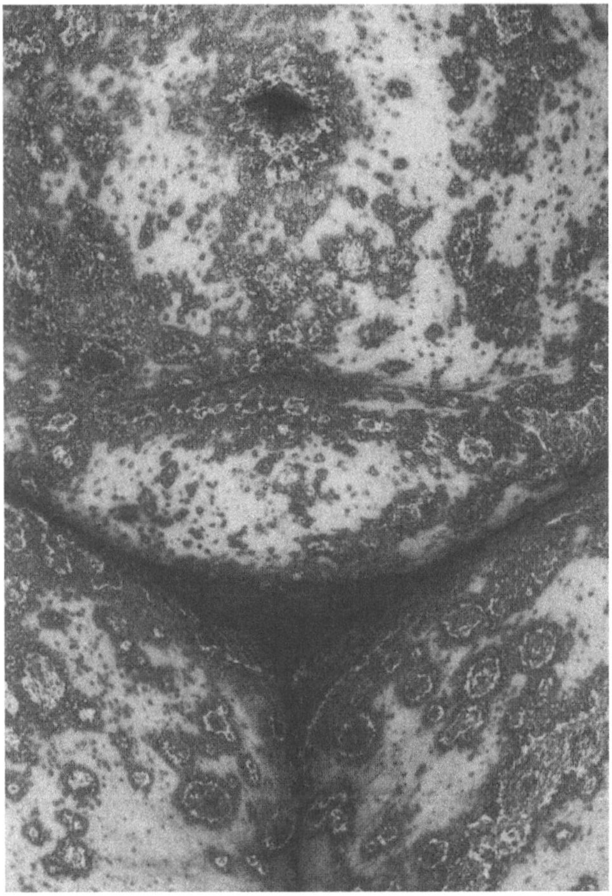

Fig. 1. Pustular and purpuric drug eruption (ampicillin)

The first example is *urticaria,* as frequently seen after penicillin intake. The main characteristic is a more or less massive edema indicated by widening of the spaces between the collagen bundles. There is a sparse mixed perivascular infiltrate around the dilated vessels of the superficial plexus.

In 1%–5% of all patients suffering from chronic urticaria, the *urticaria-vasculitis syndrome* can be suspected, and histologically it can be verified. The typical case shown in Fig. 2a was induced by indomethacin. The clinical picture shows some purpuric changes in the periphery of the wheals, histology the typical leukocytoclastic vasculitis and extravasation of red blood cells (Fig. 2b).

Another pattern of superficial dermatitis is shown in the next example, a case of *erythema multiforme* (Fig. 3a); in addition to the perivascular lymphohistiocytic infiltrate there is interface dermatitis with some vacuolar alteration of the epidermal basal cell layer and – most characteristic – single cell necrosis of keratinocytes (Fig. 3b) [6]. If the center of the lesion becomes bullous, this is due to either confluent necrosis of the epidermis or massive edema in the papillary dermis. Histopathology is very helpful in confirming the diag-

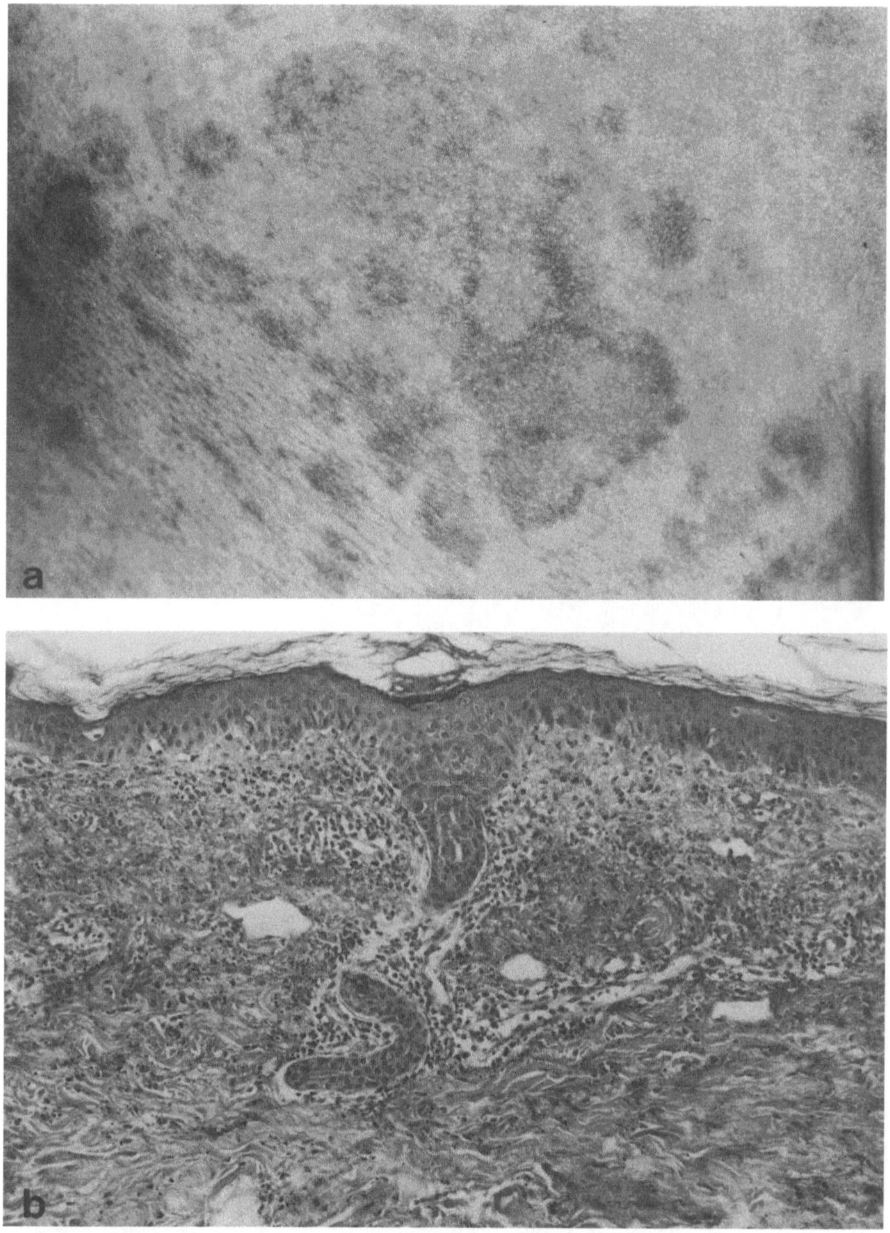

Fig. 2 a, b. Urticaria vasculitis. **a** clinical picture; **b** histological evidence of leukocytoclastic vasculitis. H & E, × 135

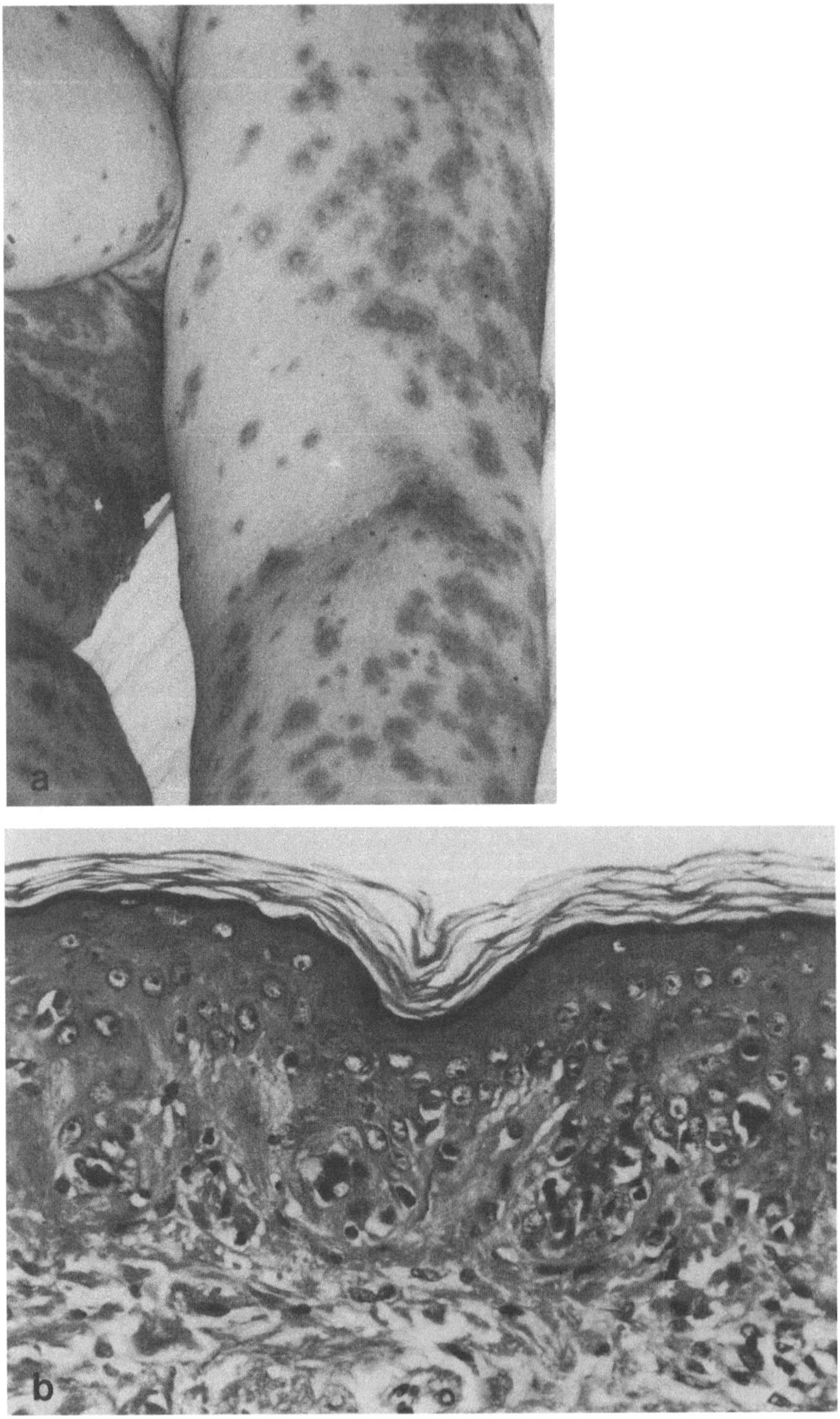

Fig. 3 a, b. Erythema multiforme. **a** typical target lesions; **b** epidermal single cell necrosis, interface dermatitis. H & E, × 350

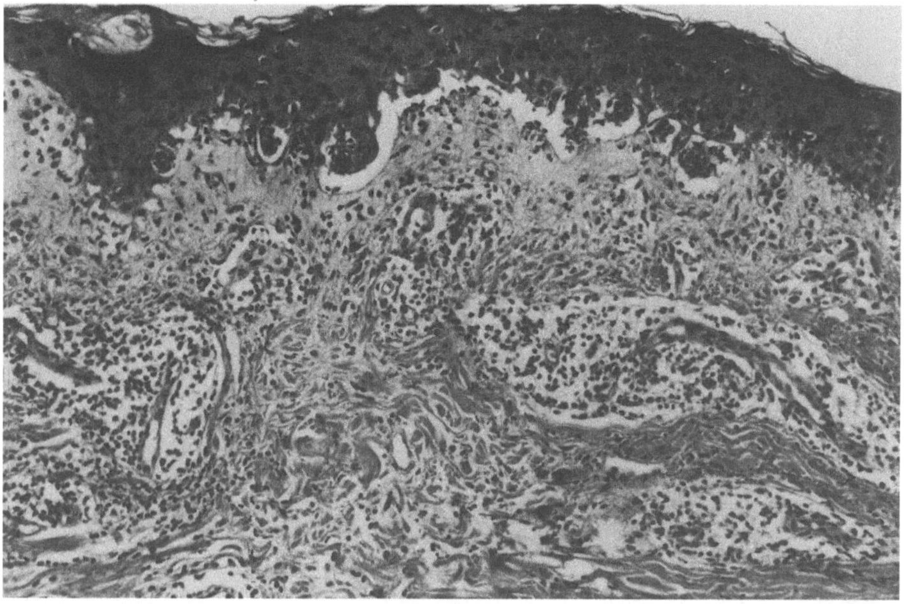

Fig. 4. Fixed drug eruption (sulfonamide). Epidermal necrosis, superficial and deep mixed inflammatory infiltrate. H & E, × 135

nosis of erythema multiforme, but again does not give clues to the many possible causes of this polyetiological skin reaction.

A rather similar pattern with epidermal single cell necrosis, sometimes confluent necrosis, and blister formation with interface dermatitis is typical of *fixed drug eruption* [7]. The infiltrate is not only superficial but also deep, comprising intermingled neutrophils, and there is pigment incontinence [13] documented by the melanophages in the upper dermis [Fig. 4]. This case of recurrent multilocular fixed drug eruption shown in Fig. 5 was caused by penicillin.

Some authors consider *Lyell's disease* (Fig. 6a) the maximal variant of erythema multiforme [1]. Histopathology does not favor this concept (Fig. 6b). The classical cases exhibit acute and complete epidermal necrosis resulting in subepidermal blister formation ("epidermal necrolysis"), almost without any interface or dermal inflammatory infiltrate [10]. Electron microscopy shows complete necrosis, as does the frozen section taken from the blister roof, which can be used for quick differential diagnosis from staphylococcal scalded skin syndrome [16]. Table 4 summarizes the differences between drug-induced and staphylococcal scalded skin syndrome. Histopathology is an essential diagnostic aid in differentiating these serious conditions.

Generally, blistering of the skin is a characteristic feature of drug eruptions of quite different pathogenesis. The case shown in Fig. 7a differs from the examples of Lyell's disease, erythema multiforme, and fixed drug eruption. This exanthema was induced by a sulfonamide. Histopathology of a subepidermal blister and the accumulation of eosinophils was suggestive of pemphigoid

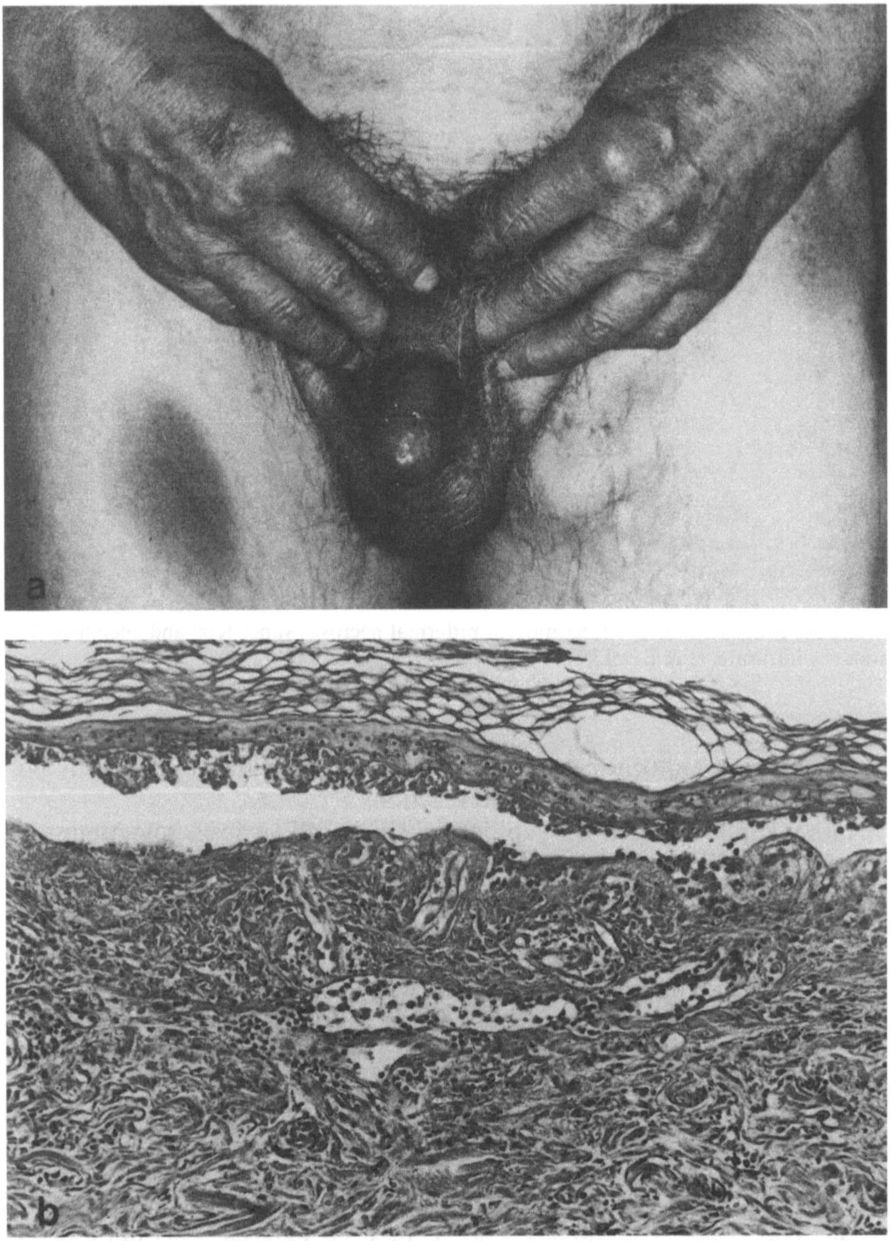

Fig. 5a, b. Multilocular fixed drug eruption (penicillin). **a** clinical appearance; **b** histopathology of a newly formed blister. H & E, × 135

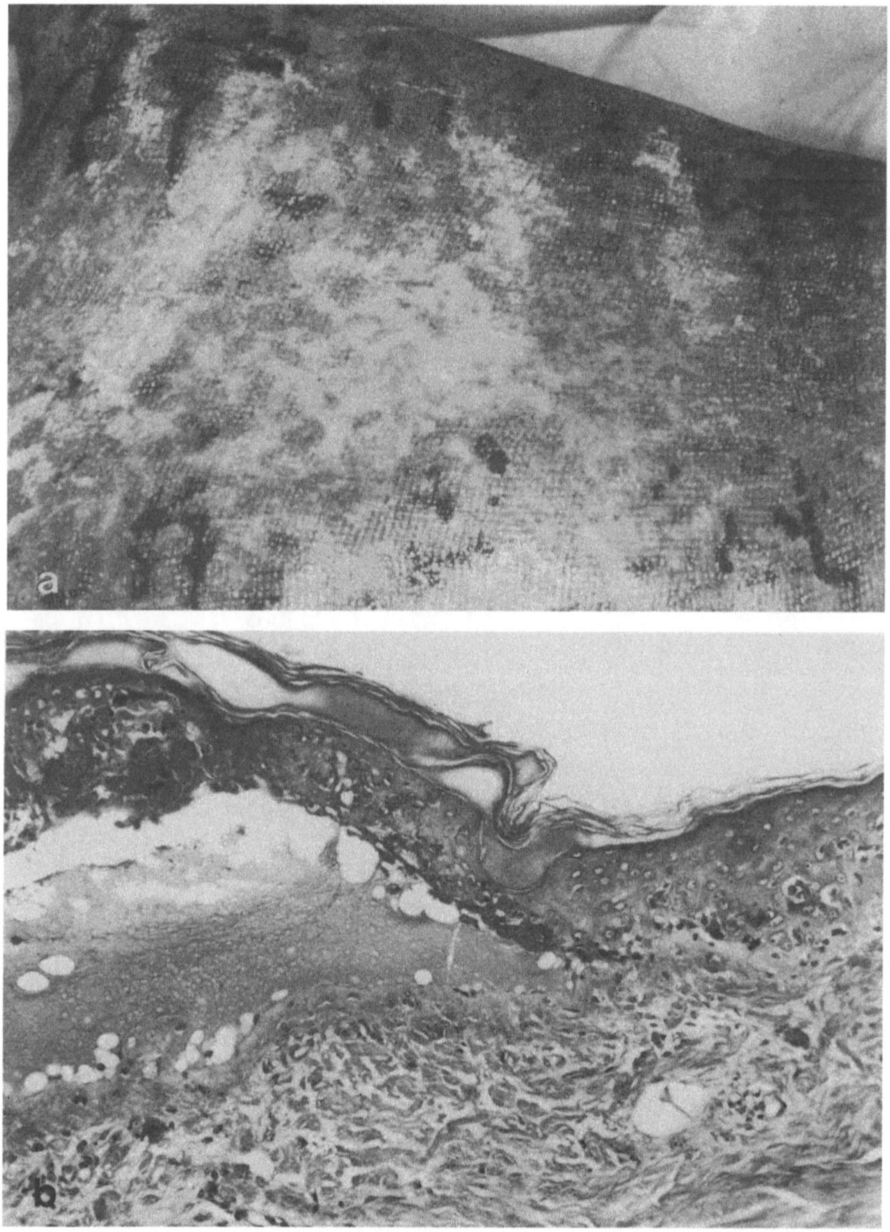

Fig. 6a, b. Lyell's disease (co-trimoxazole). **a** widespread erosions; **b** confluent epidermal necrosis, sparse dermal infiltrate. H & E, × 135

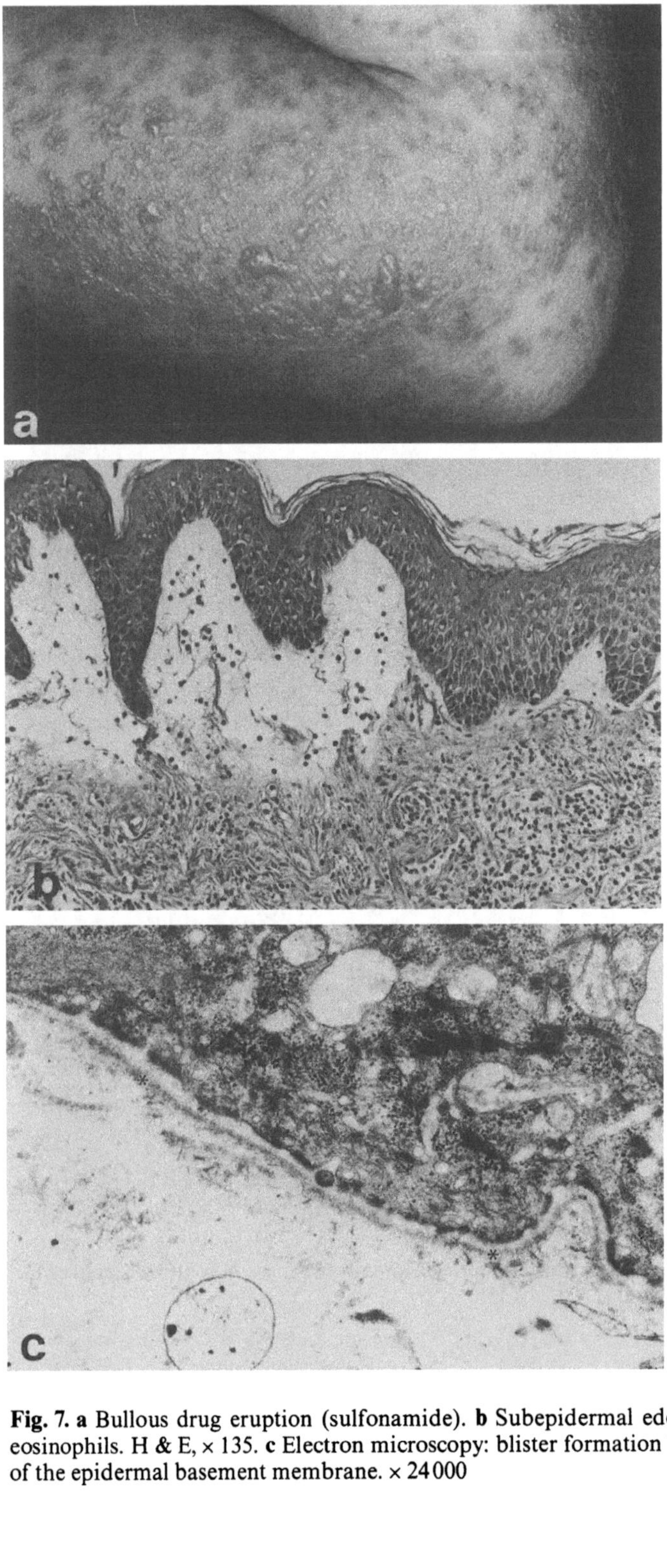

Fig. 7. **a** Bullous drug eruption (sulfonamide). **b** Subepidermal edema and blister formation, eosinophils. H & E, × 135. **c** Electron microscopy: blister formation below the lamina densa (*) of the epidermal basement membrane. × 24000

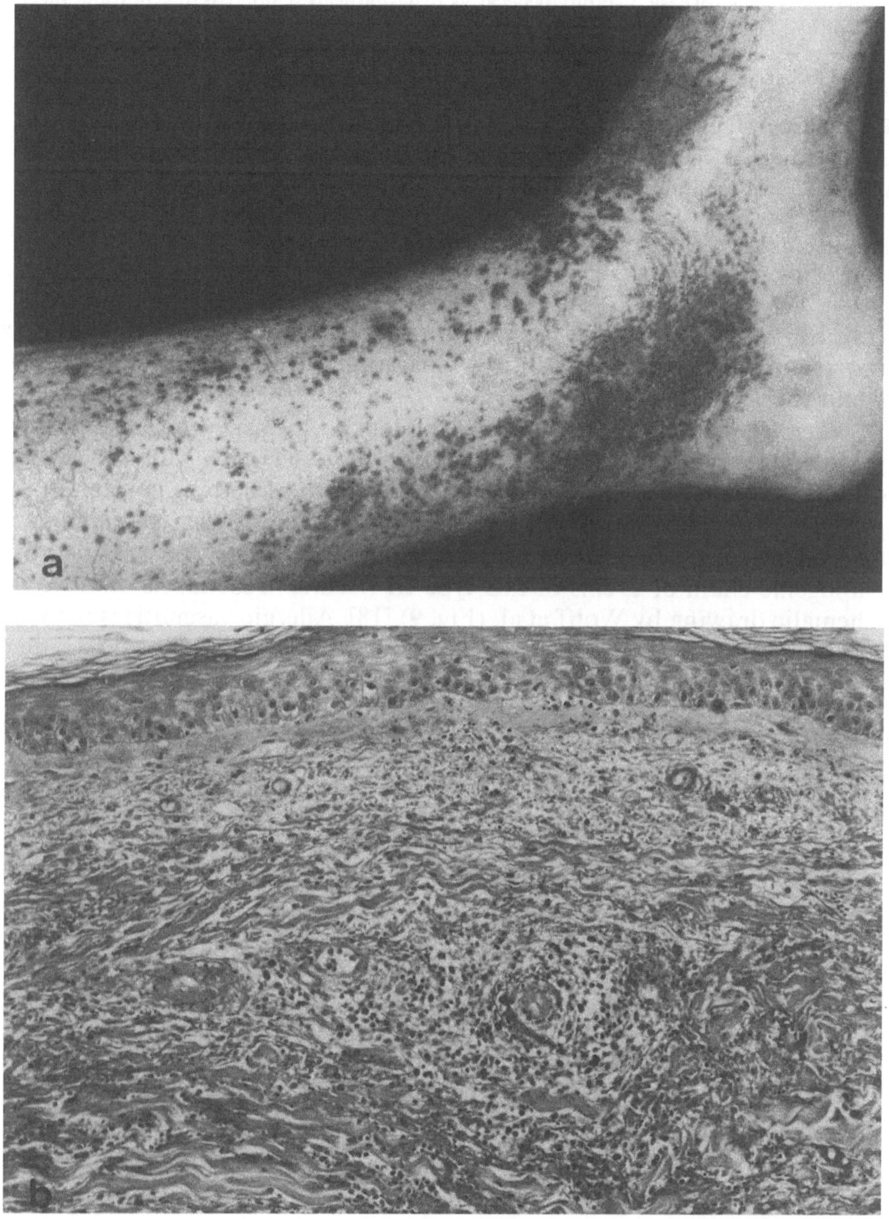

Fig. 8. a Allergic vasculitis, hemorrhagic type (oxyphenbutazone). **b** Leukocytoclastic vasculitis. H & E, × 135

Table 4. "Lyell's disease": staphylococcal vs drug-induced scalded skin syndrome (according to Wolff [16])

Staphylococcal	Drug-induced
Predominantly infants	Adults, rarely children
Staphylococcal infections	Drugs
Intraepidermal blister without necrosis	Subepidermal blister with epidermal necrosis ("necrolysis")
Prognosis quite good	Life threatening

(Fig. 7b); however, direct immunofluorescence was negative, and electron microscopy displayed no junctional separation but blister formation below the lamina densa (Fig. 7c).

Allergic vasculitis is characterized by leukocytoclasia, nuclear dust, eosinophils, erythrocyte extravasation, and fibrin in vessel walls (Fig. 8b). The clinical picture in the case illustrated (Fig. 8a) was produced by a nonsteroidal antiphlogistic (oxyphenbutazone). Direct immunofluorescence and immune electron microscopy demonstrate immune complexes within the vessel walls; the pathogenic chain of events of this type III (Arthus) reaction is outlined in the schematic drawing by Wolff et al. (Fig. 9) [18]. Allergic vasculitis is not restricted to the skin. The increasing risk after long-term allergen exposure is demonstrated by the case of a 72-year-old woman. While taking antiphlogistics, she first developed superficial allergic vasculitis, then severe necrosis of the fingertips, and finally renal failure [17].

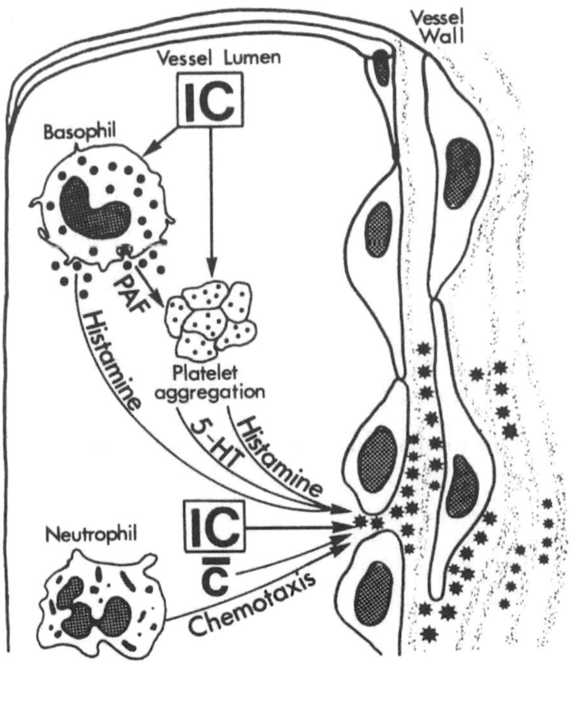

Fig. 9. Pathogenesis of allergic vasculitis. (Wolff et al. [18])

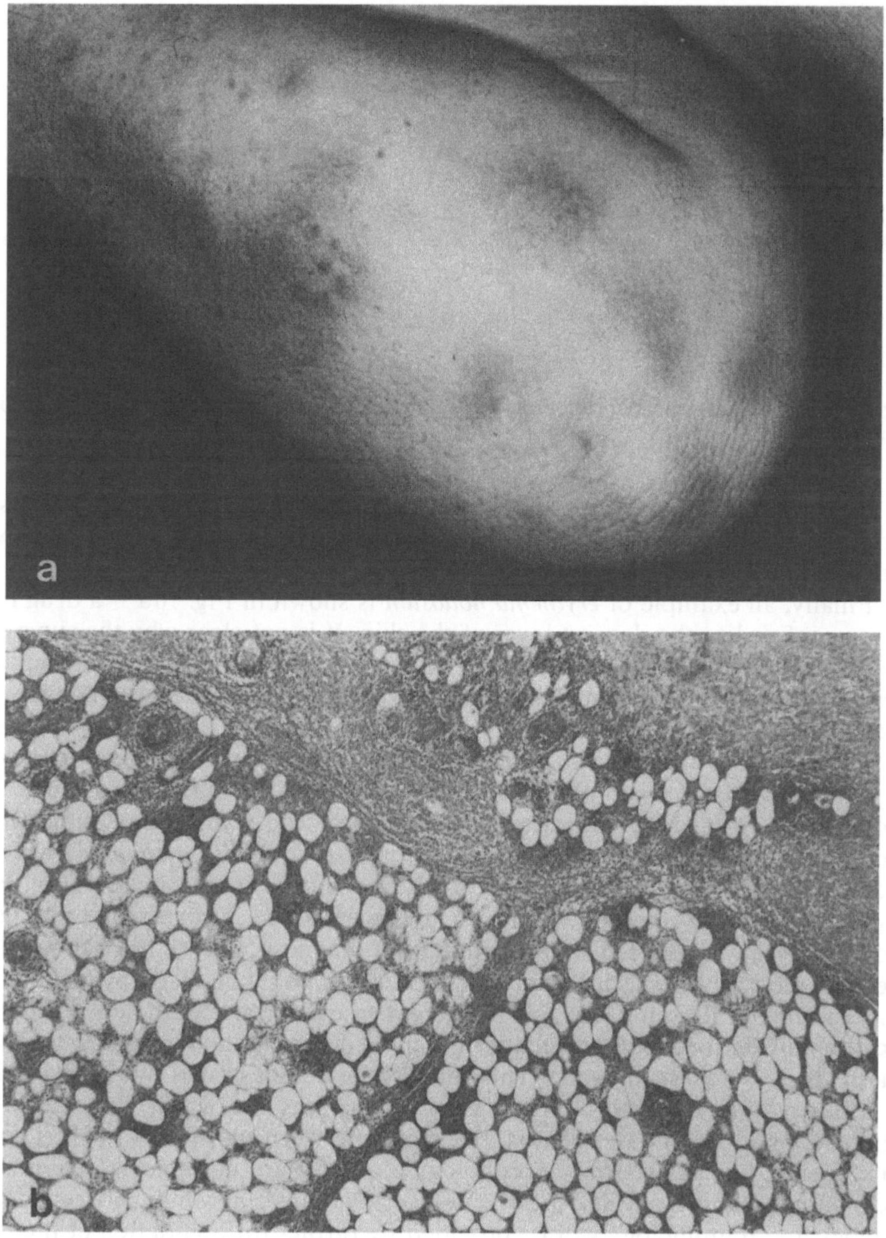

Fig. 10. **a** Erythema nodosum (analgesics). **b** Septal panniculitis. H & E, × 135

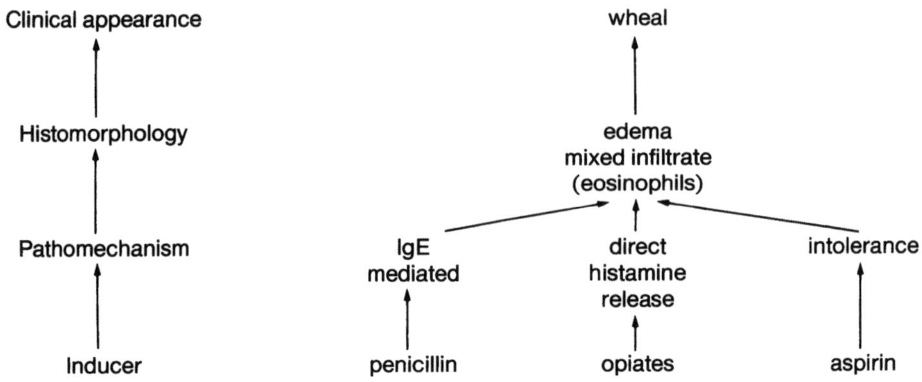

Fig. 11. The pathomechanism, histomorphology and clinical appearance of drug eruptions in urticaria

In contrast, minimal vasculitis is seen in *Schamberg's disease:* only a sparse infiltrate around small vessels of the superficial plexus (capillaritis) and extravasation of erythrocytes.

Finally, an example of *erythema nodosum* is shown in Fig. 10a – a drug reaction confined to the deepest layer of the skin. It is not clear why the superficial plexus remains unaffected in these cases. The histological pattern is that of septal panniculitis with many extravasated red blood cells and granulomatous and fibrosing features (Fig. 10b).

In conclusion, drug eruptions are characterized by a great variety of clinical appearances, even if it is probably an overstatement to claim that "any drug can produce any rash". The clinical diagnosis is based on skin lesions, subjective symptoms like itching, the course of the disease, and the anamnesis (which should place emphasis on the correlation between drug intake and onset of the rash). Nevertheless, certain clinical patterns may be recognized, and histopathology is very helpful in confirming the diagnosis. As we have shown in the examples of blisters, the exact classification can only be made by histological examination. In some cases, as in allergic vasculitis, histopathology even indicates well defined pathomechanisms but of course cannot uncover the inducer (drug? virus? or others?). This can also be demonstrated by the example of urticaria (Fig. 11): the clinician easily recognizes the wheal, and the histopathologist differentiates a broad spectrum between urticaria vasculitis and pure edema, but again, from morphology alone we are not able to determine the pathomechanism and the specific inducer. Perhaps a new link between morphology and immunology will be provided by further differentiation of the infiltrate using monoclonal antibodies [8]. However very little work has been published on this topic.

Figure 12 shows one example drawn from eight examined drug eruptions with different clinical features. In all of our cases T-helper lymphocytes are the predominant cells in the dermal infiltrate. It is too early to speculate whether this is indicative of a delayed hypersensitivity reaction.

Acknowledgment. The excellent technical assistance of Ms. G. Ackermann is acknowledged.

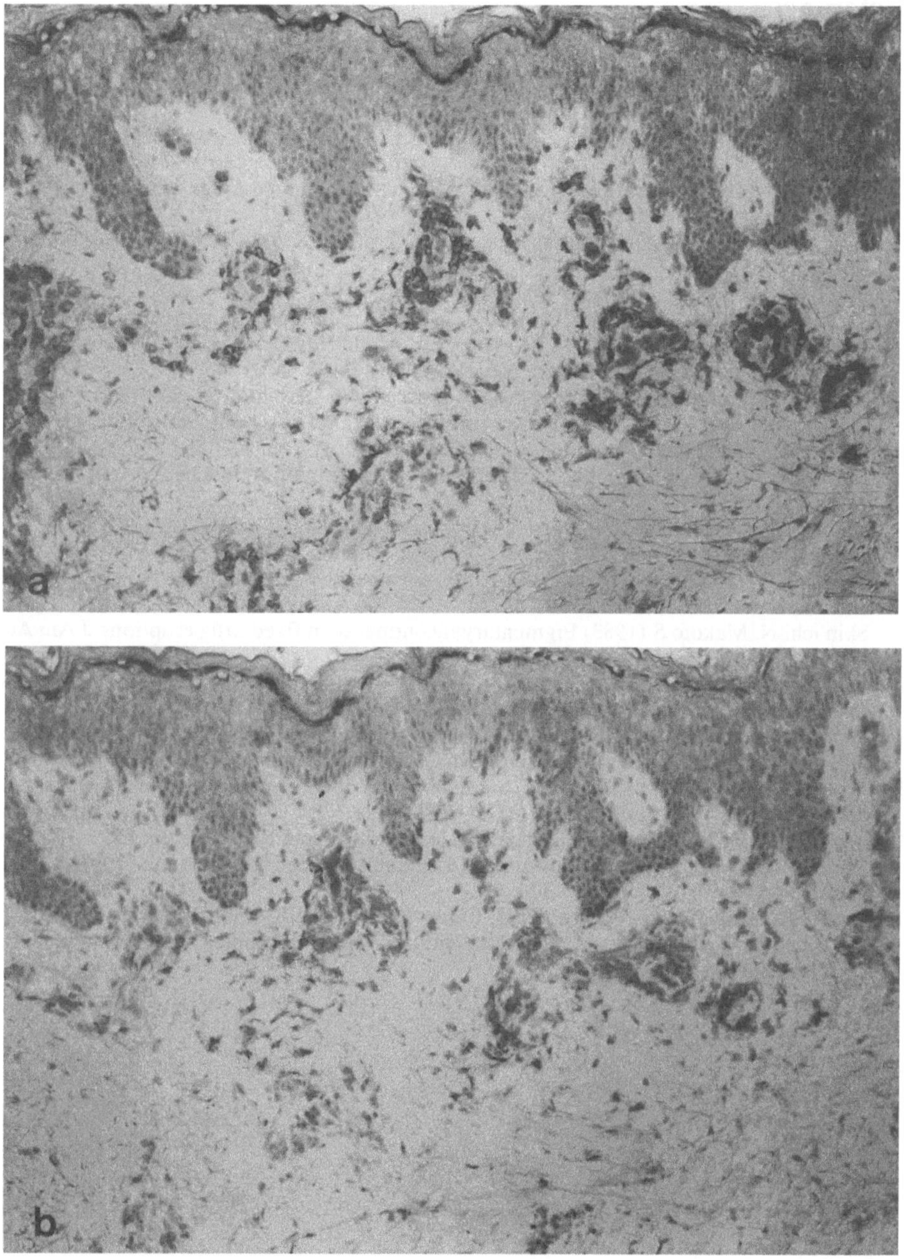

Fig. 12. Macular drug eruption (dihydrocryotamine), indirect peroxidase staining using monoclonal antibodies. **a** anti-Leu-4 (pan-T-lymphocytes). **b** anti-Leu-2 (suppressor lymphocytes). × 135

References

1. Ackerman AB (1978) Histologic diagnosis of inflammatory skin diseases. Lea and Febiger, Philadelphia, pp 188–191, 601–605
2. Albrecht G (1985) Unerwünschte Wirkungen von Lithium an der Haut. Hautarzt 36:77–82
3. Cohnen G (1985) Arzneimittelinduzierte Lupus-erythematodes-ähnliche Syndrome. Allergologie, 8 (7):282–292
4. Goerz G, Merk H (1981) Nicht allergische Arzneimittel-Reaktionen an der Haut. Dermatosen 29 (3):65–74
5. Illig L (1976) Purpura. Fortschr Med 94 (26):1379–1389
6. Kazmierowski JA, Wuepper KD (1983) Erythema multiforme: clinical spectrum and immunopathogenesis. In: Gigli IN, Miescher PA, Müller Eberhard HJ (eds) Immunodermatology. Springer, Berlin Heidelberg New York, pp 47–55
7. Korkij WK, Soltanik (1984) Fixed drug eruption. Arch Dermatol 120:520–524
8. Margolis RJ et al. (1983) Lymphocyte subsets and Langerhans cells/indeterminate cells in erythema multiforme. J Invest Dermatol 81:403–406
9. Matkaluk M et al. (1981) Penicillamine-induced pemphigus foliaceus. Arch Dermatol 117:156–157
10. Rienhoff HY (1982) Toxic epidermal necrolysis. Johns Hopkins Med J 151:326–331
11. Scherer R, Wolff HH (1979) Vasculitis allergica. Allergologie 2:62–71
12. Seehafer JR (1981) Lichen planus-like lesions caused by penicillamine in primary biliary cirrhosis. Arch Dermatol 117:140–142
13. Skin'ichi N, Makoto S (1983) Pigmentary incontinence in fixed drug eruptions. J Am Acad Dermatol 8 (4):525–532
14. Uddin MS, Lynfield Yl, Grosberg SJ, Stiefler R (1979) Cutaneous reaction to spironolactone resembling lupus erythematosus. Cutis 24:198–200
15. Wintroub BU et al. (1979) Adverse cutaneous reactions to drugs. In: Fitzpatrick TB et al. (eds) Dermatology in general medicine. McGraw-Hill, New York, pp 555–567
16. Wolff HH (1980) Lyell-Syndrom: Staphylogenes oder medikamentöses „Syndrom der verbrühten Haut". Notfallmedizin 6:272–277
17. Wolff HH (1983) Vaskulitis allergica – Klassifikation und Ätiologie. In: Braun-Falco O, Burg G (eds) Fortschritte der praktischen Dermatologie und Venerologie. Springer, Berlin Heidelberg New York, pp 297–304
18. Wolff HH, Maciejewski W, Scherer R, Braun-Falco O (1978) Immunoelectronmicroscopic examination of early lesions in histamine induced immune complex vasculitis in man. Br J Dermatol 99:13–24

*Photosensitivity Due to Nonsteroidal Antiinflammatory Drugs**

A. Galosi, B. Przybilla, J. Ring, M. Dorn, and U. Schwab

Dermatologische Klinik und Poliklinik der Ludwig-Maximilians-Universität München, 8000 Munich, Federal Republic of Germany

Abstract

Until now the number of clinically used nonsteroidal antiinflammatory drugs (NSAID) increased up to fourty. Some of these NSAID are known to exert photosensitizing effects.

In this study, different methods were used to identify the photosensitivity of the NSAID including photopatch test, photothreshold testing, oral photoprovocation test, photohaemolysis (PHT) and photo-basophil-histamine-release test (PBHRT).

177 patients with no history of exposure to NSAID were tested by photopatch test. After exposure to 15 J/cm² UV-A positive reactions occurred in about 25% to tiaprofenic acid, 24% to carprofen, 9% to aspirin, 8% to piroxicam, 7% to diclofenac and 2% to ketoprofen. The histologic pattern of biopsies taken at day 3 after UV-A irradiation mostly was photoallergic contact dermatitis.

Photo-threshold testing was performed in 7 patients with positive reactions to tiaprofenic acid. To achieve a positive photopatch test reaction the UV-A-dose needed was once 0.125 J/cm², once 0.25 J/cm², once 2.0 J/cm², once 4.0 J/cm², once higher than 4.0 J/cm² and twice higher than 7.0 J/cm².

To evaluate the phototoxic action of tiaprofenic acid, ketoprofen, diclofenac, indoprofen, ketoprofen, aspirin and tiophen (a ring structure of tiaprofenic acid) these NSAID were tested in vitro with photohemolysis (PHT) and photo-basophil-histamine-release test (PBHRT). Dilutions of the NSAID at concentrations of $10^{-3}-10^{-6}$ mol/l were examined in a modified PHT using sheep erythrocytes and in a PBHRT using peripheral human leucocytes. After exposure of cell suspensions to $1-100$ J/cm² UV-A the increase of extinction at 546 nm was determined as a percentage of total haemolysis in the PHT; the histamine release was measured as a percentage of total releasable histamine content in the PBHRT. With both test procedures, phototoxic action of carprofen and tiaprofenic acid was demonstrated. Benoxaprofen caused only weak reactions. Compared to the PHT, the PBHRT seemed to be more sensitive.

---

* Supported by Deutsche Forschungsgemeinschaft BR 147/54-6

During treatment with tiaprofenic acid a 75-year-old female patient had developed eczematous lesions in light exposed skin requiring hospital treatment. An oral photo-provocation test with 400 mg of tiaprofenic acid was performed. Before and 30, 60, 90 and 200 minutes after ingestion areas of 10 × 10 cm on the patient's back were irradiated with 50 J/cm² UV-A. At the sites having been exposed 60, 90 and 200 minutes after intake of the drug positive reactions started to develop on the next day.

The possibility has to be considered that the photosensitizing properties and the pharmacological effects of NSAID may be related. The test methods presented seem to be helpful to identify mechanisms of drug-induced photosensitivity.

Introduction

Several nonsteroidal antiinflammatory drugs (NSAID) have been reported to cause photosensitivity. The most prominent of these is benoxaprofen, which is a well-known phototoxic agent [6, 11, 12, 15, 17, 18, 25]. Increasing evidence suggests that a considerable number of other NSAID, such as azapropazone, diclofenac, diflunisal, ketoprofen, carprofen, piroxicam, tiaprofenic acid, ibuprofen, indomethacin, naproxen, oxyphenbutazone, mefenamic acid and aspirin may also exert photosensitising effects [1, 2, 4, 7, 10, 13, 14, 16, 19, 20, 22, 24]. In order to determine the photosensitising potency of NSAID we used different in vivo and in vitro methods.

Photopatch Test

Epicutaneous testing of NSAID was performed within a routine standard photopatch test series. The routine irradiation dose was 15 J/cm² UV-A; in most patients additional test series were exposed to non-erythematogenic doses of UV-B (half the minimal erythema dose or 40 mJ/cm² UV-B) and a combination of UV-B and UV-A. In the majority of tests the UV exposure was repeat-

Table 1. Reactions to NSAID in the photopatch test

Substance	Patients tested	Patients reacting at exposed sites			
		Day 3	Later than Day 3	Total	
				n	%
Tiaprofenic acid	175	36	7	43	24.6
Carprofen	86	14	7	21	24.4
Aspirin	76	5	2	7	9.2
Piroxicam	84	5	2	7	8.3
Diclofenac	75	2	3	3	6.7
Ketoprofen	53	1	1	2	3.8

ed a fortnight after the first irradiation. Test results were read routinely on the 2nd, 3rd, 16th and 17th test days.

In 60 of 177 individuals (33.9%) positive photpatch test reactions occurred to at least one of the NSAID applied. There were reactions to tiaprofenic acid in 24.6%, to carprofen in 24.4%, to aspirin in 9.2%, to piroxicam in 8.3%, to diclofenac in 6.7% and to ketoprofen in 3.8% of the tests. In 16 patients positive photopatch test reactions started to develop later than the 3rd test day (between day 7 and day 34). More detailed results are shown in Table 1. Positive test reactions in the non-exposed control series were seen occasionally with tiaprofenic acid, carprofen, aspirin and diclofenac.

Most of the positive photopatch test reactions could be elicited by UV-A alone. In some cases combined irradiation with UV-B and UV-A was necessary to yield positive results, and in a few cases positive reactions occurred exclusively with UV-B.

In seven patients with positive reactions to tiaprofenic acid after exposure to 15 J/cm^2 UV-A, photopatch threshold testing was performed. In four of these there were reactions to doses as low as 0.125, 0.25, 2.0 and 4.0 J/cm^2 UV-A respectively.

The histological examination of biopsies taken in some cases from positive photopatch test reactions revealed a pattern compatible with allergic dermatitis.

Oral Photoprovocation Test

An oral photoprovocation test was carried out in a 75-year-old female who had developed eczematous lesions on light-exposed skin during treatment with tiaprofenic acid.

Before and 30, 60, 90 and 200 min after ingestion of 400 mg tiaprofenic acid, areas on the patient's back were irradiated with 50 J/cm^2 UV-A. On the following day, positive reactions characterised by erythematous infiltrates started to develop at the sites exposed to UV-A 60, 90 and 200 min after intake of the drug. These reactions became more intense up to the 3rd day, the maximum reaction occurring in the area irradiated 90 min after ingestion. On histological examination, a pattern of lymphohistiocytic vasculitis was found. This patient also reacted to tiaprofenic acid in the photopatch test.

Photohemolysis Test and Photo-Basophil-Histamine-Release Test

Dilutions of benoxaprofen, carprofen, tiaprofenic acid, diclofenac, indoprofen, ketoprofen, aspirin and thiophene (a ring structure of tiaprofenic acid) at concentrations of $10^{-6}-10^{-3}$ mol/l were examined in a modified photohemolysis test (PHT) using sheep erythrocytes, and in a newly developed photo-basophil histamine release test (PBHRT) using peripheral human leucocytes. After exposure of the cell suspensions incubated with NSAID to doses of 1 – 100 J/cm² UV-A, the increase of extinction was determined as a percentage of the total hemolysis in the PHT and the histamine release was measured as percentage of the total releasable histamine content in the PBHRT.

In the PHT, the maximum increase of extinction induced by 100 J/cm² UV-A was found to be 1% for indoprofen, 2% for aspirin, 2% for benoxaprofen, 3% for diclofenac, 4% for carprofen, 33% for thiophene, 43% for tiaprofenic acid and 43% for ketoprofen. In the PBHRT, indoprofen induced no histamine release; the maximum amount of histamine release after UV exposure was 4%

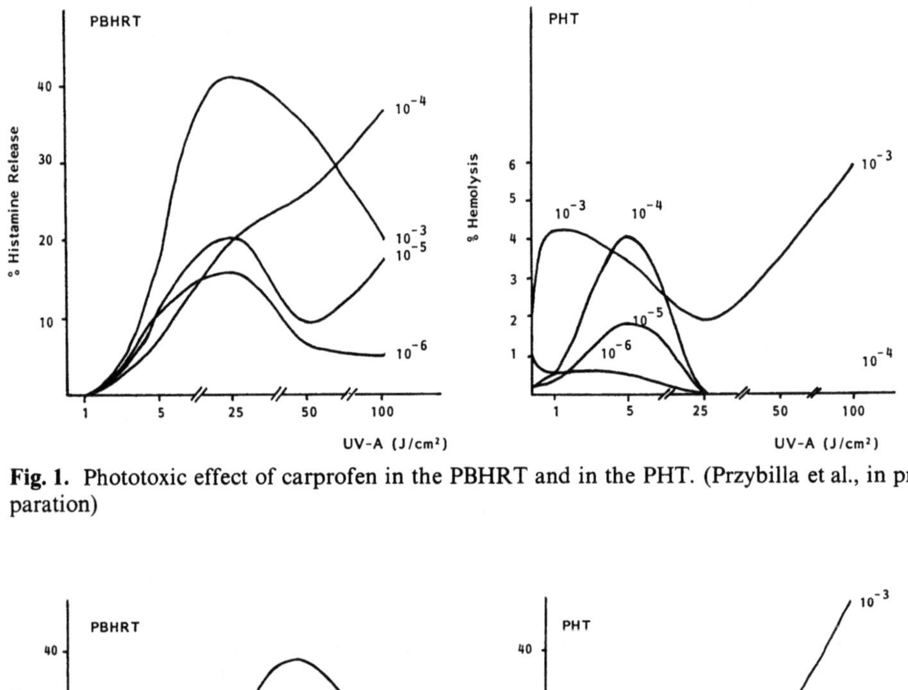

Fig. 1. Phototoxic effect of carprofen in the PBHRT and in the PHT. (Przybilla et al., in preparation)

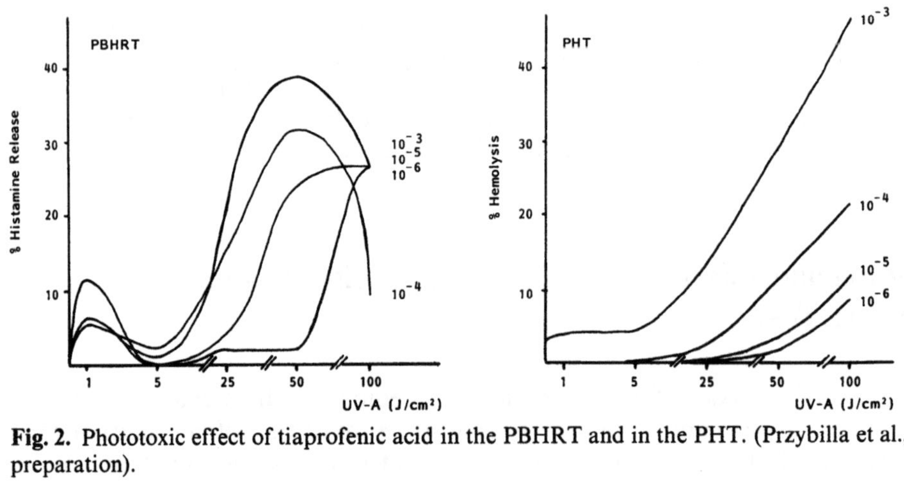

Fig. 2. Phototoxic effect of tiaprofenic acid in the PBHRT and in the PHT. (Przybilla et al., in preparation).

with aspirin, 10% with benoxaprofen, 20% with thiophene, 28% with diclofenac, 39% with tiaprofenic acid, 40% with carprofen and 55% with ketoprofen. The results obtained with carprofen and tiaprofenic acid are shown in Figs. 1 and 2.

Photosensitivity – Phototoxic or Photoallergic?

The results of in vitro phototoxicity testing and the high incidence of positive photopatch test reactions to NSAID suggest a phototoxic action of these substances. Similarly, in a recent study from Sweden a phototoxic action of several NSAID could be demonstrated by various in vitro methods [16]. However, in the light of the development of positive skin test reactions later than day 3, the histological picture seen in biopsies of test reactions, the high UV sensitivity found with photopatch threshold testing and the spreading of photopatch test reactions observed occasionally, a photoallergic mechanism has to be considered for some cases. Phototoxic reactions may possibly have promoted photoallergic sensitisation in these cases.

Clinical Relevance

Another question which remains to be answered is whether systemic treatment with NSAID will cause photosensitivity with comparable frequency. UV-induced drug reactions in vivo due to NSAID have so far been established by phototesting only for the propionic acid derivatives benoxaprofen [5, 6, 11, 15, 18, 25], carprofen [1, 10, 13, 14, 20], tiaprofenic acid [4, 8, 9, 22] and naproxen [4] and for the oxicam derivative piroxicam [4, 7, 23]. Phototoxic as well as photoallergic mechanisms seem to be involved in clinical photosensitivity to carprofen and tiaprofenic acid, whereas benoxaprofen and naproxen are phototoxic and piroxicam probably causes photoallergic reactions. The action spectra of all these photosensitising NSAID seem to lie in the UV-B as well as in the UV-A range.

Pathomechanism

Many of the NSAID exerting photosensitising effects in vivo or in vitro, i.e. benoxaprofen, carprofen, tiaprofenic acid and ketoprofen, are derivatives of propionic acid. Therefore we should like to propose a relationship between the UV-sensitising action of NSAID and the structure of propionic acid, which is an additive used to preserve some foods [21]. It has been suggested that the ingestion of propionic acid, may be related to the occurrence of photosensitivity of etiologically unknown origin, such as in polymorphic light eruption [21]. However, other structures may also be responsible for photosensitivity to NSAID. Thiophene, a heterocyclic ring system of the tiaprofenic acid molecule, was found to be phototoxic in the PBHRT and in the PHT, and alpha-terthienyl, which is composed of three thiophene rings, has been shown to exert phototoxic effects [3].

Moreover, a relationship between the pharmacological and the photosensitising action of NSAID seems possible. Such an association would be of fundamental interest with regard to the mechanism of photosensitisation. One can speculate that inhibition of cyclooxygenase by NSAID may prevent formation of protective metabolites, i.e. prostaglandin E2, which otherwise might prevent or reduce UV-induced skin damage. Furthermore, products of the lipoxygenase pathway may be involved in photosensitisation by NSAID.

Conclusion

Overall, present knowledge indicates that at least some NSAID are *proven* photosensitisers and that the whole pharmacological group should be included in the list of *possible* photosensitising agents. Further investigations are necessary to elucidate the pathomechanism of the photosensitising action of these compounds.

References

1. Bause R (1983) Photoallergische Arzneireaktion auf Carprofen. Z Hautkr 59:393
2. Bruinsma W (1972) Adverse reaction profiles of drug eruptions. Dermatologica 145:377–388
3. Chan GFQ, Prihoda M, Towers GHN, Mitchell JC (1977) Phototoxicity evoked by alpha-terthienyl. Contact Dermatitis 3:215–216
4. Diffey BL, Daymond TJ, Fairgreaves H (1983) Phototoxic reactions to piroxicam, naproxen and tiaprofenic acid. Br J Rheumatol 22:239–242
5. Fenton DA, Wilkinson JD, English HS (1981) Photosensitisation to benoxaprofen not due to ultraviolet A alone. Lancet ii:1230–1231
6. Ferguson J, Addo JA, McGill PE, Woodcok KR, Johnson BE, Frain-Bell W (1982) A study of benoxaprofen-induced photosensitivity. Br J Dermatol 107:429–442
7. Fjellner B (1983) Photosensitivity induced by piroxicam. Acta Derm Venerol (Stockh) 63:557–558
8. Galosi A, Przybilla B, Ring J, Dorn M (1984) Systemische Photoprovokation mit Surgam. Allergologie 7:143–144
9. Galosi A, Przybilla B, Ring J, Dorn M (1984) Photosensitising potential of the nonsteroidal antiinflammatory drug (NSAID) tiaprofenic acid (TPA). J Allergy Clin Immunol 73:165

10. Geißler B, Lischka (1984) Lichtsensibilisierung durch Carprofen. Akt Dermatol 10:185–187
11. Greist MC, Ozols II, Ridolfo AS, Muus JC (1982) The phototoxic effects of benoxaprofen and their management and prevention. Eur J Rheumatol Inflam 5:138–147
12. Halsey P, Cardoe N (1982) Benoxaprofen: side-effect profile in 300 patients. Br Med J 284:1365–1368
13. Hoting E, Schulz KH (1984) Photoallergische Reaktion auf Carprofen. Dermatosen 32:215–216
14. Kietzmann H, Rüther TH, Scheuer B (1984) Photosensitive Hautreaktionen auf Carprofen. Akt Dermatol 10:17–20
15. Kligman AM, Kaidbey KH (1982) Phototoxicity to benoxaprofen. Eur J Rheumatol Inflam 5:124–137
16. Ljunggren B (1985) Propionic acid-derived non-steroidal antiinflammatory drugs are phototoxic in vitro. Photodermatology 2:3–9
17. Ljunggren B, Bjellurup M, Möller H (1983) Experimental studies on the mechanism of benoxaprofen photoreactions. Arch Dermatol Res 275:318–323
18. McCormack LS, Elgart ML, Turner ML (1982) Benoxaprofen-induced photo-onycholysis. J Am Acad Dermatol 7:678–680
19. Merot Y, Harms M, Saurat J-M (1983) Photosensibilisation au Carprofène (Imadyl), un nouvel antiinflammatoire non stéroidien. Dermatologica 166:301–307
20. Przybilla B, Brunner R, Ring J, Galosi A, Dorn M (1984) Lichtinduziertes Arzneiexanthem. Auslösung durch Carprofen. Münch Med Wochenschr 126:1503–1506
21. Przybilla B, Dorn M (1984) Photosensibilisierung durch nichtsteroidale Antirheumatika. Hautarzt 35:561–562
22. Przybilla B, Ring J, Galosi A, Dorn M (1984) Photopatch test reactions to tiaprofenic acid. Contact Dermatitis 10:55–56
23. Serrano G, Bonillo J, Aliaga A, Gargallo E, Pelufo C (1984) Piroxicam-induced photosensitivity. In vivo and in vitro studies of its photosensitizing potential. J Am Acad Dermatol 11:113–120
24. Stern RS, Sachs R (1983) Phototoxic reactions to Piroxicam and other nonsteroidal antiinflammatory agents (letter). N Engl J Med 309:186–187
25. Wiskemann A (1981) Photosensibilisierung durch Benoxaprofen. Arzneimittelforsch Drug Res 31:730–732

Anaphylactoid Reactions to Mild Analgesics

B. Przybilla, A.-R. Bonnländer, and J. Ring
Dermatologische Klinik und Poliklinik der Ludwig-Maximilians-Universität München, 8000 Munich, Federal Republic of Germany

Abstract

"Mild" analgesic preparations (MAP), containing as main active compounds salicylates, pyrazolons, or p-aminophenol derivatives, are well-known elicitors of AR. The identification of the responsible agent is often difficult, as routine skin tests are only rarely conclusive.

The diagnostic value of skin tests (prick test, intracutaneous tests), challenge tests, and basophil histamine release tests was assessed in patients presenting with AR to MAP.

Prick testing with common components of MAP or commercial preparations (mostly in saturated solutions) yielded conclusive results (≥ 3 mm wheal diameter) in 19/282 patients. Positive reactions in more than 1% were observed only with the pyrazolons dipyrone (3.3%), propyphenazone (2.2%), and antipyrine (1.1%). The yield of conclusive results increased with the severity of the reactions reported in the history, reaching 25% in patients with a history of a full shock. – In 155 patients (mostly with negative prick test), *oral challenge tests* were performed. At least one conclusive positive result was obtained in 90 patients. The most frequent reactions were due to propyphenazone (in 39% of the patients tested), aspirin (23%), dipyrone (25%), acetaminophen (6%), and phenacetin (6%). In more than half of the patients with aspirin-induced AR there were additional reactions to pyrazolons and/or p-aminophenol derivatives. Among 71 patients reacting to dipyrone or propyphenazone, "cross reactivity" to both pyrazolon compounds occurred only in 12 cases. – *Intracutaneous* skin testing (ICT) with solutions of 10^{-2} M was compared with the oral challenge test results: with propyphenazone 4/6 ICT reactions proved to be false positive, and in only 2/6 patients with a positive challenge test a conclusive ICT was found. 0/4 patients with AR to dipyrone were identifiable by ICT. In 3 patients showing conclusive positive prick test reactions to propyphenazone and/ or dipyrone oral challenges with these compounds were positive. – In 19 patients with positive oral challenge tests the *histamine release* from basophils was evaluated in vitro after incubation with the eliciting compounds. Only in 1 patient reactive to propyphenazone and dipyrone a concordant clearcut positive result was obtained.

These results indicate that at present oral challenge tests are the only reliable procedure to evaluate AR to MAP. They should include a battery of different drugs, since all mild analgesics, including acetaminophen, may elicit AR. Conclusive prick test results can be obtained with some pyrazolone derivatives, especially in patients with severe reactions. They probably are then sufficient for diagnosis. ICT as described does not seem to yield any advantage and bears the risk of false positive reactions. Positive results in the basophil histamine release test may be diagnostic, however, they are only observed in rare cases.

Introduction

Salicylates, para-aminophenol derivatives, and pyrazolon derivatives belong to the group of non-narcotic, mild analgesics [23] which exert analgesic effects by interference with prostaglandin synthesis. Preparations containing these agents are widely used in the general population. Such preparations frequently contain combinations of mild analgesics, and not rarely they also include other components such as codeine, caffeine, sedatives, or vitamins. Mild analgesic preparations are well-known elicitors of anaphylactoid reactions.

Anaphylactoid reactions can either be elicited immunologically, that is by an allergy, or are due to nonimmunological idiosyncrasy (pseudo-allergy) [12]. They comprise a spectrum of symptoms from mere urticarial skin reactions as the mildest manifestation, through minor respiratory, gastrointestinal, or cardiovascular symptoms, to full shock as a possible life-threatening event. Identification of the agent responsible for anaphylactoid reactions to mild analgesic preparations is often difficult when various preparations or mixtures of various compounds have been used, and routine skin tests are inconclusive.

Pathomechanism of Anaphylactoid Reactions to Mild Analgesics

The exact pathomechanisms of anaphylactoid reactions to mild analgesics have not yet been elucidated, and several pathogenetic principles have to be discussed: IgE-mediated reactions may play a role in a number of allergic mechanisms; however, one can also speculate about short-term sensitizing antibodies or immune complex anaphylaxis. Interference of mild analgesics with arachidonic acid metabolism might be of importance as regards idiosyncrasy [2, 21]. In addition, aspirin has been shown to activate complement directly [22], but the relevance of this finding for the induction of symptoms has recently been questioned [10]. Other mechanisms, such as direct mast cell activation, enzyme defects, or other effects, may also be involved in pseudo-allergy [12]. Recently, aspirin-induced increased platelet-dependent cytotoxic reactions have been observed in patients with aspirin idiosyncrasy [1]. Currently anaphylactoid reactions to aspirin are mostly thought to be nonimmunological in origin [2, 5, 6, 8, 13, 15, 17, 21]; a pathogenetic role of the highly immunogenic aspirin anhydride has been proposed for some cases [3]. Pyrazolon derivatives may cause idiosyncratic as well as allergic reactions [2, 21], and little is known about the pathomechanism of reactions to para-aminophenol derivatives.

Considering this insufficient knowledge of the pathomechanism of anaphylactoid reactions to mild analgesics, it is not surprising that diagnostic evaluation is difficult.

Prick Tests

In a series of 282 patients with a history of drug reactions we performed prick testing with a battery of common components of mild analgesics preparations and additionally with commercial preparations, in most cases using saturated aqueous solutions [11]. Only immediate reactions with a wheal diameter of at least 3 mm were regarded as positive. In only 19 patients (7%) were positive prick tests obtained. There were 26 positive reactions to single components and 14 positive reactions to commercial analgesic preparations. Detailed results are shown in Table 1. The majority of positive reactions to single compounds occurred with pyrazolon derivatives. This is in good accordance with the general experience [2, 6, 7, 8, 18, 21]; Sometimes pyrazolon derivatives are capable of evoking contact urticaria even without scarification [7, 14]. In our patients cross-reactivity between pyrazolon derivatives was not the rule; for example of 12 patients reacting to dipyrone or propyphenazone, only 3 exhibited positive results to both agents.

Table 1. Immediate prick test reactions to components of mild analgesic preparations

Compound	Tests (*n*)	
	Total	Positive [a]
Pyrazolon derivatives		
Dipyrone	277	9 (3.3%)
Propyphenazone	276	6 (2.2%)
Antipyrine	277	3 (1.1%)
Phenylbutazone	275	2 (0.7%)
Oxyphenbutazone	276	2 (0.7%)
Para-aminophenol derivatives		
Phenacetin	277	1 (0.4%)
Other single compounds		
Phenobarbital	271	1 (0.4%)
Carbromal	274	1 (0.4%)
Vitamin B_1	273	1 (0.4%)
Commercial preparations	253	14 (5.5%)

[a] Wheal diameter ≧ 3 mm

Table 2. History and prick test reactions to components of analgesic preparations

History	Number of patients	Patients with positive prick tests		
Clear-cut anaphylactoid reactions due to analgesics:	117	15 (13%)		
Skin symptoms	41	3 (7%)		
Respiratory/cardiovascular symptoms	52	6 (12%)	$P<0.05$ [a]	$P<0.01$ [a]
Full shock	24	6 (25%)		
Uncertain history	165	4 (2%)		
Total	282	19 (7%)		

[a] Chi-square test

The poor yield of positive prick tests improves considerably when only those 117 individuals are considered who gave a clear-cut history of anaphylactoid reactions to mild analgesic preparations. Of these patients, 15 (13%) exhibited positive results and the diagnostic value of the skin test increased with the severity of anaphylactoid symptoms: positive results were found in 7% with only skin reactions, in 12% with additional minor respiratory or cardiovascular symptoms, and in 25% with full shock. Similar findings of a correlation between the yield of positive skin tests and the severity of reactions have been reported recently [6]. Positive prick tests were significantly less frequent in individuals with an uncertain history of anaphylactoid reactions to mild analgesic preparations than in those with a clear-cut history. The interdependence of prick test results and clinical history is shown in Table 2.

Oral Challenge Tests

Oral challenge tests were performed in a total of 155 patients with anaphylactoid reactions to mild analgesic preparations, only 3 of whom had had positive prick results in the standard test (see below). These challenges were done in the hospital under utmost caution. Usually incremental amounts of 10%, 50%, and 100% of the conventional dose of a single compound were applied in gelatine capsules, and occasionally commercial preparations were tested in a similar way. The 100% doses were 500 mg for aspirin, 500 mg for acetaminophen, 300 mg for phenacetin, 500 mg for dipyrone, and 200 mg for propyphenazone. In the course of the study the initial dose of propyphenazone was reduced to 2.5%, as with 10% (20 mg) a full shock had twice developed. Following positive reactions an interval of at least 72 h was allowed before the next challenge in order to avoid false-negative results during a possible refractory period [20]. If necessary, placebo controls were carried out.

At least one conclusive positive result was obtained in 90 patients. In another three individuals there were reactions to various analgesics but also to

Table 3. Oral challenge tests with analgesics

Compound	Tests (*n*)	
	Total	Positive
Salicylates		
Aspirin	142	33 (23%)
Para-aminophenol derivatives		
Acetaminophen	134	8 (6%)
Phenacetin	135	8 (6%)
Pyrazolon derivatives		
Dipyrone	132	33 (25%)
Propyphenazone	133	52 (39%)
Other single compounds	151	10 (7%)
Commercial preparations	160	15 (9%)
Total	987	159 (16%)

Table 4. Reaction pattern[a] of oral challenge tests with analgesics

Reactions to	Patients	
	n	%
Aspirin	13	15
Aspirin + pyrazolons	12	14
Aspirin + pyrazolons + para-aminophenol derivatives	8	9
Pyrazolons	48	55
Pyrazolons + para-aminophenol derivatives	6	7
Total	87	100

[a] Reactions to aspirin, dipyrone, propyphenazone, phenacetin, and acetaminophen

placebo; these patients were excluded from further evaluation. There was a total of 159 positive challenge results. Of the patients tested, 39% reacted to propyphenazone, 25% to dipyrone, 23% to aspirin, 6% to acetaminophen, and 6% to phenacetin (Table 3).

In 71 individuals challenged with both dipyrone and propyphenazone and reacting to at least one of these pyrazolon compounds, cross-reactivity between the two agents was observed in only 17%. Similarly, cross-reactivity between the para-aminophenol derivatives acetaminophen and phenacetin occurred in only 2 of 12 patients (18%).

Our standard series, including aspirin, dipyrone, propyphenazone, phenacetin, and acetaminophen, was tested in most of the patients. Eighty-seven individuals reacted to at least one of these agents. Distinctive reaction patterns can be detected. In more than 50% there were reactions exclusively to pyrazolon derivatives, in 15% only to aspirin, and in 30% to combinations of compounds of different pharmacological groups. Adverse reactions to other mild analgesics occurred in about two-thirds of patients in whom aspirin was not tolerated. Details of the reaction patterns are given in Table 4.

The doses of pyrazolon derivatives necessary to elicit reactions were significantly lower in patients responding exclusively to these compounds than in individuals reactive to aspirin as well as pyrazolon derivatives (Fig. 1). Both this difference in the eliciting dose and the distinctive reaction pattern, with multiple positive results to compounds of different pharmacological groups predominantly in patients not tolerating aspirin are in good accordance with the concept of the existence of two different pathomechanisms which has been proposed by the group of Szczeklik [2, 21]: patients reacting to aspirin and further compounds probably suffer from nonimmunological idiosyncreasy, whereas allergic mechanisms seem to play a role in exclusive reactions to pyrazolon derivatives. With the exception of three individuals all our patients had had a negative prick test. In contrast to these results it has been claimed that skin tests will be positive in all pyrazolon – allergic patients [2, 21]. This discrepancy at least partially seems due to the use of intracutaneous testing, which probably bears the risk of false-positive reactions (see below). There are findings similar to ours suggesting the existence of a skin test-negative pyrazolon-allergic group of patients [6, 9, 16].

Why is the prick test negative in patients who are probably allergic? It may be that our test solutions are inadequate with regard to solubility, concentra-

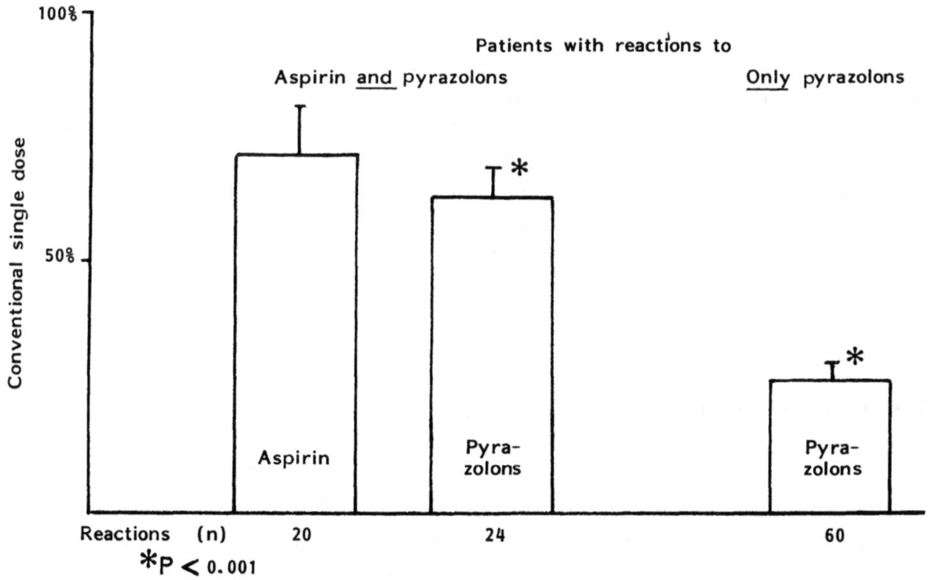

Fig. 1. Mean eliciting challenge doses for aspirin and pyrazolon derivatives in patients reacting to aspirin *and* pyrazolons and in patients reacting *only* to pyrazolons

tion, skin penetration, or protein binding of the substances. The carrier to which small hapten molecules have to bind to become allergenic may be lacking at the test site. Furthermore, the patient may be allergic not to the compound itself but also metabolites evolving in the organism after systemic application. Lastly, the poor results with skin testing may be due to the presence of non-IgE-mediated allergy.

Intracutaneous Skin Tests

Intracutaneous testing is used by some as a routine method in the evaluation of anaphylactoid reactions to mild analgesics. The recommended concentrations of test solutions range from 0.1% [2, 6] up to 10% [4]. We have compared the results of oral callenges and intracutaneous testing with 10^{-2} M (0.23%) solutions of propyphenazone (Table 5). Of positive intracutaneous reactions, 50% proved to be false, and in only 2 of 12 patients were concordant positive results found. When tested intracutaneously, four of the six patients reacting in the challenge test did not exhibit a positive result; at least two of these four individuals exhibited at challenge the "allergic pattern of reaction" as proposed above. None of five patients with anaphylactoid reactions to dipyrone (two individuals were presumably allergic) could be identified by intracutaneous testing with a 10^{-2} M (0.35%) solution. These results suggest that intracutaneous testing in this form is not yet a reliable test procedure. Titration studies with increasing concentrations of dipyrone and decreasing concentrations of propyphenazone will show whether there is a more appropriate concentration for intracutaneous testing. However, at least for propyphenazone, intracutaneous testing does not seem to be a good diagnostic tool as there were both false-positive and false-negative reactions at the concentrations now used.

The poor correlation between oral challenges and intracutaneous testing prompted us to ask how reliable prick testing is. Thus we have recently started to challenge patients with positive prick test results. Up to now three patients showing positive prick test reactions to propyphenazone and/or dipyrone have been investigated: oral challenges with the skin test-positive compounds were positive in all of them.

Basophil Histamine Release Tests

Routine in vitro test methods are not available for the diagnosis of anaphylactoid reactions to mild analgesics. We have assessed the value of a basophil histamine release test: The patients' peripheral blood leukocytes were washed and incubated with $10^{-5}-10^{-3}$ M of aspirin, acetaminophen, phenacetin, dipyrone, or propyphenazone for 30 min. The histamine released was

Table 5. Intracutaneous tests and oral challenge tests with propyphenazone in 12 patients

Intracutaneous test	Oral challenge test	Patients	
		n	%
+	+	2	17
+	−	6	50
−	+	4	33
Total		12	100

+ = positive reaction; − = negative reaction

Table 6. Results of the basophil histamine release test in 18 patients with positive challenge tests

Compound	Positive challenges (*n*)	% histamine release (HR) in 4 patients with HR > 5%			
		Pat. 1	Pat. 2	Pat. 3	Pat. 4
Aspirin	5	5.4 [a]			
Acetaminophen	2				
Phenacetin	2		6.9 [a]		
Dipyrone	8				51.5
Propyphenazone	10			9.4 [a]	53.5

[a] Cannot be regarded as diagnostic (see text)

determined spectrofluorometrically using an automated analyzing technique [19]. A release of more than 5% of the total histamine content with compounds positive at challenge was observed in only 4 of 18 patients (Table 6). However, the values found with aspirin, propyphenazone, and phenacetin in three of these patients cannot be regarded as diagnostic as individuals tolerating these agents exhibited similar results. Only in one patient reacting to dipyrone and propyphenazone at challenge was a concordant and conclusive result with a histamine release of more than 50% obtained.

Conclusions

Positive prick test reactions can be obtained with pyrazolon derivatives, especially in patients with severe reactions. Further investigations are needed to show whether such prick test results are sufficient for diagnosis – at present they are thought to be. Intracutaneous testing with at least propyphenazone does not seem to yield more advantage, as both false-positive and false-negative results occurred at moderate concentrations. The diagnostic value of intracutaneous testing has to be evaluated for further compounds by correlation with challenge test results. Skin testing may be more effective with analgesic compounds conjugated to large carrier molecules to overcome their hapten character. A multicenter study using such conjugates is currently being conducted by the European Group for Drug Allergy (EGDA). Using conjugates in vitro testing may also be more promising. Positive results in the basophil histamine release test may be diagnostic; however, they are only observed in rare cases and thus are not suitable for routine diagnostics. As long as the basic pathomechanisms of anaphylactoid reactions to mild analgesics have not been elucidated, the challenge test remains the only reliable diagnostic procedure. It should include a battery of different drugs, since all mild analgesics, including acetaminophen (which is claimed by some to be safe without testing), may elicit anaphylactoid reactions.

Acknowledgments. The authors would like to thank Mrs. Leilani Oberbauer, Mrs. Angelika Ruf, and Mrs. Franziska Sedlmeier for excellent technical assistance.

References

1. Capron A, Ameisen JC, Joseph M, Auriault C, Tonnel AB, Caen J (1985) New functions for platelets and their pathological implications. Int Arch Allergy Appl Immunol 77:107–114
2. Czerniawska-Mysik G, Szczeklik A (1981) Idiosyncrasy to pyrazolone drugs. Allergy 36:381–384
3. De Weck AL (1971) Immunological effects of aspirin anhydride, a contaminant of commercial acetylsalicylic acid preparations. Int Arch Allergy 41:393–418
4. Gottmann-Lückerath I, Steigleder GK (1974) Nachweis von Arzneimittelallergien durch Hauttests. In: Werner M, Ruppert V (eds) Praktische Allergiediagnostik. Methoden des direkten Allergennachweises. Thieme, Stuttgart, pp 115–128
5. Illig L (1982) Pseudo-allergische (anaphylactoide) Reaktionen der Haut auf Lebensmittelfarbstoffe. Allergologie 5:193–198
6. Kleinhans D (1985) Reaktionen vom Soforttyp auf Analgetika-Wirkstoffe: Allergie und Intoleranz. Allergologie 8:254–259
7. Maucher OM, Fuchs A (1983) Kontakturtikaria im Epikutantest bei Pyrazolonallergie. Hautarzt 34:383–386
8. Merk H, Goerz G (1983) Analgetika-Intoleranz. Z Hautkr 58:535–542
9. Patriarca G, Venuti A, Bonini W (1973) Allergy to pyramidon (aminopyrine). Ann Allergy 31:84–86
10. Pleskow WW, Chenoweth DE, Simon RA, Stevenson DD, Curd JG (1983) The absence of detectable complement activation in aspirin-sensitive asthmatic patients during aspirin challenge. J Allergy Clin Immunol 72:462–468
11. Przybilla B, Ring J, Harle R (1984) Evaluation of anaphylactoid reactions (AR) to "mild" analgesics. J Allergy Clin Immunol 73:164 (Abstract)
12. Ring J, Laubenthal H, Meßmer K (1982) Incidence and classification of adverse reactions to plasma substitutes. Klin Wochenschr 60:997–1002
13. Samter M, Beers RF (1968) Intolerance to aspirin. Clinical studies and consideration of its pathogenesis. Ann Intern Med 68:975–983
14. Sertoli A, Marliani A, Lombardi P, Panconesi E (1980) Immediate sensitization to methamizole verified by patch tests. Contact Dermatitis 6:294
15. Settipane GA (1983) Aspirin and allergic diseases: a review. Am J Med 74 (6A):102–109

16. Scheuer B (1983) Dermatologische Nebenwirkungen von Propyphenazon. Allergologie 6:450–453
17. Schlumberger HD (1980) Drug-induced pseudo-allergic syndrome as exemplified by acetylsalicylic acid intolerance. In: Dukor P, Kallós P, Schlumberger HD, West GB (eds) PAR. Pseudo-allergic reactions. Involvement of drugs and chemicals, vol 1. Karger, Basel, pp 125–203
18. Schulz KH (1979) Stellenwert und Aussagekraft von Testmethoden bei allergischen Arzneiexanthemen. In: Braun-Falco O, Wolff HH (eds) Fortschritte der praktischen Dermatologie und Venerologie, vol 9. Springer, Berlin Heidelberg New York, pp 71–80
19. Siraganian RP (1976) Histamine release and assay methods for the study of human allergy. In: Rose NR, Friedmann H (eds) Manual of clinical immunology. American Society for Microbiology, Washington, pp 603–615
20. Stevenson DD, Pleskow WW, Curd JG, Simon RA, Mathison DA (1982) Desensitization to acetylsalicylic acid (ASA) in ASA-sensitive patients with rhinosinusitis/asthma. In: Dukor P, Kallós P, Schlumberger HD, West GB (eds) PAR. Pseudo-allergic reactions. Involvement of drugs and chemicals, vol 3. Karger, Basel, pp 133–156
21. Szczeklik A, Gryglewski RJ, Czerniawska-Mysik G (1977) Clinical patterns of hypersensitivity to nonsteroidal anti-inflammatory drugs and their pathogenesis. J Allergy Clin Immunol 6:276–284
22. Voigtländer V, Hänsch GM, Rother U (1980) Effect of aspirin on complement in vivo. Int Arch Allergy Appl Immunol 61:145–149
23. Woodbury DM, Fingl E (1975) Analgesic-antipyretics, anti-inflammatory agents, and drugs employed in the therapy of gout. In: Goodman LS, Gilman A (eds) The pharmacological basis of therapeutics. Macmillan, New York, pp 325–358

Immune Complex Anaphylaxis Induced by Dextran and Its Elimination by Hapten Inhibition

A. W. Richter

Department of Biomedical Research Pharmacia AB, 75182 Uppsala, Sweden and Department of Immunology, University of Stockholm, 10401 Stockholm, Sweden

Abstract

Purpose: To elucidate the mechanism of the rare anaphylactic reactions elicited by i.v. infusion of Macrodex® and Rheomacrodex® and to find measures for their elimination.

Methods: Hapten inhibition in vitro and in dextran anaphylaxis in guinea pigs and dogs.

Human serology: Complement profiles; IgE assays: RAST, PCA in monkeys, RCLAAR*; estimation of dextran reactive antibodies (DRA) by gel diffusion, passive hemagglutination, RCLAAR for IgG and subclasses, IgA, IgM, IgD; ELISA for IgG. Histopathology of human lung specimens. Clinical trials in five countries to assess efficacy of hapten inhibition.

Summary of results: Dextran anaphylaxis (incidence 0.05%) occurs upon *the first* infusion of a few ml of clinical dextran. Severity of anaphylaxis positively correlates with IgG-DRA levels (especially IgG_2) reaching conc of 1 mg/ml. High titers of specific IgA and IgM were also found *but no IgE* or IgD. C1q levels were low. Lung histopathology of fatal cases disclosed obstruction of vessels with globuli of fibrinlike material, aggregated platelets and leukocytes. The naturally occurring DRA which cause anaphylaxis originate from immunization with ingested wild type dextran or cross-reactive bacterial polysaccharides. Since dextran anaphylaxis in animals could be prevented or reduced by hapten inhibition, and a dextran fraction of M_w 1000 (Promit®) proved to be non-eliciting and safe, clinical trials were started. 130000 patients were treated with injection of 1.5 or 3 g of Promit® 2 min prior to clinical dextran infusion. The 3 g dose reduced the incidence of anaphylaxis about 20 times. This was confirmed by a two years post-marketing surveillance period in Sweden.

---

* Red cell linked antigen antibody reaction.

Conclusions: Dextran anaphylaxis is an immediate type, IgG-mediated reaction comparable to anaphylaxis in patients with deficiency of IgA or factor VIII. Hapten inhibition could be successfully applied to eliminate life-threatening dextran reactions by injecting monovalent hapten-dextran (Promit®) prior to infusion of Macrodex®/Rheomacrodes®.

Introduction

In recent years the worldwide use of pharmaceuticals with established medical value has imposed increased demands on their safety. Among plasma substitutes the efficacy of dextran is well documented. Its additional blood flow improving and thromboprophylactic effects are widely used. Although severe adverse reactions to clinical dextran preparations are rare [1], they occur with an estimated incidence of 1:2000 patients [2]. The elimination of such reactions was therefore made the aim of studies begun in Uppsala in 1968. Since then, many workers have joined the research program and formed collaborating study groups in Munich, Uppsala, and Vienna. Many publications have reflected the progress of the project [3–24; for reviews see 14, 21, 22, 24, 43]. The stepwise elucidation of the mechanism of dextran anaphylaxis in man, the study of animal models of dextran anaphylaxis, and its successful prevention by hapten inhibition, as well as the production of monovalent hapten-dextran on a large scale [18] enabled us to begin clinical trials of hapten prophylaxis in humans in 1978. The trials grew into large multicenter multinational studies, which ended in 1982 and were published in a series of articles [24, 33–40]. Results show that the incidence of severe dextran-induced anaphylactic reactions (DIARs) is greatly reduced by preinjection of hapten-dextran in a dose-dependent manner, conferring greater safety to dextran infusion therapy. In this chapter I shall outline the course of the research program and the present data from the combined clinical trials and subsequent postmarketing surveillance in Sweden (1983–1984). The role of IgG-mediated anaphylactic reactions, as opposed to IgE-mediated ones, will also be discussed.

Historical Background

Dextran of $\bar{M}_w$ 70000 was introduced into medicine as plasma substitute in 1947 by Ingelman and Grönwall [6]. It was prepared from a branched type of native dextran and quite frequently caused mild allergic reactions. Change to a more linear dextran reduced the incidence of allergic reactions [25]. This dextran produced by the *Leuconostoc mesenteroides* NRRL B 512 strain is still used today.

Gelin and co-workers showed that dextran of $\bar{M}_w$ 40000 increased the suspension stability of blood and improved blood flow in the microcirculation [26]. This led to the introduction of Rheomacrodex as a blood flow-improving agent [27]. In the 1960s an additional effect of dextran 70 was found, i.e., that it reduced the incidence of postoperative pulmonary embolism [28]. This thromboprophylactic effect is now the most frequent medical indication for dextran 70. The increased worldwide use of clinical dextran led to a considerable number of reported adverse reactions in spite of the low incidence of such reactions.

Immunology of Dextran

The immunogenicity of B 512 dextran in man is molecular weight dependent [29]. Whereas native and very high molecular weight dextrans are immunogenic in humans, dextran 70 and 40 are nonimmunogenic [21]. From the immunological point of view, a dextran infusion with 30–100 g represents an "overwhelming" dose. In animals corresponding doses lead to immunological unresponsiveness. Like other polysaccharides, dextran induces a thymus-independent IgM response in mice [21]. However, dextran can be converted to a thymus-dependent antigen by covalent coupling to protein [5]. Such conjugates elicit a strong IgG antidextran response upon immunization of carp, mice, guinea pigs, rabbits, sheep, and horses. We have utilized this fact to raise antidextrans in rabbits and dogs for use in our anaphylaxis models and for analytical purposes [5, 8]. Most people have natural dextran-reactive antibodies (DRAs) in their sera. They may have been induced by native, high molecular weight dextran ingested as food contaminant, produced by bacteria of the gastrointestinal tract, or produced by other cross-reactive microbial polysaccharides [30; for review see 21].

Table 1. Scale of severity of clinical symptoms of adverse reactions to colloidal infusion solutions (Rind and Meßmer [14], Laubenthal [36])

Grade of severity	Clinical symptoms
I	Skin manifestations: flush, erythema, urticaria
II	Measurable, but not life-threatening hemodynamic reaction (blood pressure fall, 20–60 mmHg). Dyspnea, nausea, vomiting
III	Shock (blood pressure fall exceeding 60 mmHg). Life-threatening bronchospasm
IV	Cardiac and/or respiratory arrest

Serology in Humans

Antibodies

Analysis of sera of dextran reactors and nonreactors, accumulated over many years, with various standardized procedures for measuring DRAs, gave the following results. Circulating DRAs occur in low titers in the majority of human populations; high titers are only found in a small percentage of individuals. Geographical variations in titer distribution do occur [23]. All patients with severe DIAR of grades III and IV (see Table 1 for classification) have high or very high titers of circulating DRA before the reaction. No IgE class DRAs could be found in 100 dextran reactors with different methods [7]. When Ig classes and subgroups were studied by RCLAAR and ELISA in reactors and nonreactors to dextran, high titers of IgG, especially of IgG_2, usually accompanied by IgA and IgM, were found in reactors, whereas nonreactors had small amounts of mostly IgM class DRAs [11, 19]. An excellent correlation was found between the grade of severity of DIAR and the titer of IgG class DRAs, implying that large amounts of immune complexes are formed in the circulation of patients with the most severe reactions [19].

Complement

Complement profiles were established in dextran reactors [7]. The most important finding was a significant decrease in the levels of $C1_q$ in severe DIAR. Concentrations of the other complement proteins and of the anaphylatoxin inactivator were normal. These results show that the classical pathway is activated in dextran reactors by immune complexes. The findings are in accord with the occurrence of high titers of IgG class DRAs in patients with severe DIAR.

Studies of the Chemical and Pharmaceutical Manufacturing Procedure

Dextran is a polysaccharide produced by the action of *Leuconostoc mesenteroides* NRRL B 512 on sucrose in the presence of nutrients. Thus, a careful purification process is necessary to manufacture clinical dextran preparations of defined molecular weight and molecular weight distribution. Since macromolecular contaminants may sensitize patients, we tested the immunogenicity of dextran from the early stages of the manufacturing process. No evidence for immunogenic impurities could be demonstrated [5]. Later, it was found that a soluble macromolecular component of *Leuconostoc* bacteria reacted with anti-yeast mannan antibodies. As such a *Leuconostoc*-derived component could be a potentially sensitizing agent in clinical dextran, an immunochemical test for its detection and quantitation was developed [31]. By improved purification, its concentration in clinical dextran was reduced to 10 ppm or less. Comparison of the incidence of adverse reactions to clinical dextran before and after introduction of the *Leuconostoc* RSRI purity test provided no evidence for a causal role of this contaminant in eliciting DIAR, but suggested an elicitor role of the dextran molecule itself.

Hapten Inhibition In Vitro

Haptens cannot induce antibody formation but do bind to antibodies of corresponding specificity. They may be poly-/or monovalent with regard to the number of antigenic determinants. Whereas a polyvalent hapten forms immune complexes with antibodies, a monovalent hapten binds to individual combining sites of antibodies only, and cannot join together antibodies by bridging. In the B 512 dextran-antidextran system, monovalent isomalto-oligosaccharides (IOS) inhibit the precipitation of antidextran by large dextran molecules [32]. Their inhibitory power increases strongly from isomaltose to isomaltopentaose with little further increase for isomalto-hexaose and isomalto-heptaose. These results were confirmed by indirect single radial immunodiffusion [5]. A dextran fragment of 6 glucose units ($\bar{M}_w$ 990) was judged suitable as a monovalent hapten for in vivo experiments. Thus, dextran 1 with $\bar{M}_w$ 1000 was prepared on a large scale by prolonged acid hydrolysis of B 512 dextran with subsequent fractionation and purification [18]. It is a mixture of IOS with 2–13 glucose units. Its molecular size distribution is controlled by gel chromatography. Dextran 1 is used clinically as a sterile 15% solution delivered in 20-ml vials.

Animal Experiments on Anaphylactic Shock

Hapten Inhibition of Cytotropic Passive Dextran Anaphylaxis in Guinea Pigs

The most important findings show that 100% protection from anaphylactic death can be achieved by admixture of low molecular hapten-dextran to the challenging high molecular dextran or by injection of hapten-dextran prior to challenge [3]. The protective effect is dose dependent and a significant reduction in mortality is observed when the hapten is present in a molar excess of 3–7, corresponding to an admixture of 10%–50% w/w to the challenging dextran [3, 4]. For the hapten, a $\bar{M}_w$ range of 1000 was found to be optimal in terms of both protective effect and safety requirements [5]. No elicitor action is present upon challenge with such a hapten, even at maximal degrees of sensitization. Since the basic bridging (elicitor) mechanism in anaphylaxis appears to be shared by all mammals, these considerations should also apply to humans, both for IgE- and IgG-mediated reactions.

Hapten Inhibition of Active Dextran Anaphylaxis, i.e., Immune Complex (Aggregate, IgG-Mediated) Anaphylaxis in Dogs

Most important is the fact that in this active anaphylaxis model circulating DRAs are induced (by immunization with edestin-dextran) in a titer pattern roughly comparable to that of humans [8]. In both conscious [9, 15] and anesthetized dogs [13], DIARs of varying degree of severity could be elicited and followed by measurements of hemodynamics, blood cell numbers, and DRA titers. Hapten-dextran of M_w 1000 given either before or admixed to the challenging dextran 60 significantly reduced both the number and the severity of DIAR [13].

Comparison of Cytotropic and Aggregate or Immune Complex Anaphylaxis in Monkeys

Different cardiorespiratory patterns of shock were observed in aggregate anaphylaxis (AA) and cytotropic anaphylaxis (CA), reflecting different biological actions of IgE and IgG class antibodies. A decrease in cardiac output and concomitant hypotension was seen in AA and CA. During AA, intense pulmonary vasoconstriction was initially important in depressing cardiac output; peripheral blood pooling was the main mechanism in CA. The respiratory reaction limited gas transport over the lungs greatly in CA but not in AA. Decreased pulmonary compliance in AA was due to pulmonary congestion, whereas in CA it was due to constriction of bronchial smooth muscle. The differences between AA and CA might be explained by the fact that platelets were activated only in AA. Apparently, vasoconstricting mediators predominate in AA and vasodilating ones in CA [12, 16].

Multicenter Clinical Trials of Hapten Prophylaxis in Five Countries

Prospective open clinical trials began in 1978 and ended in 1982. Physicians at 80 clinics in Finland, Sweden, Norway, Germany, and Switzerland participated. It was apparent that a large number of patients would be required to assess a reduction in the incidence of severe DIAR. From a large amount of historical control material comprising reports on DIAR in Sweden [2], the incidence of severe DIAR (grades III and IV) was estimated to 0.05%, i.e., 1:2000 patients. This represents a minimum figure, and thus the number of severe DIARs expected to occur in 100000 patients infused with dextran 70 and hapten could be about 50. Therefore, the inclusion of a large control group was considered unethical. Results of clinical trials in Germany [24, 33, 36], Switzerland [34, 35], and Scandinavia [37–40] have been reported elsewhere. For combined clinical trials, see Table 2. Among 37626 patients receiving dextran 70 after injection of 10 ml hapten-dextran, 0.029% (i.e., 29 per 100000) reacted with severe DIAR. This was not satisfactory, and in further trials the hapten dose was doubled to 20 ml, since hapten inhibition in animal models is a dose- dependent phenomenon. And indeed, among 79951 patients receiving dextran 70 after injection of 20 ml hapten-dextran, only 0.00375% reacted with severe DIAR (grade III only). This would correspond to 3.75 per 100000. The protective effect of the 20 ml dose is 7.8 times better than that of the 10 ml dose. With regard to the "historical" control figure for severe DIAR (0.05% per patient), the 10 ml dose decreased the incidence by 42% and the 20 ml dose by 93%. Instead of an incidence of severe DIAR of 1 : 2000 patients before use of hapten-dextran, we now have an incidence of 1 : 27000 according to results of 80000 protocolled patients receiving preinjection of 20 ml dextran 1.

Table 2. Prophylaxis against DIARs by administration of dextran 70 after injection of either 10 ml or 20 ml hapten-dextran

Country	Patients	DIARs	No. of DIARs, grade of severity				
	(*n*)	(total no.)	I	II	III	IV	V*
10-ml studies							
Germany	6113	13	8	3	2	0	0
Switzerland	2280	3	1	0	2	0	0
Scandinavia	29233	61	41	13	6	1	0
	37626	77	50	16	10	1	0
					0.0292% (III–IV)		1 of 3421 patients
20 ml studies							
Germany	24513	24	16	6	2	0	0
Switzerland	14339	14	9	5	0	0	0
Scandinavia	41099	72	56	15	1	0	0
	79951	110	81	26	3	0	0
					0.0038%		1 of 27000 patients

* grade V = lethal outcome

Postmarketing Surveillance of Hapten Prophylaxis in Sweden, 1983–1984

The Scandinavian multicenter clinical trials of hapten prophylaxis of DIAR ended in September 1981. They showed a 14-fold reduction in the incidence of severe DIAR. In November 1982 hapten-dextran was registered as a drug in Sweden under the name of Promiten (dextran 1, Pharmacia AB, Uppsala, Sweden) for the prophylaxis of severe DIAR. A preliminary survey based on spontaneous reports of DIAR to the health authorities and the producer has been compiled [41] and is presented here (Table 3). As in the clinical trials, each case report has been evaluated regarding causality and severity. The nomenclature used by the health authorities was adapted for causality classification: P = dextran is the probable or possible cause, N = the elicitation of the reaction by dextran is not probable or not assessable. In many instances, classification was facilitated by access to serum samples taken before the reaction and estimation of DRAs by passive hemagglutination or ELISA. The use of clinical dextran in Sweden has increased: during 1983–84, 424858 units were sold, as well as 205408 units of Promiten. This suggests that the prophylaxis concept has been accepted by the great majority of physicians, since for each dextran 1 unit, about 2.1 units of clinical dextran have been used. Therefore prerequisites are fulfilled for a valid estimation of the efficacy of Promiten prophylaxis during this time period, especially since the reporting of severe and lethal drug reactions is mandatory in Sweden (see Table 3). Compared to the control period of 1975–79, when clinical dextran was used without hapten [2], the incidence of severe DIAR (grades III, IV, and V) was reduced at least 16 times. One fatal reaction occurred in a patient with sepsis accompanied by an

Table 3. Findings regarding postmarketing surveillance of hapten prophylaxis in Sweden, 1983–1984 [41]

Period	No. of dextran bottles used	DIARs (total no.)	DIARs, grade of severity: I	II	III	IV	V
1975–1979 (no hapten)	647756	300	61	94	78	44	23
Incidence (%):					0.0224 (III–V)		
						0.0103 (IV–V)	
1983–1984 (with hapten)	424858	53	34	13	5	0	1
Incidence (%):					0.0014 (III–V)		
						0.0002 (IV–V)	
Decrease of incidence in %:		74	15	79	90	100	94
Reduction of incidence:							15 times
						45 times (IV–V)	
					16 times (III–V)		

Table 4. Mitigated severe DIAR reflecting a beneficial hapten effect (suspected DIAR in post-marketing study 1983 – 1984)

1	2	3	4	5	6[a]	7[b]	8
Code	Sev-erity	P, NP	DRA titer pass hem	IgG DRA assay titer	ELISA (OD, 410 nm)	Prec. DRA (mg/ml)	Classification (clin. and immun. data)
E	I	P	512	800	0.163		True grade I DIAR
G	I	P	512	50000	>2.000		Mitigated severe DIAR
H	V	NP	128	1000	0.134		Not antibody mediated
K	II	P	512	400000	>2.000	0.5	Mitigated severe DIAR
M	I	P	128	400	0.047		True grade I DIAR
O	III	P	2048	200000	>2.000	0.7	Mitigated severe DIAR
P	II	P	512	1600	0.175		True grade II DIAR
Q	V	P	2048	1600000	>2.000	2.4	True grade V DIAR
R	III	P	1024	400000	>2.000	1.1	Mitigated severe DIAR

[a] Column 6: All sera screened at a dilution 1:400
[b] Column 7: Estimation of precipitating DRA by RSRI

extremely high titer of DRA of IgG class (2.4 mg IgG/ml serum) (see Table 4). In this patient the hapten dose was not sufficient or was not distributed evenly in the circulation due to circulatory insufficiency.

The incidence of severe DIAR in the surveillance period is 1 : 33000 patients, a figure well in accord with that of the combined 20 ml clinical trials of dextran 1. The effect of hapten is also exemplified in Table 4, showing cases from the surveillance study with mild DIAR exhibiting extremely high titers of IgG class DRAs. These cases have been classified by clinical and immunological data as "mitigated severe DIAR," contrasting to "true" mild reactions accompanied by low titers of IgG class DRAs.

Conclusions

Dextran-induced anaphylactic reactions in humans are classified as IgG-mediated immune complex anaphylaxis. This is evident from the presence of mg/ml concentrations of specific antibody, complement activation via the classical pathway, and pathological changes in lungs conforming to the picture of immune complex (IgG) but not cytotropic (IgE) anaphylaxis in monkeys. Severe DIARs occur upon the first infusion of a few milliliters of clinical dextran. Dextran reactors have thus not been sensitized by clinical dextran but they are high responders to dextran and have high titers of preformed naturally occurring DRA in their sera. Though IgE anaphylaxis appears to dominate in humans, DIARs are not the only example of IgG-mediated anaphylactic reactions. Another well documented example is anaphylaxis in IgA-deficient patients upon repeated infusion of IgA-containing blood or plasma [42]. The regular occurrence of DRA in severe DIAR and the possibility of large – scale production of a monovalent hapten [18] led to the successful application of hapten inhibition in preventing dextran anaphylaxis. In the era before hapten prophylaxis, the estimated incidence of severe DIAR was 1 : 2000 patients [2]. In clinical trials with 10 and 20 ml Promiten the incidence was 1 : 3400 and 1 : 27000 respectively. In the postmarketing surveillance of about 200000 patients the incidence was 1 : 33000 patients. The incidence of lethal DIAR was 1 : 15000 patients without hapten and 1 : 200000 with 20 ml hapten-dextran.

It should be pointed out that an estimated number of 2000000 patients have hitherto received hapten-dextran worldwide. The risk of giving dextran should be compared with its beneficial effect when used as a thromboprophylactic agent [28]. In Sweden an estimated number of at least 200 patients were protected from fatal lung embolism in a 2-year period, compared with one fatal anaphylactic dextran reaction [41].

Participants in the Research Program

Sweden: Richter W, Hedin H, Granath K, Ingelman B, Perlman P, Stålenheim G, Smedegård G, Ljungström KG, Renck H, Revenäs B, Saldeen T
Germany: Messmer K, Ring J, Seemann-Mendler C, Laubenthal H, Peter K, Selbmann HK, Schwartz JA, Gregori M
Austria: Kraft D, Rumpold H, Scheiner O, Steinbereithner K
Great Britain: Devey M, Stanworth D
USA: Müller-Eberhard HJ et al.
Switzerland: Gruber U, Allemann U, Gerber H, Wettler H
Japan: Takamoto H

Acknowledgments. Thanks are due to our laboratory technicians and to the staff and personnel of the 80 hospitals which made possible the successful performance of the clinical trials.

References

1. Furhoff AK (1977) Anaphylactoid reactions to dextran – a report of 133 cases. Acta Anaesth Scand 21:161–167
2. Ljungström KG, Renck H, Strandberg K, Hedin H, Richter W, Widerlöf E (1983) Adverse reactions to dextran in Sweden 1970–1979. Acta Chir Scand 149:253–262
3. Richter W (1971) Hapten inhibition of passive antidextran dextran anaphylaxis in guinea pigs. Int Arch Allergy 41:826–844
4. Richter W (1973) Built-in hapten inhibition of anaphylaxis by the low molecular weight subfractions of a B 512 dextran fraction of $\bar{M}_w$ 3400. Int Arch Allergy 45:930–936
5. Richter W (1973) Immunological in vivo and in vitro studies of the dextran antidextran system. Thesis, University of Uppsala
6. Ingelman B (1947) Dextran and its use as a plasma substitute. Acta Chem Scand 1:731–738

7. Hedin H (1977) Dextran-induced anaphylactoid reactions in man. Immunological in vitro and in vivo studies. Thesis, University of Uppsala
8. Seeman C, Hedin H, Richter W, Ring J, Stippig S, Messmer K (1978) Haptenhemmung der Dextran-induzierten anaphylaktischen Reaktion beim Hund. Allergologie 1:185
9. Schwarz JA, Raschack M (1978) Verhinderung Antikörperbedingter Dextran-Nebenwirkungen durch Hapten-Hemmung – eine experimentelle Pilotstudie am wachen Hund. Allergologie 1:184
10. Hedin H, Smedegård G (1979) Complement profiles in monkeys subjected to aggregate (immune complex) anaphylaxis and following injection of soluble and particulate polysaccharides. Int Arch Allergy Appl Immunol 60:286–294
11. Hedin H, Kraft D, Richter W, Scheiner O, Devey M (1979) Dextran-reactive antibodies in patients with anaphylactoid reactions to dextran. Immunobiology 156:289–290
12. Smedegård G (1980) Anaphylactic shock. Pathophysiology of aggregate and cytotropic anaphylaxis in the monkey. Thesis, Acta Univers Upsala, p 548
13. Mendler C (1980) Hapten-Hemmung der Dextran-induzierten anaphylaktischen Reaktion beim Hund. Thesis, Ludwig-Maximilians-University Munich
14. Ring J (1976) Anaphylaktoide Reaktionen nach Infusion natürlicher und künstlicher Kolloide. Thesis for habilitation, Ludwig-Maximilian-University Munich
15. Schwarz JA, Rother U, Koch W, Raschack M, Till G (1981) Verhinderung Antikörper-bedingter Dextran-Nebenwirkungen durch Haptenhemmung mit Dextran 1 am Hund. Anaesthesist 30:297–303
16. Revenäs B, Smedegård G, Saldeen T, Fredholm BB, Strandberg K (1981) Anaphylactic shock in monkeys passively sensitized with human reaginic serum. II. Respiratory mechanics, hematology and metabolism. Acta Physiol Scand 111:249–257
17. Schwarz JA, Koch W, Bühler V, Kaumeier S (1981) Pharmacokinetics of low molecular (monovalent) dextran (Dx 1) in volunteers. Int J Clin Pharmacol Ther Toxicol 19:358–367
18. Richter AW, Ingelman B, Granath K (1982) An isomalto-oligosaccharide product for medical use. Abstract, poster presentation, 11th international carbohyd symposium, Vancouver, BC
19. Kraft D, Hedin H, Richter W, Scheiner O, Rumpold H, Devey ME (1982) Immunoglobulin class and subclass distribution of dextran reactive antibodies in human reactors and nonreactors to clinical dextran. Allergy 37:481–489
20. Hedin H, Richter W (1982) Pathomechanism of dextran-induced anyphylactoid/anaphylactic reactions in man. Int Arch Allergy Appl Immunol 68:122–126
21. Richter AW, Hedin HI (1982) Dextran hypersensitivity (a review). Immunol Today 3:132–138
22. Richter W, Hedin H (1983) Solutions and emulsions used for intravenous infusions. In: de Weck AL, Bundgaard H (eds) Allergic reaction to drugs. Springer, Berlin Heidelberg New York Tokyo (Handbook of experimental pharmacology, vol 63)
23. Messmer K, Richter W, Takaori M (1984) Prinzip der Haptenhemmung zur Prophylaxe der Dextrananaphylaxie: immunologische Aspekte. Beitr Anaesth Intensivmed 3:15–27
24. Laubenthal H, Peter K, Richter W, Kraft D, Selbmann HK, Messmer K (1983) Anaphylaktoide/anaphylaktische Reaktionen auf Dextran. Pathomechanismus und Prophylaxe. Diagnostik Intensivtherapie 8:4–14
25. Kabat EA, Turino GM, Tarrow AB, Maurer PH (1957) Studies on the immunochemical basis of allergic reactions to dextran in man. J Clin Invest 36:1160–1170
26. Gelin LE (1956) Studies in anemia of injury. Thesis, University of Gothenburg. Acta Chir Scand Suppl 210
27. Gelin LE, Ingelman B (1961) Rheomacrodex – a new dextran solution for rheological treatment of impaired capillary flow. Acta Chir Scand 122:294–302
28. Bergentz SE (1978) Dextran in the prophylaxis of pulmonary embolism. World J Surg 2:19–25
29. Kabat EA, Bezer AE (1958) The effect of variation in molecular weight on the antigenicity of dextran in man. Arch Biochem Biophys 78:306–318
30. Hehre EJ, Neill JM (1946) Formation of serologically reactive dextrans by streptococci from subacute bacterial endocarditis. J Exp Med 83:147–163

31. Richter AW (1980) A new immunochemical purity test for clinical dextran. Methodology and studies on clinical dextran preparations. Int Arch Allergy Appl Immunol 61:457–466
32. Kabat EA (1961) Inhibition reactions. In: Kabat EA, Mayer MM (eds) Experimental immunochemistry, 2nd edn. Thomas, Springfield
33. Messmer K, Ljungström KG, Gruber UF, Richter W, Hedin H (1980) Prevention of dextran-induced anaphylactoid reactions by hapten inhibition. Lancet 1:975
34. Gruber UF, Allemann U, Gerber H, Wettler H (1982) Erster direkter Vergleich der allergischen Nebenwirkungen des Dextrans mit und ohne Hapten. Schweiz Med Wochenschr 112:605–612
35. Gruber UF, Wettler H, Allemann U, Gerber H, Laubenthal H, Messmer K (1982) Prophylaxe allergischer Dextran-Reaktionen durch Vorinjektion von 20 ml Hapten bei 12000 Patienten in der Schweiz. Schweiz Rundschau Med (Praxis) 71:1092–1100
36. Laubenthal H (1983) Dextrananaphylaxie. Pathomechanismus und Prophylaxe durch Haptenhemmung. Ergebnisse einer multizentrischen, klinischen Studie. Thesis for habilitation, Ludwig-Maximilian-University, Munich
37. Ljungström KG, Renck H, Hedin H, Richter W, Rosberg B (1983) Prevention of dextran-induced anaphylactic reactions by hapten inhibition. I. A Scandinavian multicenter study on the effects of 10 ml dextran, 15%, administered before dextran 70 or dextran 40. Acta Chir Scand 149:341–348
38. Renck H, Ljungström KG, Rosberg B, Dhuner KG, Dahl S (1983) Prevention of dextran-induced anaphylactic reactions by hapten inhibition. II. A comparison of the effects of 20 ml Dextran 1, 15%, administered either admixed to or before dextran 70 or dextran 40. Acta Chir Scand 149:349–353
39. Renck H, Ljungström KG, Hedin H, Richter W (1983) Prevention of dextran-induced anaphylactic reactions by hapten inhibition. III. A Scandinavian multicenter study on the effects of 20 ml Dextran 1, 15%, administered before dextran 70 or dextran 40. Acta Chir Scand 149:355–360
40. Ljungström KG, Renck H (1983) Säkrare dextranterapi med hapteninhibition. Stor skandinavisk studie. Läkartidningen 80 (1–2):26–27
41. Ljungström KG, Renck H, Hedin H, Richter W, Wiholm BE (1985) Hapteninhibition minskade biverkningarna vid dextran-användning. Läkartidningen 82:2772–2773
42. Leikola J, Koistinen J, Lethinen M, Virolainen M (1973) IgA-induced anaphylactic transfusion reactions: a report of four cases. Blood 42:111–119
43. Ring J (1982) Zur Problematik der Dextran-Unverträglichkeit und ihrer spezifischen Prophylaxe durch Haptenhemmung. Fortschr Med 100:1917–1921

Immunotherapy

Standardization of Allergenic Extracts

H. Løwenstein

The Protein Laboratory, University of Copenhagen, Sigurdsgade 34, 2200 Copenhagen, Denmark

Abstract

The purpose of allergen standardization is to make proper allergenic material available for use in diagnosis and treatment. The performance of standardization requires the presence of standards. The subcommittee on allergen standardization of the International Union of Immunological Societies (I.U.I.S.) has prepared a number of international standards (IS) available through WHO. The IS were selected allergen specialists on the basis of detailed specifications to ensure typical and representative materials. The usefulness and assessibility of standards were confirmed through the performance of international collaborative studies. Comparison between preparations relative to the IS gave results which within limits were independent of method, time and laboratory. These IS are recommended for use as callibrators (i.e. standards for measurements of relative potency) and are not recommended for use as prototypes (i.e. materials to which an extract is to be matched in all respects). The activity of each standard is defined in arbitrary international units (IU) and one IU of a specific standard preparation is not related to the unit activity of another preparation although it may be similar. The IS preparations may be utilized as callibrators for determination of total allergenic activity and/or as callibrators in determination of individual components of allergenic extracts. A number of methods have been shown to be useful for this purpose, but any method giving relevant information on the potency and quality of allergenic extracts can be used. Current international collaborative studies have shown that standardization relative to an IS is possible. Depending on requirements from various national control authorities and the technical ability of allergen extract manufacturers, in the near future only standardized allergenic extracts should be used – for the benefit of allergic patients.

Introduction

Standardization of allergenic extracts has been increasingly required by allergologists and control authorities ever since the introduction of these substances for specific diagnosis and immunotherapy. Possibilities were at first limited by the low level of knowledge about allergenic extracts, which only included skin testing for potency measurement and some rather rough physicochemical data such as weight/volume and PNU. During the last 15 years, however, extensive knowledge about allergenic extracts has been gained and in vitro methods developed which are more accurate than the former in vivo methods for potency measurements. Furthermore, methods have been developed which allow detailed characterization of allergenic extracts according to the composition and allergenic significance of the antigens.

With this level of knowledge, the question is no longer: "Is standardization possible?", but "How do we organize it and implement it?".

Standardization requirements from legal authorities differ from country to country and may include, for example, a potency determination performed by a specified method, a concentration determination for some well-defined allergenic molecules, "complete" molecular characterization of any molecular components, or any combination of these principles. Other requirements may be described, such as tolerated minimum or maximum amounts of certain molecules or certain relationships between characteristic components.

Another controversial point is unitage, where more recent proposals have been based upon, for instance, histamine equivalence by in vivo testing, specific IgE equivalence by in vitro testing, absolute content of allergenic molecules, or just arbitrary units.

The degree of complexity is further increased by the fact that many companies are multinational. However, any cooperative effort in the direction of more standardized legal requirements for allergenic extracts will clearly be beneficial for manufacturers and control authorities, but above all for patients insofar as the use of irrelevant or even uncontrolled allergenic extracts can be avoided.

The aim of this presentation is to give the scientific background to standardization of allergenic extracts, to report the progress in international allergen standardization, and to emphasize some outstanding problems in standardization.

Allergens and Patient Response

The allergenic molecules isolated from quite different sources have been thoroughly analyzed. The conclusion from the general molecular characterization and the activity/confirmation dependence of allergens is that they do not exhibit any specific known features which should facilitate the induction and production of IgE, giving rise to clinical symptoms in allergic patients. However, they mostly seem to include proteins in a certain molecular range which have properties that are stable under natural conditions of exposure of the patient. The lower molecular weight limit is determined by the molecular capability to be structurally complex enough to be immunogenic. The upper limit is determined by the molecular capability to penetrate mucosal membranes. It is important to add that a significant contribution to the generation of an allergen is made by the genetic capability of the individual Ig-producing system to recognize the allergen in a limiting low dosage [1, 2].

Allergenic extracts are complex mixtures of a number of antigenic components. The number of detectable antigens varies considerably and might well be underestimated due to limited sensitivity of the analysis performed. In general, the most simply composed extracts seem to be those from animal dander, the number of antigens being between 10 and 20. Extracts derived from the various house dust mites have been shown to contain between 20 and 40 antigens, and most pollen extracts are even more complicated, containing between 30 and 50 detectable antigenic components. The most complicated known allergenic extracts are those from molds, where the number of antigens detected has been as high as 80 [3].

Patients' responses to allergenic molecules reveal individuality, both in intensity and specificity. Any antigen binding the patient's IgE is an allergenic molecule. We use the term major allergen for an antigen against which more than 50% of a selected group of patients (allergic to the allergen source in question) react in CRIE and against which half of these patients have specific IgE of high-binding capacity [3]. For most allergenic extracts analyzed, the number of defined allergens detected is between one-quarter and one-half of the total number of antigens, whereas the number of major allergens is normally one to three [4].

Diagnostic and Therapeutic Extracts

The requirements regarding allergenic extracts for diagnostic use are therefore that they should include all potential allergens in relevant ratios and in native forms and that all irrelevant material should be excluded. The "potential allergens" are those components against which some patients within the patient population allergic to the allergen source in question have IgE. "Relevant ratios" means that the proportions between extracted components must be similar to the proportions in which the same molecules would have appeared during natural exposure and extraction on their way to the patient's immunosystem. The requirement "native form" means that the allergic molecules should remain in their native form, identical to that form to which natural exposure occurs. The "irrelevant material" comprises those molecules against which patients will have no immunological reactions but which may cause nonspecific, nonimmunological reactions.

The use of allergenic extracts for specific immunotherapy presupposes that, in order to avoid the appearance of new allergies and to minimize the antigenic competition, treatment should only be performed with those components against which the patient has specific IgE. However, a number of recent studies have shown that the appearance of new allergies is not influenced by current specific immunotherapy [e.g., 5]. On the other hand, it has also been shown [5] that treatment will influence only the level of those IgE specifities where patients are treated with the corresponding allergenic molecules, thus indicating the specificity of the treatment. Against this background, it seems obvious that individual patients should be treated with specially tailored extracts corresponding to their individual IgE responses. A proposal in this direction has indeed been made, but at present this is not a practical solution. More relevant is the use of partially purified allergenic extracts which on the one hand include all the relevant (from a statistical point of view) allergenic molecules, and on the other exclude all molecules against which patients extremely seldom react. Several double-blind clinical investigations support this solution [6, 7], the basis of which is that the partially purified allergenic extract must be controlled for the presence of a number of important components.

Progress in International Allergen Standardization

As is evident from the above discussion, allergen standardization is complicated due to the complex composition of allergenic extracts and patient response to these. Consequently, one single international working group including allergologists, scientists dealing with allergen chemistry, manufacturers, and control authorities has been created in order to promote concrete measures of standardization.

Naturally the first goal was to develop a number of standards, three of which (timothy, short ragweed, and the house dust mite *Dermatophagoides pteronyssinus*) are available from WHO [8–10] and a further five (birch pollen, bermuda grass pollen, dog, *Alternaria*, and cat) of which can be expected within the near future. This development has already indirectly influenced the quality of extracts from some companies. Strict requirements from various national control authorities – hopefully internationally coordinated – can soon be expected and will directly force standardization.

The next step was to develop recommendations for use of the standards. This included both overall potency and concentration of individual allergens. The standards were arbitrarily given international units (IU). Currently produced allergenic extracts can now be standardized relative to the WHO standards and assigned a number of IU. Unfortunately such unitage depends upon the methods used for comparison with the standard, and consequently the method chosen for comparison – and in some respects calibration – has to be assigned too. This present solution to the problem of standardization of allergenic extracts is not ideal, but it is a necessary compromise due to the complex nature of the allergenic extracts. It would only be possible to assign international unitage which really means the same potency if all existing extracts were identical in composition and the same methods were used for the determination of potency. Nevertheless, the present solution will have several practical effects, ensuring better reproducibility of extracts, and control of potency or concentration with relevant methods. It will allow rough comparisons between

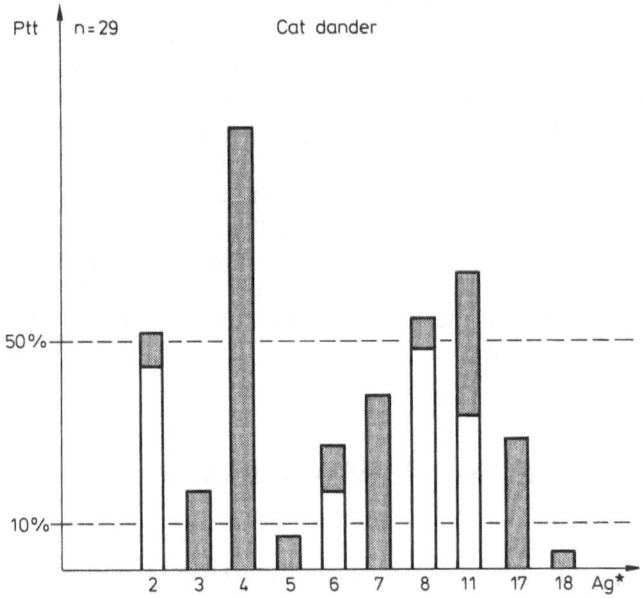

Fig. 1. Allergogram for antigens of cat dander based upon sera from 29 patients allergic to cats. Specific Ig binding to the individual allergens (*abscissa*) was obtained by means of CRIE. *Hatched columns* indicate high IgE binding. For further details see [11]

Table 1. Relative quantities (as assessed by QIE) of verified cat allergenic molecules in various preparations, using Cat 0580 as a standard and normalizing the cat albumin content (modified from [11])

Allergen no.	Cat 0580	Cat 206	Cat 149	Cat 160	Cat saliva
2	100	3.3	0.46	3.67	820
3 (Cat alb)	100	100	100	100	100
4 (Cat ag 1)	100	0.32	1.44	1.48	68
5	100	<0.1	0.12	0.27	5152
6	100	0.19	<0.1	0.51	<0.1
7	100	<0.1	0.62	<0.1	488
8	100	<0.1	0.21	0.59	1578
Cat ag 1/Cat alb (%, W/W)	67	0.24	1.20	2.33	46

extracts from various manufacturers. This is obviously an advantage, but might be misused if too much attention is given to the potency and insufficient care is taken with regard to the quality (e.g., composition of the extract, ratio between important components, exclusion of nonallergenic components, etc.). The significance of the quality of extracts is exemplified by comparing the allergogram of a cat dander extract (Fig. 1) and the relative quantities of cat dander allergens in various preparations (Table 1). The control of only a few components or the total allergenic activity allows an extreme and perhaps dangerous variability between the components which will be significant for a number of patients.

It is not difficult today to produce a quite strong allergenic extract. However, in some cases it can be difficult to produce an extract which includes all potential allergens in reasonable ratios and in a native form. However, with the presence of the international standards, no manufacturer can say that he is not aware of the problem and does not have the tools to control the composition of his extract.

The third step in the standardization process is the requirements placed on allergenic extracts by the legal authorities. As we now have standards which can be used as calibrators and a great number of relevant methods, the know-how is available for standardization. Requirements can be expressed in a number of different ways, and traditions vary from nation to nation. In my opinion these requirements should include the following points: (a) all potential allergenic molecules should be included, (b) extracts should be available at relevant potency levels, (c) there should be relevant ratios between allergenic molecules, and (d) the allergenic molecules should be in a native form.

If standardization of allergenic extracts is performed, the most probable impact will be the exclusion of irrelevant extracts and ensurance of relevant levels of potency resulting in relevant composition of extracts. This would give rise to a safer specific diagnosis and immunotherapy.

There will be a need for allergenic extracts in allergy practice in the future. Whatever the treatment is – avoidance, symptomatic treatment, or specific immunotherapy – the need for exact knowledge of the cause of the allergy will exist. We will not be able to solve the patient's problem without access to such material. The problem today is not the possibility of standardization of allergenic extracts, but when it can be performed and the requirements to be placed on allergen standardization. On the other hand, if standardization is not performed, confidence in allergologists will disappear, and allergy practice will become merely a part of general practice – a development which from the patient's viewpoint would be unsatisfactory.

References

1. Løwenstein H (1985) Molecular characteristics of allergens. Allergy [Suppl, 3] 40:10–12
2. Marsh DG (1975) Allergens and genetics of allergy. In: Sela (ed) The antigens, vol 3. Academic, New York, pp 271–359
3. Løwenstein H (1978) Quantitative immunoelectrophoretic methods as a tool for the analysis and isolation of allergens. Prog Allergy 25:1–62
4. Løwenstein H (1983) Purification and standardization of allergens. Proceedings, XII congress of the European academy of allergology and clinical immunology. O.I.C. Medical, Firenze
5. Osterballe O, Ipsen HH, Weeke B, Løwenstein H (1983) Specific IgE response towards allergenic molecules during perennial hyposensitization. J Allergy Clin Immunol 71:40–46
6. Osterballe O (1982) Immunotherapy with grass pollen major allergens. Clinical results from a prospective 3-year double blind study. Allergy 37:379–388

7. Sundin B, Lilja G, Graff-Lonnevig V, Hedlin G, Heilborn H, Norrlind K, Pegelow KO, Løwenstein H (1986) Immunotherapy with partly purified and standardized animal dander extracts. I. Clinical results from a double-blind study on patients with animal dander asthma. J Allergy Clin Immunol 77:488–496
8. Gjesing B, Jager L, Marsh DG, Løwenstein H (1985) The international collaborative study establishing the first international standard for Timothy (*Phleum pratense*) grass pollen allergenic extract. J Allergy Clin Immunol 75:258–267
9. Helm RM, Gauerke MB, Baer H, Løwenstein H, Ford A, Levy DA, Norman PS, Yunginger JW (1984) Production and testing of an international reference standard of short ragweed pollen extract. J Allergy Clin Immunol 73:790–800
10. Ford A, Seagroatt V, Platts-Mills TAE, Løwenstein H (1985) A collaborative study on the first international standard of *Dermatophagoides pteronyssinus* (house dust mite) extract. J Allergy Clin Immunol 75:676–686
11. Løwenstein H, Lind P, Weeke B (1985) Identification and clinical significance of allergenic molecules of cat origin. A part of the DAS 76 study. Allergy 40:430–441

Allergen Extracts from Animals for Diagnosis and Immunotherapy

U. Wahn
Universitätskinderklinik, Heubnerweg 6, 1000 Berlin 19/West

Abstract

Animals are multiallergenic systems. During the last years considerable information on their allergens has been accumulated. They may be present in epidermal tissues, saliva, urine, serum, milk, and faeces. Several allergenic proteins from horses, cats, dogs, cows, rodents, and mites have been identified, their allergenic activity has been evaluated by immunoelectrophoretic methods, RAST, or histamine release from leukocytes.

Human IgE responses to animal allergens have been demonstrated to be heterogeneous. However, there is a small number of "major allergens" in most species, to which the great majority of an allergic population is sensitive.

Using peptide fragments of allergens some studies have focused on the allergenic structure and the distribution and quality of epitopes binding to human IgE-antibodies. The complete aminoacid sequence of some allergens is known.

Several controlled studies have investigated the clinical efficacy of immunotherapy with biologically standardized allergen extracts from animals (cats, dogs, mites). They suggest, that immunotherapy with partially purified extracts and a defined concentration of major allergens is immunologically effective and reduces the sensitivity of allergic airways. The results may be improved by using extracts containing a more specific spectrum of allergenic proteins for each patient.

Introduction

Allergic diseases resulting from exposure to animals have long been recognized. Apart from house dust mites, domestic animals are the most important allergenic sources in house dust. They have become a serious problem especially for atopic children. The true incidence of domestic animal hypersensitivity is unknown. In a Swedish study the prevalence of allergy to furred animals has been estimated to be 5.3% [12].

In addition to these problems in the domestic setting, allergic reactions to allergens from laboratory animals have become a major occupational health hazard for individuals who work with experimental animals. It has been estimated that

Table 1. Incidence of laboratory animal allergy

Author(s)	Exposed	Sensitive	%
Lincoln et al. [13]	238	27	11.3
Lutsky and Neuman [18]	1293	191	14.7
Newman-Taylor [22]	144	27	19
Gross [8]	399	59	15
Davies and McArdle [6]	585	113	19.5
Cockcroft et al. [5]	179	49	27
Schumacher [27]	121	39	32

the number of workers or scientists exposed to experimental animals exceeds 35000 in the United States alone. A number of studies on the prevalence of allergy to laboratory animals have been performed during recent years. In general they have been cross-sectional in design, and only provide information on those working with animals at the time of the study, a "survivor population" [22]. Results of longitudinal studies have not yet been reported. The majority of the studies suggest that the prevalence of allergic airway symptoms and urticaria in individuals working with laboratory animals is between 10% and 30% (Table 1). It appears that subjects with a history of seasonal rhinitis tend to become more easily sensitized to animals and develop higher levels of specific IgE serum antibodies.

For a long time it was assumed that allergy to animals results from sensitization to parts of their skin like hair, fur, scales, etc. Commercial skin test preparations in general are prepared from fur, epidermal scrapings, or whole pelts, and several studies on allergic diseases in response to laboratory or domestic animals have used pelt-derived materials for diagnostic and therapeutic purposes. However, during the last few years it has become evident that in some species there are even more potent allergenic sources than the epidermis, e.g., saliva or urine, which are obviously the primary sources of allergenic molecules. In these animals the allergenic activity of the epidermis may at least partly be due to contamination [7, 9, 11, 21, 37].

During the last decade considerable information has been accumulated on the protein content of various tissues of and materials from animals, and especially the content of allergenic molecules. Precise information on the distribution and concentration of allergens in tissues and secretions is an important prerequisite for the production of appropriate allergenic extracts for diagnostic and therapeutic use.

Cat

Aqueous extracts prepared from cat hair and dander have been demonstrated by crossed immunoelectrophoresis to contain at least 18 different proteins, 12 of which bind to IgE antibodies of cat-sensitive individuals [15]. Among these 12, the most important allergen, cat allergen I (CA I), is the only major allergen

[23]. The protein has a molecular weight of 32000 and an isoelectric point of its major component of 3.8. Besides CA I a number of other proteins may be responsible for hypersensitivity reactions in some allergic individuals, acting as minor allergens. Among these albumin has been demonstrated to be of some relevance in a minority of cat-sensitive patients. Using an immunohistological technique with monospecific anti-CA I we were able to demonstrate that CA I is produced by mucous salivary glands (Gl. sublingulis), and in addition by sebaceous glands [1]. CA I is also present in cat urine. Recently it has been demonstrated that the ratio of CA I to cat albumin depends on the extract source, being highest in saliva and dander. Therefore a standardized cat extract should be quantitated for both cat antigen I and cat albumin [4, 16, 24].

Dog

Among domestic animals dogs are the second most common sensitizers (cats being the most common). An allergen extract prepared from dog epidermis contains 11 allergenic proteins as demonstrated by crossed radioimmunoelectrophoresis [15]. Among these [11] there appears to be no dominating protein leading to sensitization in the majority of dog-allergic patients. A number of studies during recent years have focussed on the allergenic significance of dog serum albumin using the skin prick test, RAST, and leukocyte histamine release [20]. From these studies it became clear that dog serum albumin is a potent allergen, but only for a minority of dog-allergic individuals, leading to sensitization in 10% [31] or 20%, as we were able to demonstrate by leukocyte histamine release. Breed specificity to allergy to dogs has long been assumed. Blands and co-workers [2], however, have shown that various allergenic extracts of different dog breeds contain the same allergens, although in different concentrations. There is some cross-reactivity between serum-derived and epidermal allergens from cats and dogs [32, 38].

Horse

An epidermal allergen extract of horses contains up to 15 proteins which have the capacity to bind IgE antibodies from the sera of sensitized humans. The individual spectra of sensitization vary from one patient to another [36]. Five of the most important allergens have recently been isolated and purified. By means of crossed radioimmunoelectrophoresis and histamine release from washed leukocytes the allergens 6, 9, and 11 have been demonstrated to be major allergens. These proteins are present in an epidermal allergen extract at the highest concentrations. There are, however, considerable quantitative differences in the capacity of horse allergens to bind human IgE and to trigger basophils for histamine release (Fig. 1), and it appears that the most sensitive horse-allergic individuals tend to react to a larger number of allergens, including serum proteins.

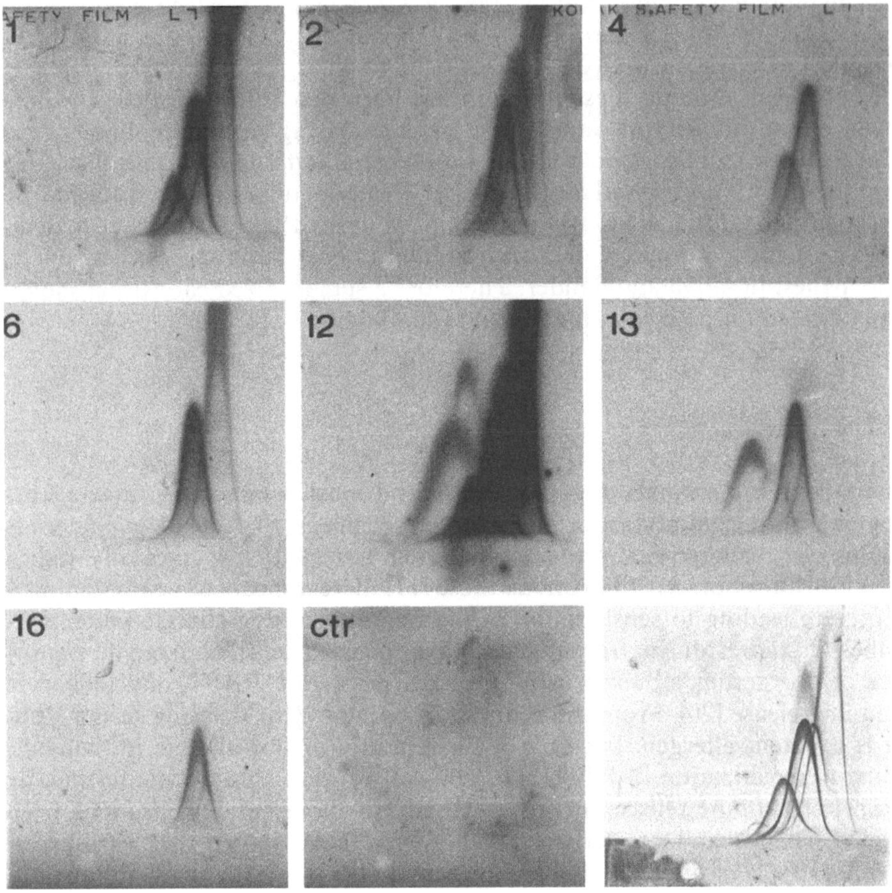

Fig. 1. Allergoprints for seven horse-allergic children, pool of sera from 1000 normal individuals (control = *ctr*), together with the CIE reference plate with identified important allergens (*bottom right*) [36]

Table 2. Urinary allergens from rats and mice

	Molecular weight	Isoelectric point	Reference
Rat			
Prealbumin	16000–18000	5.4, 5.6, 5.8	14
alpha$_2$-Euglobulin	20000–21000	5.4, 4.6	14
Serum albumin	68000		34
Mouse			
Prealbumin ("MUP complex")	20000	4.2	14, 26
Serum albumin	67000		28

Cow

An epidermal allergen extract from cows has been demonstrated to contain 11 allergens which induce IgE responses in humans. None of these proteins meet the criteria of a major allergen, although some of the molecules show strong IgE binding in a minority of patients. Three of the most potent allergens have been isolated and purified [25]. Some of the epidermal proteins like IgG are present in serum too. Bovine serum albumin (BSA) may induce IgE responses in patients highly sensitive to cows [35]. Like bovine IgG, it is present in bovine whey, where it may lead to anaphylactic reactions in infants and young children with cows' milk allergy.

Rat

Rats, like mice, have a physiological proteinuria. The amount of the protein excreted with the urine depends on the age and sex of the animals. The allergenicity of rat fur or epithelia appears to result largely from contamination with urine or rat saliva. Some of the urinary proteins have been shown to be major allergens, becoming airborn after contamination of dust from the animal cages [21].

Two proteins from rat urine, an α_2 euglobulin and a prealbumin, seem to have allergenic activity in the majority of rat-sensitive people [14] (Table 2). Serum albumin, which is present in rat urine only in low concentrations, releases histamine from leukocytes in about 24% of all rat-sensitive patients [34].

Utilizing RAST-inhibition experiments, Lutsky and co-workers [19] were unable to detect any strain specificity among urinary antigens from rats.

Mouse

The composition of mouse urine seems to be less complex. Its protein consists almost entirely of a prealbumin component with a molecular weight of approximately 20000 and an isoelectric point of 4.2–4.4. This major urinary protein (MUP) complex [26] shows almost complete cross-reactivity between different mouse strains. At least part of the allergenicity of mouse pelt material results from its content of components of this MUP complex. However, a larger allergen with a molecular weight of 67000, most probably serum albumin, induces histamine release from leukocytes in about 30% of mouse-sensitive patients [28].

Serum Albumins as Allergens

As pointed out before, serum proteins of a number of animals are present in epidermal allergen extracts, where they may serve as allergens. Among them, serum albumin, although in general a minor allergen, is an excellent model for studies of allergenic properties and structure. The complete amino acid of some serum albumins like BSA is known, and albumins from different species have been shown to be structurally similar. Structural studies performed by Brown [3] indicate that the BSA molecule consists of nine separate disulfide-bonded loops connected by peptide links of 11 – 26 residues. These loops define three domains.

In order to study the allergenic structure of albumins, we performed histamine release studies with large fragments of BSA and rat serum albumin (RSA), which had been produced by limited proteolytic treatment of the native albumin molecule. Such fragments appear to retain much of the conformation which they have in the intact molecule (Table 3).

The leukocytes of eight RSA-allergic patients were challenged with RSA and two peptic fragments of the molecule. The cells from five patients responded to both peptic fragments of RSA with histamine release. Therefore there are at least two separate determinants on each of the two fragments RSA-P_{306} and RSA-$P_{307-581}$. The sum of the total allergenic activity recovered in both fragments was low, ranging from 0.09% to 31%. This indicates that 70% – 99% of the allergenic activity was lost by the cleavage of the RSA molecule in the middle of the second domain. Out of eight patients, two did not recognize either determinant on RSA-$P_{307-581}$, and one recognized one (haptenic) determinant (Fig. 2). Clearly there is no single immunodominant site on the molecule which is important for all RSA-sensitive patients [34].

Histamine release experiments with basophils from rabbits immunized with BSA indicated that there are at least two separate allergenic determinants on each of the fragments BSA-P_{1-306}, BSA-$P_{307-582}$, and BSA-$T_{377-582}$. However, little of the activity of the BSA was recovered in the different fragments. The sum of their activities ranged from less than 6% to 20% of the activity of BSA. In three patients who were found to be sensitive to BSA, the amount of the activity recovered in the peptide fragments was even less [35].

The loss of activity of the BSA molecule on proteolytic cleavage into two halves could be due to the brake up of the molecule in the middle of the third domain with a loss of allergenic sites; it might further be due to minor conformational changes in the fragments as compared with the intact molecule. Our data suggest the presence of at least four IgE-binding sites on the BSA molecule.

We desensitized rabbit basophils for histamine release with the peptide fragments to test for the presence of IgE antibodies recognizing unique or homologous sites. Desensitization occurs when the cells are exposed to an antigen under nonoptimal conditions like the absence of calcium. With rabbit basophils desensitization is antigen specific. As expected, cells desensitized with BSA-P_{1-306} failed to release histamine when rechallenged with the desensitiz-

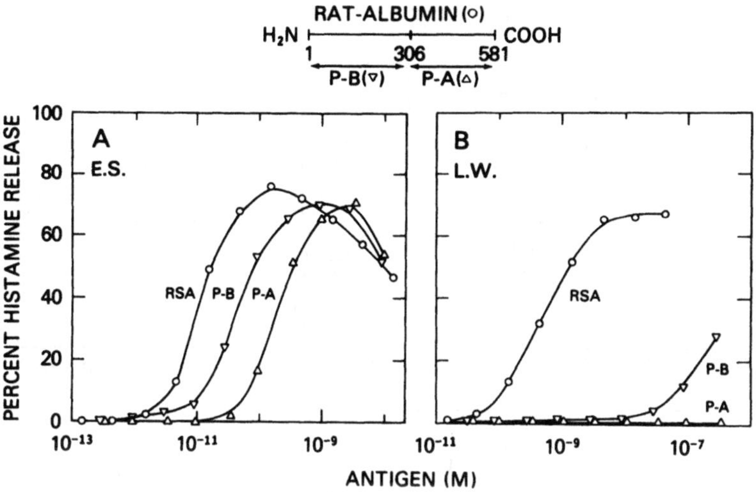

Fig. 2. Histamine release by RSA and fragments from the leukocytes of two patients allergic to rats

Table 3. Serum albumin and peptide fragments

Fragment [a]	Molecular weight
Rat serum albumin (RSA)	66500
RSA-P_{1-306}	35000
RSA-$P_{387-581}$	31500
Bovine serum albumin (BSA)	66340
BSA-P_{1-306}	34950
BSA-$P_{307-582}$	31390
BSA-$T_{377-582}$	23270
BSA-$P_{505-582}$	8620

[a] P refers to the peptides prepared with pepsin, and T with trypsin

ing antigen (Fig. 3). There was also reduced reactivity on the desensitized cells when they were incubated with the other fragments. Desensitization with BSA-$P_{307-582}$ resulted in unresponsiveness to the desensitizing fragment without any change in the BSA-P_{1-306} induced histamine release. These data indicate that there are unique IgE-reactive antigenic sites on each half of the BSA molecule. However, some of the sites on the COOH terminal half cross-reacted with antibodies directed toward the NH_2 terminal part of the molecule.

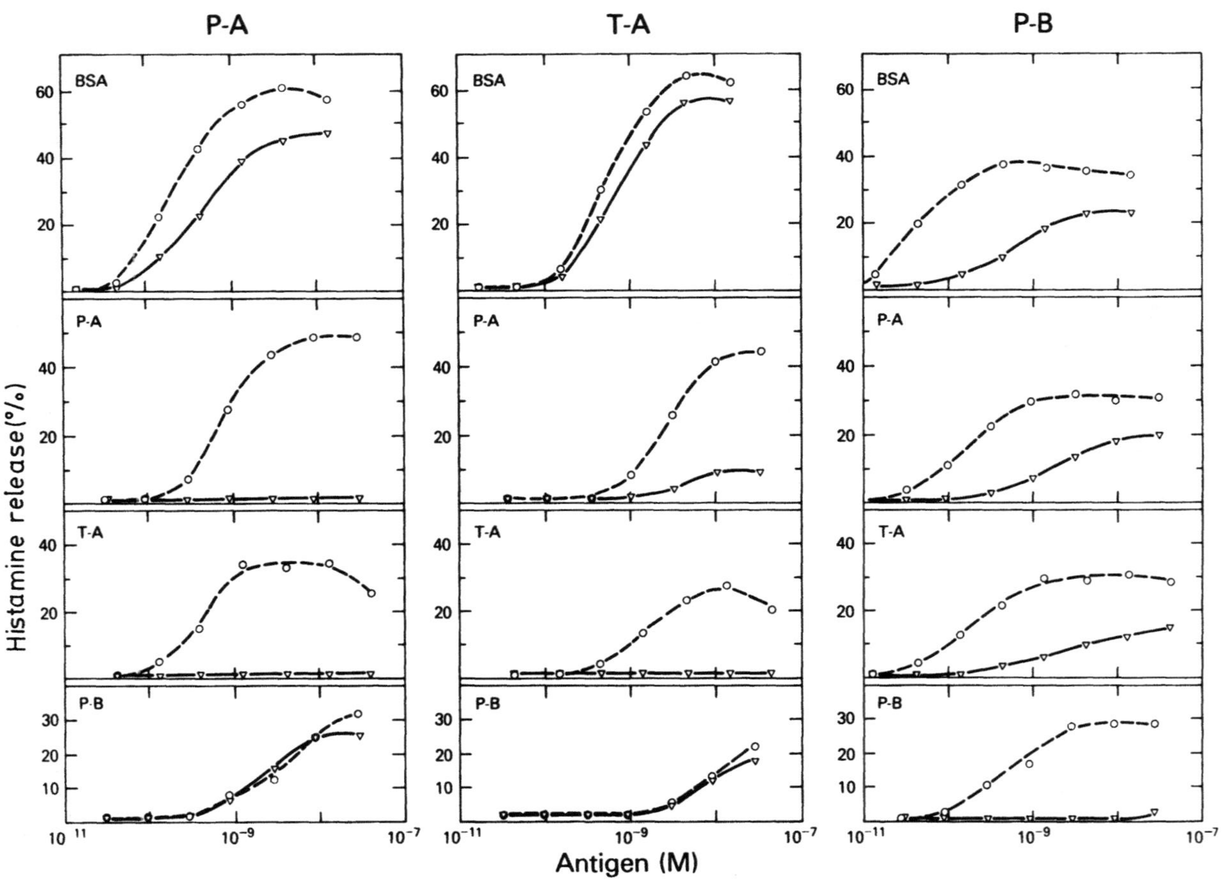

Fig. 3. Specificity of IgE-reactive antigenic determinants on BSA. Rabbit basophils were desensitized by incubation with BSA-$P_{307-582}$ (*first panel*), BSA-$T_{377-582}$ (*second panel*) or BSA-P_{1-306} (*third panel*). Control cells were preincubated in medium. After 60 min the cells were washed twice and challenged with BSA and the three fragments. (▽ – ▽, desensitized cells; ○ – ○, cells incubated in medium)

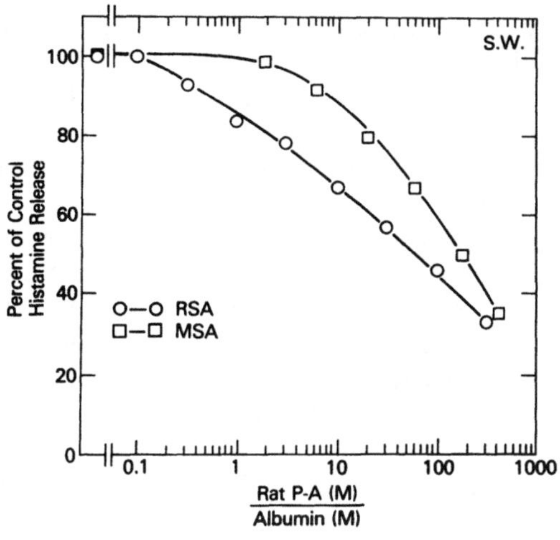

Fig. 4. Inhibition of RSA- and MSA-induced histamine release by the RSA-$P_{307-581}$ fragment

Cross-reactivity Between Animals

Multiple sensitizations of various mammals are a common phenomenon. There is experimental evidence for the hypothesis that this is at least partly due to real cross-reactivity. It has been proposed that serum proteins like serum albumin from different animals, such as cats and dogs or rats and mice, cross-react, binding with some of their epitopes to an identical IgE antibody population of a sensitized individuum [15, 32, 38].

We found the leukocytes of all RSA-sensitive patients to release histamine with mouse serum albumin (MSA), too. Utilizing the haptenic peptide RSA-$P_{307-581}$ for inhibition of serum albumin-induced histamine release, we were able to show that besides RSA, MSA-induced histamine release was inhibited at only slightly higher molar concentrations of the inhibiting fragment (Fig. 4). These experiments clearly show that at least one allergenic determinant on the serum albumins of rats and mice is identical or at least similar. In contrast, a haptenic fragment from BSA specifically blocked histamine release induced by BSA, but not by MSA or RSA.

Immunotherapy

The efficacy of immunotherapy with animal extracts has been questioned in the past. Since avoidance of contact with domestic or laboratory animals sometimes may be difficult, several studies on the value of immunotherapy with animal allergen extracts have been performed using poorly defined allergen extracts without a control group. They gave conflicting results. Using nonpurified allergen extracts from the whole pelt of laboratory animals (mouse, rat, rabbit) in an uncontrolled study, we were able to demonstrate that immunotherapy was effective in causing an increase in blocking antibodies, which appeared to be specific. The antibody level correlated with the cumulative allergen dose injected during therapy [33].

Using a characterized and standardized cat allergen extract for hyposensitization, Ohman et al. [24] were able to demonstrate a reduction in specific bronchial sensitivity in cat-allergic asthmatics. The efficacy of immunotherapy with a standardized dog extract was investigated in a double-blind study in children by Valovirta et al. [30]. After 1 year of therapy they found a significant decrease in conjunctival sensitivity to dog extract, but not a decrease in bronchial sensitivity.

A multicenter study on immunotherapy with partially purified and standardized animal extracts from cats and dogs, which was placebo controlled, recently reported a significant decrease in bronchial sensitivity toward cats but not toward dogs after 1 year of treatment [29]. In the actively treated group of patients the skin prick test reactions decreased continuously, the decrease being the first sign of an immunological effect of the therapy. IgG and IgG_4 levels showed an increase in the allergen-treated patients. The authors found no correlation between these parameters and the patients' own subjective evaluation or the allergen bronchial challenge test [10].

For the cat allergen-treated group the specificities of IgG antibodies were directed against cat antigens number 2, 3 (cat albumin), 4 (CA I), and 7, and for the dog allergen-treated group against dog antigens number 2 (dog albumin), 13, and 20. The most significant changes in the levels of allergen-specific IgE antibodies were found for the dander proteins, whereas IgE levels to cat or dog serum albumin did not change very much. The authors conclude from their study that allergenic extracts from animals used for immunotherapy should contain a high percentage of dander protein like CA I [17].

References

1. Bartholomé K, Baer H, Kopietz-Schulte E, Wahn U (1985) Where does cat allergen I come from? J Allergy Clin Immunol 76:503–506
2. Blands J, Løwenstein H, Weeke B (1977) Characterization of extracts of dog hair and dandruff from six different dog breeds by quantitative immunoelectrophoresis. Identification of allergens by crossed radioimmunoelectrophoresis (CRIE). Acta Allerg 32:147–169
3. Brown JR (1977) Serum albumin: amino acid sequence. In: Rosenoor VM, Oratz M, Rothschild MA (eds) Albumin structure, function and uses. Pergamon, Oxford, p 27
4. Brown PR, Leitermann K, Ohman JL Jr (1984) Distribution of cat allergen 1 in cat tissues and fluids. Int Arch Allergy Appl Immunol 74:67–70
5. Cockcroft A, McCarthy P, Edwards J, Andersson N (1981) Allergy in laboratory animal workers. Lancet 1:827–830
6. Davies GE, McArdle LA (1981) Allergy to laboratory animals: a survey by questionnaire. Int Arch Allergy Appl Immunol 64:302–307

7. Didierlaurent A, Foglietti MJ, Guérin B, Hewitt BE, Percheron F (1984) Comparative study on cat allergens from fur and saliva. Int Archs Allergy Appl Immunol 73:27–31
8. Gross NJ (1980) Allergy to laboratory animals: epidemiologic, clinical and physiologic aspects, and a trial of cromolyn in its management. J Allergy Clin Immunol 66:158–165
9. Guerin B, Hewitt B (1981) A comparative study of allergen extracts from cat fur, cat pelt and cat saliva. Ann Allergy 46:127–131
10. Hedlin G, Graff-Lonnevig V, Heilborn H, Lilja G, Norrlind K, Pegelow KO, Sundin B, Løwenstein H (1986) Immunotherapy with cat and dog dander extracts. II. In vivo and in vitro immunological effects observed in a 1-year double blind placebo study. J Allergy Clin Immunol 77:488–496
11. Hoffman DR (1980) Dog and cat allergens: urinary proteins or dander proteins? Ann Allergy 45:205–206
12. Kjellman B, Petterson R (1983) The problems of furred pets in childhood atopic disease. Allergy 38:65
13. Lincoln TA, Bolton NE, Garrett AS (1974) Occupational allergy to animal dander and sera. J Occup Med 16:465–469
14. Longbottom JL (1983) Characterization of allergens from the urines of experimental animals. In: Kerr JW, Ganderton MA (eds) Proceedings of the 11th International congress of allergology and clinical immunology. Macmillan, London pp 525–529
15. Løwenstein H (1981) Allergene von Katze, Hund, Rind und Pferd. Allergologie 4:265–269
16. Løwenstein H, Lind P, Weeke B (in press) Identification and clinical significance of allergenic molecules of cat origin. A part of the DAS 76 study. Allergy
17. Løwenstein H, Graff-Lonnevig V, Hedlin G, Heilborn H, Lilja G, Norrlind K, Pegelow KO, Sundin B (1986) Immunotherapy with cat and dog dander extracts. III. Allergen-specific Ig-responses in a 1-year double blind placebo study. J Allergy Clin Immunol 77: 497–504
18. Lutsky I, Neuman I (1975) Laboratory animal dander allergy. I. An occupational disease. Ann Allergy 35:201
19. Lutsky I, Fink JN, Kidd J, Dahlberg MJE, and Yunginger JW (1985) Allergenic properties of rat urine and pelt extracts. J Allergy Clin Immunol 75:279–284
20. McLean AC, Glovsky MM, Hoffman DR, Ghekiere LM (1980) Identification of allergens in dog dander extract. I. Clinical and immunological aspects of allergenic activity. Ann Allergy 45:199–204
21. Newman-Taylor A, Longbottom JL, Pepys J (1977) Respiratory allergy to urine proteins of rats and mice. Lancet 2:847–849
22. Newman-Taylor AJ (1982) Laboratory animal allergy. Eur J Respir Dis 63:123:60–64
23. Ohman JL, Baer H, Anderson MC, Leiterman K, Brown P (1983) Surface washes of living cats: an improved method of obtaining clinically relevant allergen. J Allergy Clin Immunol 72:288–293
24. Ohman JL, Findlay SR, Leitermann KM (1984) Immunotherapy in cat induced asthma. Double blind trial with evaluation of in vivo and in vitro responses. J Allergy Clin Immunol 74:230
25. Prahl P, Bucher D, Plesner T, Weeke B, Løwenstein H (1982) Isolation and partial characterisation of three major allergens in an extract from cow hair and dander. Int Arch Allergy Appl Immunol 67:293–301
26. Schumacher MJ (1980) Characterization of allergens from urine and pelts of laboratory mice. Mol Immunol 17:1087–1095
27. Schumacher MJ, Tait BD, Holmes MC (1981) Allergy to murine antigens in a biological research institue. J Allergy Clin Immunol 68:310–318
28. Siraganian RP, Sandberg AL (1979) Characterization of mouse allergens. J Allergy Clin Immunol 63:435–442
29. Sundin B, Lilja G, Graff-Lonnevig V, Hedlin G, Heilborn H, Norrlind K, Pegelow KO, Løwenstein H (1986) Immunotherapy with partially purified and standardized animal dander extracts. I. Clinical results from a double blind study on patients with animal dander asthma. J Allergy Clin Immunol 77:478–487
30. Valovirta E, Koivikko A, Vanto T, Viander M, Ingeman L (1984) Immunotherapy in allergy to dog: a double blind clinical study. Ann Allergy 53:85–88

31. Vanto T, Viander M, Schwartz B (1982) Dog serum albumin as an allergen. Int Arch Allergy Appl Immunol 69:311–315
32. Viander M, Valovirta E, Vanto T, Koivikko A (1983) Cross-reactivity of cat and dog allergen extracts. Int Arch Allergy Appl Immunol 71:252–260
33. Wahn U, Siraganian RP (1980) Efficacy and specificity of immunotherapy with laboratory animal allergen extracts. J Allergy Clin Immunol 65:413–421
34. Wahn U, Peters T, Siraganian RP (1980) Studies on the allergenic significance and structure of rat serum albumin. J Immunol 125:2544–2549
35. Wahn U, Peters T, Siraganian RP (1981) Allergenic and antigenic properties of bovine serum albumin. Mol Immunol 18:19–28
36. Wahn U, Herold U, Danielsen K, Løwenstein H (1982) Allergoprints in horse allergic children. Allergy 37:335–343
37. Walls AF, Longbottom JL (1985) Comparison of rat fur, urine, saliva, and other rat allergen extracts by skin testing, RAST, and RAST inhibition. J Allergy Clin Immunol 75:242–251
38. Wüthrich B, Guerin B, Hewitt BE (1985) Cross-allergenicity between extracts of hair from different dog breeds and cat fur. Clin Allergy 15:87–93

Allergoids, Mechanisms and New Developments

A. W. Wheeler and B. G. Overell

Bencard Pharmaceuticals, Yew Tree Bottom Road, Epsom, Surrey KT18 5XQ, England

Abstract

"Allergoids" are allergens that have been modified in order to eliminate reactivity with specific IgE but have a maintained capacity to induce an immunological response, particularly in terms of allergen specific IgG antibody. Such materials have been used clinically for over a decade with varying degrees of success. Both clinical and laboratory properties of these will be discussed critically. However, the term "allergoid" can now be extended to cover other preparations of allergens, modified in such a way as to eliminate certain immunological properties whilst maintaining or enhancing others.

Introduction

Hyposensitisation treatment with aqueous vaccines, though effective, can be accompanied by adverse reactions. In attempts to overcome this problem, various formulations have been designed to reduce the immediate bioavailability of the allergen and yet maintain or enhance the immunological stimulus and effectiveness of therapy (Fig. 1). Water-in-oil emulsions, suspensions of aluminium hydroxide and more recently tyrosine crystals have all been used for this purpose.

An alternative approach was adopted as early as 1935 by Carter, who used formaldehyde to modify chemically allergens used in hyposensitisation therapy. Renewed efforts by David Marsh demonstrated that modified ragweed, rye and other pollen extracts had a reduced ability to release mediators from mast cells sensitised with appropriate human IgE, yet still retained immunological activity as indicated by the induction of IgG antibody. Such materials were named "allergoids".

- **Series of Aqueous Injections**
- **Depot forms**
  - Emulsions
  - Aluminium Gels
  - L-Tyrosine
- **Allergoids**

Fig. 1. Allergen presentation forms

The Bencard group studied a vast number of modifying agents before selecting the reagent glutaraldehyde to modify pollen allergens to produce allergoid materials. The pollens of grass, ragweed, *Parietaria*, olive, and a mixture of birch, hazel and alder have been treated in this way to produce allergoid vaccines currently used for therapy.

In the development of these products it could be shown very readily that 1° NH_2 groups were progressively lost from allergenic proteins in pollen extracts with increasing concentrations of glutaraldehyde (Fig. 2). This decrease in 1° NH_2 content is accompanied by loss of skin test activity, indicating that the extracts should be safer than unmodified counterparts if used for therapy. However, it is of importance that other immunological activity is not impaired by the treatment.

As is shown in rats, although at low degrees of modification IgG antibody induction is maintained, as modification of the extract is increased, eventually immunogenicity is compromised (Fig. 3). Therefore, a level of glutaraldehyde is chosen for modification commensurate with loss of reactivity with IgE but with retained IgG antibody-inducing ability. Thus a product is made that has a reduced activity to react with human IgE in a RAST inhibition system (Fig. 4), and yet induces antibody in experimental animals as effectively as does unmodified extract, whether it is injected in Freund's adjuvant, adsorbed into tyrosine crystals or just in an aqueous form (Fig. 5).

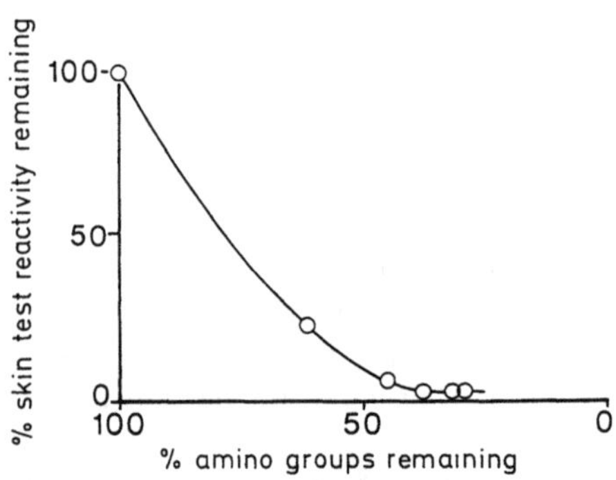

Fig. 2. Loss of skin test reactivity on glutaraldehyde modification of mixed grass pollen extract

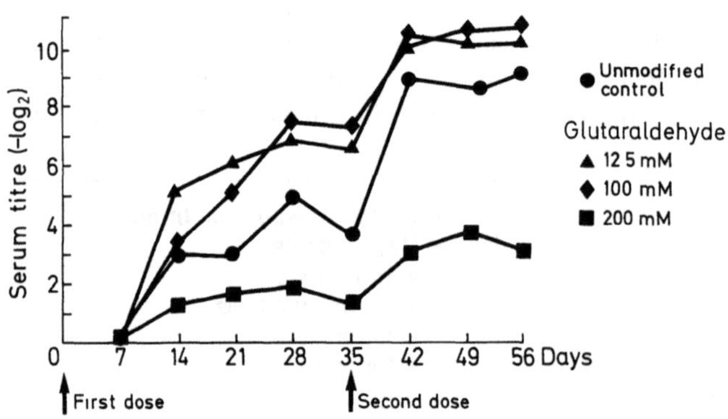

Fig. 3. Immunogenicity of glutaraldehyde-modified grass pollen extracts in rats

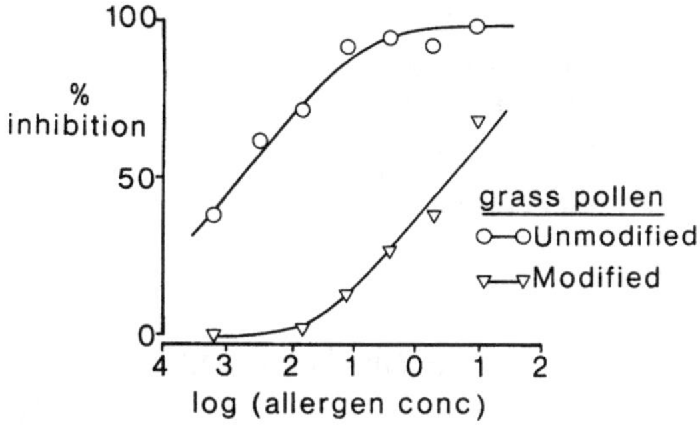

Fig. 4. Inhibition of RAST by glutaraldehyde-modified mixed grass pollen

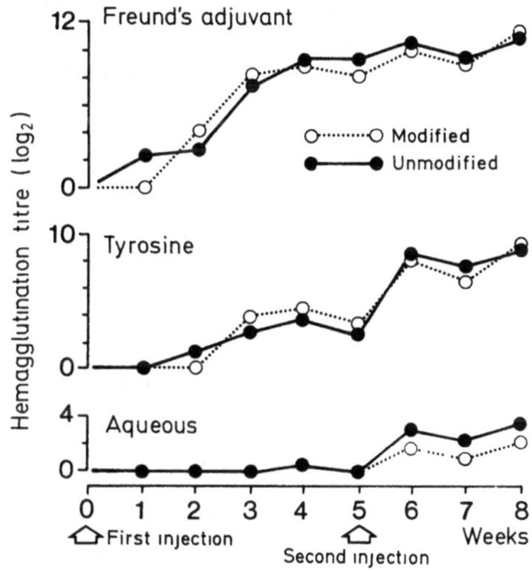

Fig. 5. Antibody production in rats after injection of modified and unmodified extracts using different adjuvants

Clearly, modified allergens with the properties described were worthy of progression to the clinic. There are various ways in which the safety bonus conferred by modification can be exploited. Firstly, patients can be treated with higher allergen concentrations. This approach has been suggested by some workers following the rationale that a greater allergen mass injected leads to more successful therapy. Bencard, on the other hand, elected to use allergoids to extend the options available, and give the clinician more choice in the type of product he can prescribe, by introducing a convenient, safer and short-course product. Vaccines of this type, using naturally occurring and relatively insoluble L-tyrosine to form depot preparations, have been made for the treatment of grass, tree, ragweed, *Parietaria* and olive pollen allergies (Fig. 6), products usually consisting of three injections of increasing allergen strength followed by optional maintenance injections at the top concentrations.

These allergoid products have been used successfully in many investigators' hands; for example, Fig. 7 shows the results of a placebo-controlled study of the Bencard ragweed allergoid product. Symptom scores, not shown, were less in those patients treated with the active material, and, as can be seen, medications

- Tyrosine allergoid grass pollen (with rye pollen)
- Tyrosine allergoid tree pollen
- Pollinex R (ragweed)
- Pollinex (*Parietaria*)
- Pollinex (olive)

Fig. 6. Glutaraldehyde allergoid products

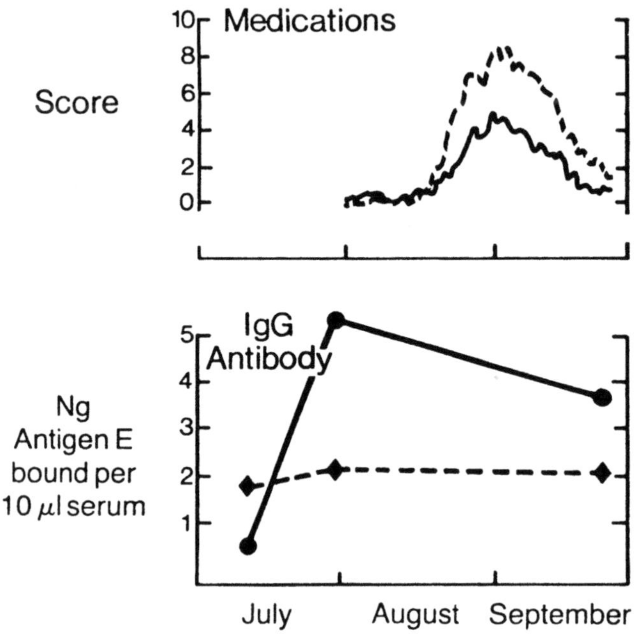

Fig. 7. Glutaraldehyde-modified ragweed/tyrosine clinical trial [Cockroft et al. (1977) J Allergy 60:56]

taken to control symptoms during the pollen season were also less. The product was also seen to induce IgG antibody specific for antigen E.

Generalised reactions with this product were minimal, in agreement with the results presented in Fig. 8. Skin test activity of the ragweed extract, as shown in this figure for three different batches, was reduced to almost undetectable levels by glutaraldehyde treatment. Subsequently other workers, and in particular Patterson, have also shown in clinical trials that glutaraldehyde-modified pollen extracts can bring about safely the required therapeutic effect.

Although IgG antibody induction during hyposensitisation therapy is possibly not directly responsible for the amelioration of allergic symptoms, it is currently regarded as an indicator of the required immunological activity of a vaccine.

Figure 9 shows that Tyrosin Allergoid Gräserpollen induces an IgG antibody response to three of the major allergens of grass pollen, R 7, R 14a and R 14b, which is our nomenclature for allergens contained within Marsh's rye allergen groups 1, 2 and 3. Similarly, from Fig. 10 it can be seen that *Parietaria*-

specific IgG antibody can be induced by treatment of patients with a course of glutaraldehyde-modified tyrosine-adsorbed *Parietaria* pollen extract.

It would appear that developments towards intrinsically safer and more convenient vaccine forms are highly desirable. The evidence is promising that this can be achieved by empirical chemical modification approaches. Therefore no doubt allergoids will continue to take their place amongst specific hyposensitisation vaccines and make a significant contribution towards the management of respiratory allergy.

So where do we go from here with the "allergoid" story? Clearly, even though new allergoids may be produced, and new clinical schedules may be devised, it is unlikely that these types of modified materials will be any more effective than unmodified ones, though, as already described, they may be used for more convenient and safer therapy.

We feel at Bencard that perhaps we could now add another word to the language of allergology, that is T'allergoid. By this we mean an allergen with reduced reactivity with specific IgE, but maintained ability to stimulate various subpopulations of allergen-specific T cells.

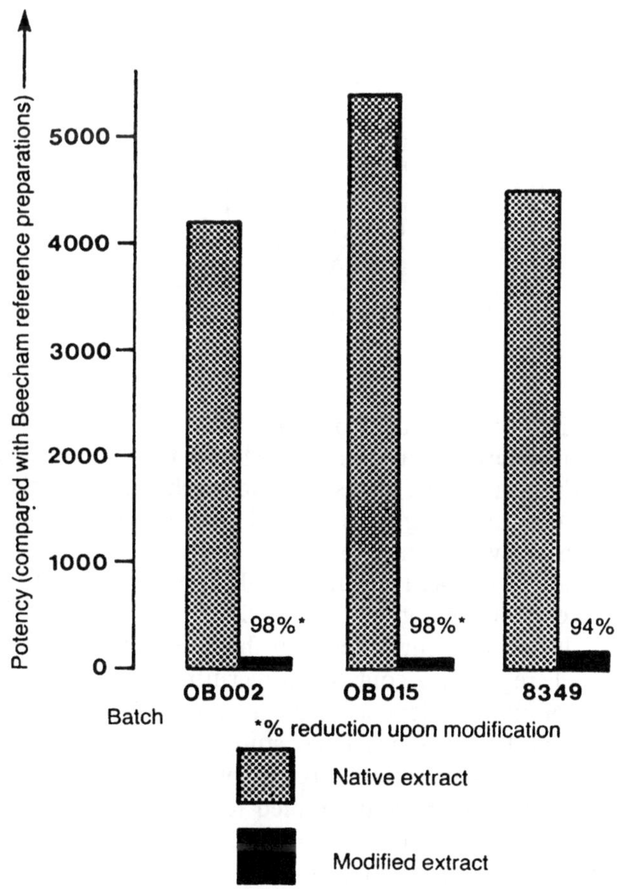

Fig. 8. Reduction of skin test activity of short ragweed by modification with glutaraldehyde

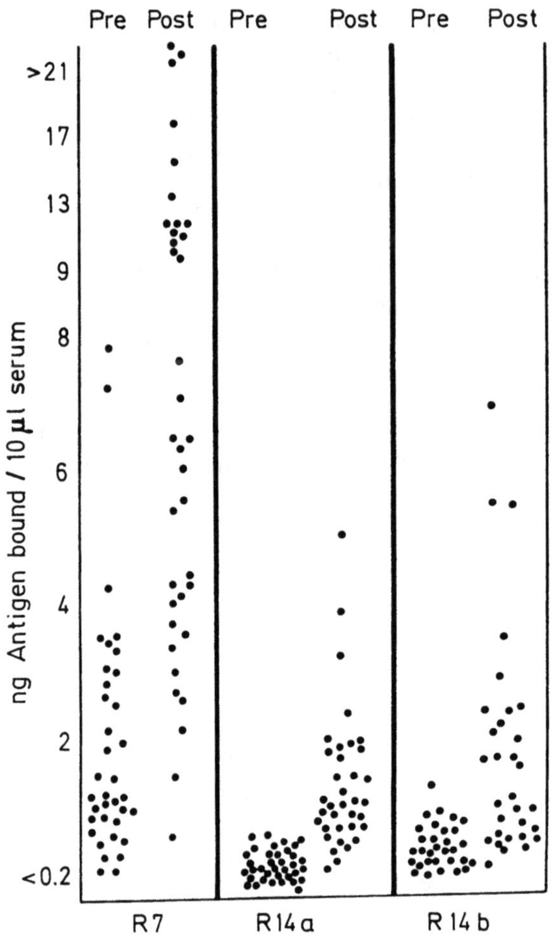

Fig. 9. IgG antibodies to R 7, R 14a and R 14b pre- and post-treatment (Pollinex)

The consequences of manipulating the immune response of patients with such materials could only be shown by clinical experimentation (Fig. 11), but might clearly give us insight into mechanisms involved in hyposensitisation.

Already allergens modified with polysarcosine, PEG and poly DGL have been shown at least in model systems, to modulate IgE production via suppressor T cell activation, though appropriate clinical schedules to exploit such materials have not yet been devised.

It has been suggested that the late reaction of allergy may also be subject to T cell regulatory control, so recruitment of eosinophils and basophils into the site of allergen deposition might very well be modulated by T'allergoids. In this context Bencard has been studying not only polysarcosine-conjugated allergens as IgE-suppressing agents but also allergens fragmented by chemical and enzymatic means and coupled to various biologically active peptides. The results cannot be discussed in detail here; however, our laboratory data are encouraging, and we already have materials that have lost reactivity with IgE and

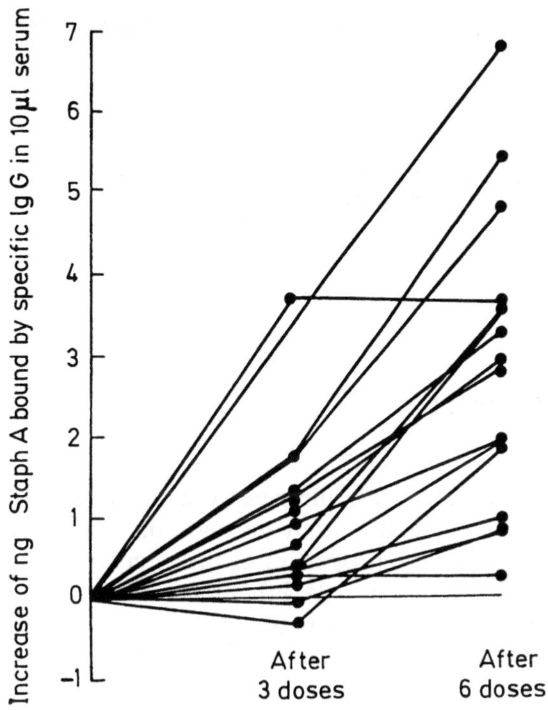

Fig. 10. *Parietaria*-specific IgG after Bencard *Parietaria* (Spain 1984/5) increases in antibody

- IgE suppression
- Modulation of late-phase reaction
- Expansion of helper cell pool
- Modulation of delayed hypersensitivity
- Unknown?

Fig. 11. Possible consequences of therapy with T′ allergoids

are poor antibody inducers but have propensities to react with different T cell populations such as those concerned with helper activity and delayed hypersensitivity.

It remains to be seen whether such innovations will ever fulfil their promise, and although work continues on these and other speculative options, it would seem that consolidation and optimisation of current clinical practices should be the immediate targets.

mPEG-Modified Allergen Preparations

S. Dreborg

Department of Pediatrics, University Hospital, 58185 Linköping, Sweden, and
Pharmacia AB, 75182 Uppsala, Sweden

Abstract

Modification of allergens was introduced with two aims: to decrease allergenicity and thereby decrease the reactivity of patients during treatment and to change the properties of the allergen and thereby decrease the IgE-response in atopic individuals. IgE suppression has only been possible to induce in animals, not in allergic patients.

Preclinical documentation of new modified allergen products should include the study of the toxicity, allergenicity, immunogenicity and pharmacokinetic properties of the preparation.

Human studies using mPEG-allergen extracts have shown clinical efficacy, reduced reaction rate with especially less risk of immediate general reactions. Furthermore, both IgE and IgG immune responses are induced to all relevant allergens.

Thus, PEG-modified allergens seem to be a promising, new alternative for immunotherapy with a reduced risk for general reactions and maintained clinical efficacy.

Introduction

Monomethoxy polyethylene glycol (mPEG)-modified allergens are produced by covalent coupling of the PEG molecule to amino groups on the allergen molecule. If "tails" of PEG (3000 – 5000 daltons) are attached to the surface of the allergen, these tails will partly cover reactive determinants and the properties of the allergenic molecule will be changed.

All modified allergens, like mPEG-modified allergens, were primarily produced to induce suppression of the specific IgE antibody response in the allergic patient.

In the first double-blind placebo-controlled study comparing mPEG-modified ragweed with placebo [1], it was clearly shown that no marked IgE suppression could be obtained in humans (Fig. 1). However, mPEG-modified allergens are less allergenic than nonmodified allergens. A major problem in immunotherapy is the risk of immediate general reactions which are potentially life-threatening. It therefore seemed important to develop PEG-modified allergen preparations.

Like all new pharmaceutical products, modified allergens have to be investigated thoroughly before clinical trials are started. Thus the toxicology of the PEG, the allergen and the mPEG-modified allergen has been studied in two animal species. The allergenicity of the preparation has been compared in vivo and in vitro with that of the same but unmodified allergen preparation. The al-

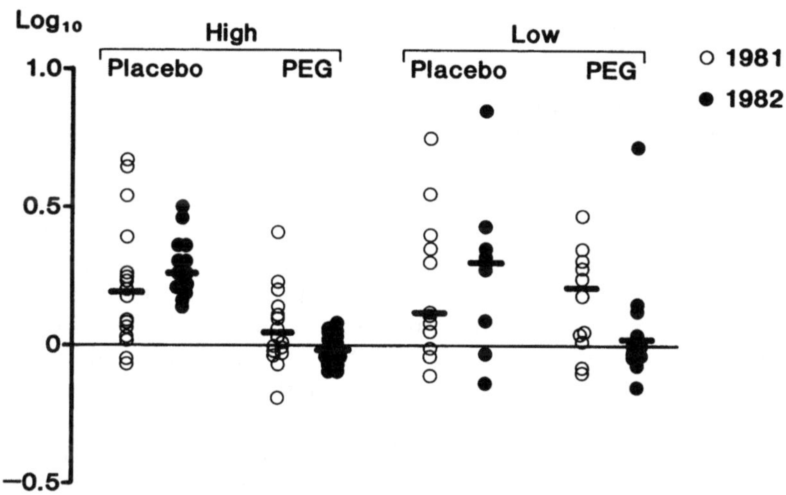

Fig. 1. Changes in ragweed-specific IgE in 36 patients with high clinical sensitivity and 26 patients with low clinical sensitivity. Each group was divided into two subgroups, one receiving mPEG-modified ragweed and one placebo. [1]

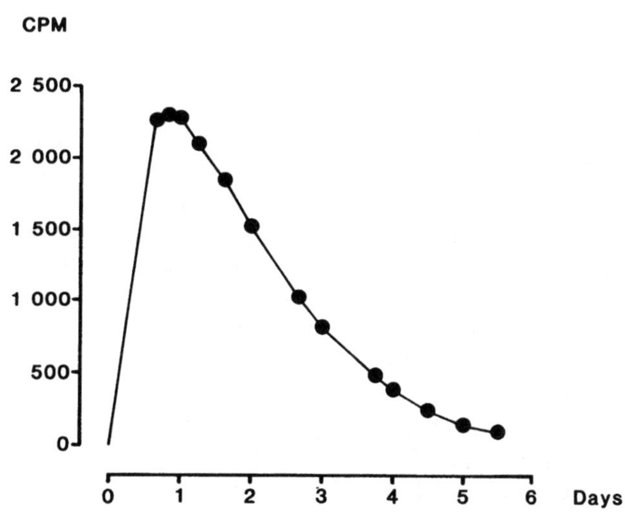

Fig. 2. Serum levels of radioactivity after subcutaneous injection of radiolabelled mPEG-modified HBV in rabbits. [2]

Table 1. Clinical trials with mPEG-modified preparations

Investigators	Material	Comparison	Reference
Norman et al.	PEG-AgE	Other modified preparations	[7]
Juniper et al.	mPEG-ragweed	Placebo	[1]
Juniper et al.	mPEG-ragweed	Two dose schedules	[3]
Öhman et al. Nordvall et al.	mPEG-HBV	Open	[4, 5]
Müller et al.	mPEG-HBV	HBV	[6]

lergenicity was reduced to less than 1%. In addition, the pharmacokinetic properties have been studied [2]. The results indicate that PEG-modified honey bee venom (HBV) is released slowly from the injection site and is present in the circulation for longer than unmodified allergens, which are readily excreted in the urine (Fig. 2). Such studies are of the greatest importance for the proper clinical use of the product. So far, published reports are available regarding the effect of mPEG-modified ragweed and mPEG-HBV (Table 1). Juniper et al. reported on the clinical and immunological effects of two different dose schedules, using mPEG-ragweed vs placebo [1]. Statistically significantly less symptoms were registered in patients given active treatment than in those given placebo treatment. The specific IgE was not suppressed to any great extent. However, the specific IgG was raised in most patients. A very rapid dose increase and a slow dose increase were compared in another trial by the same group [3]. The slow dose increase was better tolerated. Thus, the first experience with mPEG-modified pollen extracts show promising results.

mPEG-HBV has also been used in published clinical studies. In a pilot study, Öhman and co-workers [4, 5] treated 14 patients who had a clinical history indicating systemic IgE-mediated allergic reactions to bee stings, positive skin prick tests, and positive RASTs. These patients reached a top dose of 200 µg in 4 weeks. Later the dose was increased to 400 µg. The treatment was then changed to unmodified HBV. Twelve patients tolerated 200 µg, whereas two tolerated 100 µg but reacted to higher doses. Eight of 14 patients tolerated accidental honey bee stings. The IgE increased but reached pretreatment values within a few months. Specific IgG increased rapidly but then decreased. The ratio of specific IgG to specific IgE remained at a high level. The crossed radioimmunoelectrophoresis (CRIE) and immunoblotting techniques were used to study the IgE and IgG response to specific allergens. Production of antibodies directed against all relevant allergens was stimulated, indicating that the modified preparation had the capacity to induce an immune response to all relevant components.

In a double-blind study, Müller et al. [6] studied 24 patients; 12 were given unmodified and 12 modified HBV. The highest dose of HBV was 100 µg and of mPEG-modified HBV 200 µg (Fig. 3). Two patients treated with HBV experienced several severe general reactions, preventing them from reaching 100 µg HBV. Therefore they were excluded. Six patients had general reactions to HBV

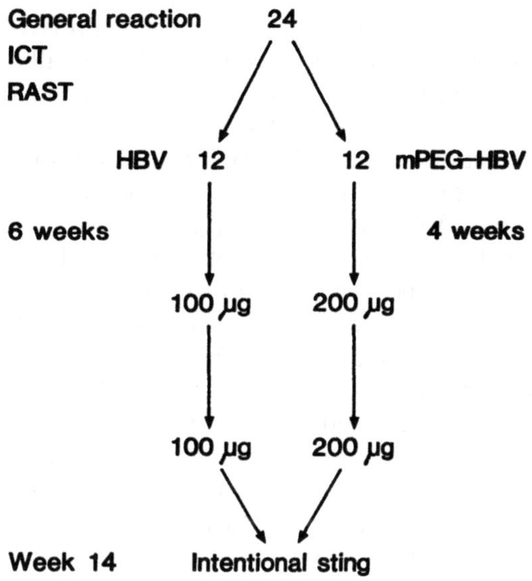

Fig. 3. Trial design. [6]

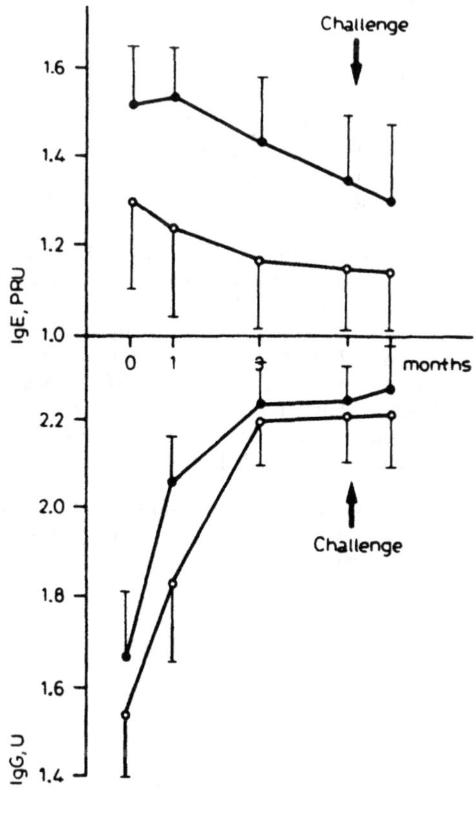

Fig. 4. Changes in specific IgE and IgG during treatment with HBV (●) and mPEG-modified HBV (○). [6]

and one had a general reaction to mPEG-HBV. Four maintenance doses were given. Then all patients were intentionally stung. One HBV-treated patient and three mPEG-HBV-treated patients reacted. One of the latter patients did not show true IgE-mediated reactivity at reevaluation. All patients who reacted to intentional stings showed an increase of the total specific IgG (Fig. 4). However, they did not show a specific IgG response to one allergen important to the individual patient (IgG CRIE). In summary, three patients in each treatment group were not protected by the treatment, indicating that higher doses are needed for full protection.

In conclusion, experience so far indicates that mPEG-modified allergens are easy to produce, yield reproducible results, are well tolerated, and induce increased specific tolerance in treated patients. However, the top dose needs to be slightly increased; by how much will be shown in ongoing studies comparing the effect of several dose levels of unmodified allergen preparation to that of several dose levels of mPEG-modified allergens. The mPEG-modified allergen preparations are a promising alternative treatment for allergic reactions to potent allergen preparations, as they combine a low rate of immediate reaction with maintained efficacy.

References

1. Juniper E, Roberts R, Kennedy L, O'Connor J, Syty-Golda M, Dolovich J, Hargreave F (1985) J Allergy Clin Immunol 75:578–585
2. Åkerblom E, Ahlstedt S, Björkstén B (1982) Allergenic and immunogenic properties of monomethoxypolyethylene glycol (mPEG) modified honey bee venom (HBV) (abstract). XI International Congress of Allergology & Clinical Immunology, London, p 153
3. Juniper E, O'Connor J, Dolovich J, Hargreave F (1984) PEG allergens ragweed immunotherapy. J Allergy Clin Immunol 73:118
4. Öhman S, Björkander J, Dreborg S, Lanner Å, Malling H-J, Weeke B (1986) A preliminary study of immunotherapy with a monomethoxy polyethylene glycol modified honey bee venom preparation. Allergy 41:81–88
5. Nordvall L, Uhlin T, Öhman S, Björkander J, Malling H-J, Weeke B, Dreborg S, Lanner S, Einarsson R (1986) IgG and IgE antibody patterns after immunotherapy with monomethoxy polyethylene glycol modified honey bee venom. Allergy 41:89–94
6. Müller U, Lanner Å, Schmid P, Bischof M, Dreborg S, Hoigné R (1985) A double blind study on immunotherapy with chemically modified honey bee venom: monomethoxy polyethylene glycol-coupled versus crude honey bee venom. Int Arch Allergy Appl Immunol 77:201–203
7. Norman PS, King TP, Alexander JF, Kagey-Sobodka A, Lichtenstein LM (1984) Immunologic responses to conjugates of antigen E in patients with ragweed hayfever. J Allergy Clin Immunol 73:782–789

Pharmacotherapy

Pharmacological Modulation of Immunoregulatory Lymphocyte Functions: The Adenosine Immunoregulatory System

S. H. Polmar and R. E. Birch

Division of Allergy and Immunology, Department of Pediatrics,
Washington University School of Medicine, St. Louis, MO 63178, USA

Abstract

During the last ten years there has been a rapid expansion in our understanding of immunoregulatory processes. Advances in two important areas have been particularly significant:

1. the delineation of lymphocyte subpopulations through the application of monoclonal antibody technology and
2. the development of a better understanding of the ways in which hormones and other intercellular communicators modulate cell behaviour.

In this presentation the interplay between immunoregulatory lymphocyte subpopulations and endogenous intercellular communicators (i.e. autacoids) will be discussed.

Histamine and prostaglandins are well-known examples of autacoids with immunoregulatory properties. Adenosine is a less well-known autacoid which also possesses impressive immunoregulatory properties. Histamine is known to suppress lymphocyte proliferation, cytotoxicity and lymphokine secretion. This action appears to be mediated by a soluble factor termed histamine suppressor factor, HSF. HSF is produced by H_2 histamine receptor-bearing T cells and acts upon macrophages resulting in secretion of immunosuppressive prostaglandins. Studies from our own laboratory indicate that mechanisms of histamine-induced immunoregulation are more complex than previously thought. We have found that histamine may produce both stimulatory as well as inhibitory lymphokines and that the control of lymphokine production is mediated by different histamine receptors. While histamine-induced lymphokines are capable of modulating lymphocyte proliferation, other histamine-induced immunoregulatory effects are not mediated by these soluble factors.

The nucleoside adenosine also has been shown to have potent immunoregulatory properties. Adenosine is liberated from cells under conditions of ischemia and hypoxia and thus may represent a cellular injury signal. Adenosine has its effects on a subpopulation of T helper/inducer lymphocytes. Adenosine acts on cells bearing specific adenosine receptors and causes the activation of suppressor cells from within the T helper/inducer lymphocyte subpopulation. The adenosine induced suppressor system has a major effect upon B cell differentiation and immunoglobulin synthesis. In addition an adenosine induced lymphokine which suppresses lymphocyte proliferation has recently been identified in our laboratory. The biochemical mechanisms involved in adenosine mediate immunoregulation, as well as the possible role of adenosine in normal immunohomeostasis and human disease states are discussed.

Introduction

The immune system in man and other mammals consists of diverse yet interacting cell populations and their products. In recent years there has been considerable progress in the elucidation of the regulatory mechanisms controlling the immune system, in large measure due to the application of monoclonal antibody techniques to the identification of lymphocyte populations and subpopulations [1]. In their explorations of the complex networks of cellular interactions and the diverse activities of lymphokines and monokines which regulate immune function, immunologists occasionally lose sight of the fact that cells of the immune system are subject to the influences of substances which do not originate exclusively from cells of the immune system. It is now clear from the work of Besedovsky and others that the lymphoid system may be influenced by the neuroendocrine system [2]. The products of allergic and inflammatory reactions, histamine [3], prostaglandins [4], and more recently leukotrienes [5, 6], have also been shown to modulate immune function and in some instances have direct effects upon immunoregulatory lymphocytes. Recently, Holgate et al. [7] have suggested that adenosine may be an important mediator of bronchoconstriction in asthma and that a major portion of theophylline's therapeutic effect may be as an antagonist of adenosine receptor mediated bronchospastic events rather than as an inhibitor of phosphodiesterase activity. Studies from our laboratory during the past 7 years have shown that adenosine has impressive immunoregulatory properties which may be of considerable importance in both normal and pathological states.

Adenosine Modulates the Expression of Subset-Specific Antigens on Human T-lymphocytes

The development of monoclonal antibodies to antigens on human T cells has permitted the identification and isolation of functionally distinct T-lymphocyte subsets. Virtually all mature T-lymphocytes express the T3 antigen, which has recently been shown to be noncovalently linked to the T-cell receptor for antigen [8]. T-lymphocyte subpopulations bearing the T3 and T4 antigens provide helper/inducer function for the differentiation of B-lymphocytes into immunoglobulin-secreting plasma cells as well as for the induction of suppressor

Table 1. Effect of adenosine (ADO) upon the surface characteristics of unfractionated, helper/inducer and cytotoxic/suppressor human T-lymphocytes

T cells	% lymphocytes ± SEM			*P*
	Marker	Control	1 μM ADO	
Unfractionated	Fc_γ	13.8 ± 1.4	22.3 ± 4.7	<0.05
	OKT3	92.9 ± 1.1	93.9 ± 0.9	NS
	OKT4	50.5 ± 1.2	22.6 ± 4.8	<0.02
	OKT8	21.5 ± 2.3	37.9 ± 4.0	<0.01
Helper/inducer				
(OKT8 depleted)	Fc_γ	10.4 ± 1.3	24.4 ± 0.6	<0.02
	OKT4	79.1 ± 5.0	32.5 ± 2.6	<0.02
	OKT8	2.4 ± 0.3	11.6 ± 2.2	<0.005
Cytotoxic/suppressor				
(OKT4 depleted)	Fc_γ	13.0 ± 1.5	16.8 ± 2.8	NS
	OKT4	16.3 ± 5.8	11.8 ± 2.9	NS
	OKT8	56.3 ± 5.7	48.1 ± 1.1	NS

and cytotoxic effector cells. Within the T3+ T4+ helper/inducer population, other monoclonal antibodies delineate T cells which facilitate B cell differentiation (T3+ T4+ TQ1 − Leu8−) versus those that induce suppressor activity (T3+ 4+ TQ1 + Leu8+) [9, 10]. T3+ T8+ lymphocyte populations contain subpopulations, distinguishable by monoclonal antibodies, which are cytotoxic effector cells and suppressor effector T cells.

Adenosine was found to modulate rapidly the expression of selected antigens and receptors on the surfaces of human T-lymphocytes [11 − 13]. Brief exposure of T-lymphocytes to 1 μM adenosine for 30 min at 37 °C causes a significant increase in expression of the T8 antigen and receptors for the Fc portion of IgG (Fc_γ receptors) and a marked loss of T4 antigen expression (Table 1). Alteration in cell surface phenotype is restricted to the T3+ T4+ helper/inducer (T_I) subpopulation; T8+ lymphocytes and B cells are unaffected by exposure to adenosine. Cell surface phenotype modulation is selective; T4, T8, and Fc_γ receptors are modulated but the T3, T5, and Ia (HLA-Dr) antigens as well as sheep erythrocyte receptor expression are unaltered by adenosine. Kinetic studies have shown that the adenosine-induced decline in T4 expression is very rapid and is maximal within 5 min of exposure of T cells to adenosine. The increases in T8 antigen and Fc_γ receptor expression occur more slowly and are maximal after 30 − 60 min. Changes in cell surface antigens and receptors were found to be stable in culture for at least 24 h after the removal of adenosine.

Adenosine Effects upon Helper/Inducer T-lymphocyte Function

The same conditions which caused alterations in T-lymphocyte surface antigen expression were found to modify the helper/inducer activity of T4+ cell populations [14]. Exposure of T4-enriched cell preparations to 1 μM adenosine for 30 min at 37° C followed by removal of the nucleoside resulted in a marked decrease in the ability of these cells to facilitate the differentiation of isolated B cells into plasma cells or the production of IgG and IgM in pokeweed mitogen- or tetanus toxoid-stimulated cultures. Adenosine exposure did not alter viability of the cells. Adenosine-treated helper/inducer cells (T_IA) were found to suppress the development of plasma cells in pokeweed mitogen-stimulated cultures containing B cells and untreated T_I cells. Moreover, depletion of Fc_γ-bearing cells from T_IA cell preparations was found to restore completely the ability of the T_IA cells to provide helper function for B cell differentiation [14]. The T_IA-Fc_γ+ cells which have been removed were found to be highly suppressive. These data indicate that adenosine activates a subset within the T4+ helper/inducer subpopulation to express suppressor activity, while the remaining T_I cells, even after exposure to adenosine, are capable of providing help once these suppressor cells are removed.

It should be noted that adenosine effects upon T-lymphocytes appear to be mediated by adenosine receptors. Adenosine receptors of the Ra and Ri type are inhibited by methylxanthines and require an intact ribose moiety on adenosine for their activity [15]. Both the adenosine-induced changes in surface antigen expression and the development of T suppressor cell activity are blocked by theophylline and isobutylmethylxanthine, and ribose-modified adenosine analogues are not effective inducers of these events.

Properties of an Adenosine-Induced Immunosuppressive Lymphokine

Another well studied pharmacological immunoregulatory system is the histamine-induced suppressor system. According to Rocklin and co-workers [16], histamine, in the presence of interleukin-1, acts upon H_2 histamine receptor-bearing T8+ lymphocytes which then secrete a lymphokine, histamine suppressor factor (HSF). They have shown that HSF inhibits lymphocyte proliferation and T cell cytotoxicity as well as antibody synthesis and expression of Ia/Dr antigens on activated T cells. HSF appears to act directly upon monocytes which then synthesize increased amounts of prostaglandins and thromboxanes which themselves mediate most of the suppressive actions of HSF.

We have recently found that adenosine induces a suppressive lymphokine which we have termed adenosine suppressor factor (ASF) [17]. ASF is produced by incubating 2×10^6 macrophage-depleted T-lymphocytes or isolated T4+ cells with 1 μM adenosine for 45 min at 37° C. Adenosine is then removed, the cells are incubated for 24 h, and the culture supernatants are collected. These ASF-containing culture supernatants suppress phytohemagglutinin (PHA) and tetanus toxoid-stimulated lymphocyte proliferation (Table 2). Preliminary molecular weight characterization indicates that ASF has a molecular weight between 10000 and 30000. Unlike HSF, ASF does not inhibit pokeweed

Table 2. Effects of adenosine suppressor factor (ASF) on phytohemagglutinin (PHA-) and tetanus toxoid (TT-) stimulated lymphocyte proliferation and pokeweed mitogen-driven in vivo immunoglobulin (Ig) synthesis

a) *Lymphocyte proliferation*

	Thymidine incorporation (cpm)			
Factor added	PHA	% Sup.[a]	TT	% Sup.
Control	81 328 ± 4 098	–	22 274 ± 1 920	–
ASF	59 554 ± 4 509	27	14 579 ± 3079	44

b) *In vitro immunoglobulin synthesis*

	Ig synthesis (ng/ml)			
Factor added	IgG	% Sup.	IgM	% Sup.
Control	13 880 ± 3 872	–	2 993 ± 1 031	–
ASF	19 363 ± 2013	–39	2 705 ± 828	9

[a] % Suppression; negative suppression represents enhancement of a function

mitogen-driven in vitro immunoglobulin synthesis (Table 2). However, the cells from which ASF was produced were found to be potent suppressors of both pokeweed mitogen- and antigen (tetanus toxoid)-stimulated IgG and IgM synthesis. In contrast, these adenosine-treated T cells did not inhibit PHA or antigen-stimulated lymphocyte proliferation.

Thus, the adenosine-induced immunoregulatory system involves not only adenosine receptor-mediated generation of suppressor cells, but also the production of an immunosuppressive lymphokine. In contrast to the histamine-induced immunosuppressive system, there is a striking dichotomy between the actions of ASF and adenosine-activated suppressor T cells; ASF inhibits only cell proliferation while activated suppressor cells inhibit only in vitro B-lymphocyte differentiation and immunoglobulin synthesis. The mechanisms whereby ASF and adenosine-activated T-suppressor cells exert their immunoregulatory functions are currently under investigation in our laboratory.

The Possible Physiological and Pathophysiological Importance of the Adenosine Immunoregulatory System

The physiological role of the adenosine immunoregulatory system is a matter of speculation. We have proposed that this system may be an important immunohomeostatic mechanism which limits immune responses to self-tissue antigens under pathological circumstances in which tissue damage is occurring [18] (Fig. 1). Adenosine is principally maintained within cells in the form of nu-

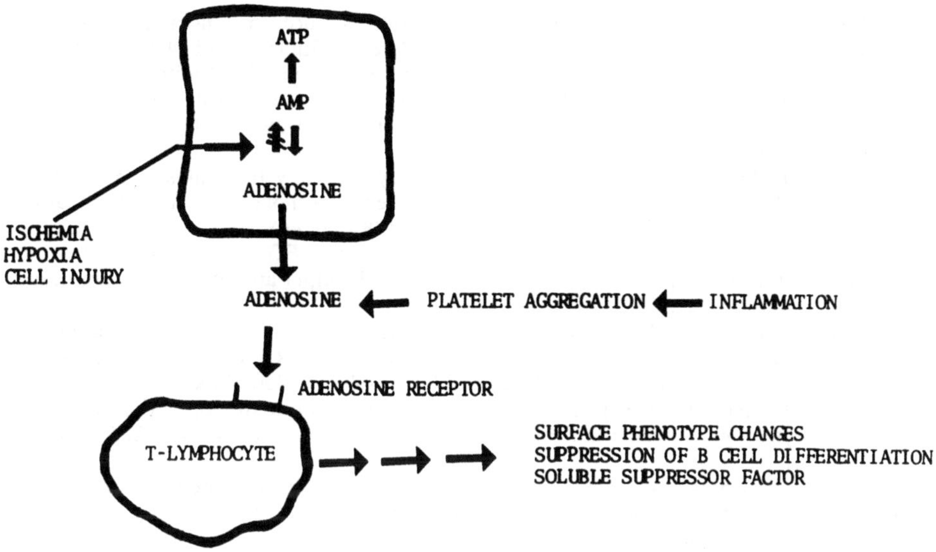

Fig. 1. The pathophysiological significance of adenosine-induced immunosuppression

cleotides by energy-dependent phosphorylation. When cells are subjected to ischemia and hypoxia, oxidative phosphorylation decreases and adenosine is released from cells [19]. Adenosine is also derived from nucleotides released by aggregating platelets through the action of nucleotidases and from damaged vascular endothelial cells in the course of inflammatory and allergic reactions [20]. As shown in Fig. 1, adenosine may represent a tissue injury signal and adenosine-induced immunosuppression may be a mechanism to impair antibody synthesis as well as other immune responses against autologous tissue antigens.

References

1. Reinherz EL, Schlossman SF (1980) Regulation of the immune response: inducer and suppressor T-lymphocyte subsets in human beings. N Engl J Med 303:370–373
2. Besedovsky HO, del Rey A, Sorkin E (1983) Neuroendocrine immunoregulatory circuits. In: Hadden JW, Chedid L, Dukor P, Spreafico F, Willoughby D (eds) Advances in Immunopharmacology, vol 2. Pergamon, Oxford, p 457
3. Beer DJ, Rocklin RE (1984) Histamine-induced suppressor activity. J Allergy Clin Immunol 73:439–452
4. Goodwin JS, Webb DR (1980) Regulation of the immune response by prostaglandins. Clin Immunol Immunopathol 15:106–122
5. Rola-Pleszczynski M, Borgeat P, Sirois P (1982) Leukotriene B_4 induces human suppressor lymphocytes. Biochem Biophys Res Commun 108:1531–1537
6. Atluru D, Goodwin JS (1984) Control of polyclonal immunoglobulin production from human lymphocytes by leukotrienes: Leukotriene B_4 induces an OKT8(+) radiosensitive suppressor cell from resting OKT8(–) T-cells. J Clin Invest 74:1444–1450

7. Holgate ST, Mann JS, Cushley MJ (1984) Adenosine as a bronchoconstrictor mediator in asthma and its antagonism by methylxanthines. J Allergy Clin Immunol 74:302–306
8. Meuer SC, Hussey RC, Cantrell DA, Hodgdon JC, Schlossman SF, Smith KA, Reinherz EL (1984) Triggering of the T3-Ti antigen-receptor complex results in clonal T-cell proliferation through an interleukin 2 dependent autocrine pathway. Proc Natl Acad Sci USA 81:1509–1513
9. Reinherz EL, Moriomoto C, Fitzgerald KA, Hussey RE, Daly JF, Schlossman SF (1982) Heterogeneity of human T4+ inducer T-cells defined by a monoclonal antibody that delineates two functional subpopulations. J Immunol 128:463–468
10. Gatenby PA, Kansas GS, Xian CY, Evans RL, Engelman EG (1982) Dissection of immunoregulatory subpopulations of T-lymphocytes with helper and suppressor sublineages in man. J Immunol 129:1997–2000
11. Polmar SH, Birch RE (1980) Regulation of Fc receptors on T-lymphocyte subsets mediated by adenosine and histamine receptors. In: Krakauer RS, Cathcart MK (eds) Immunoregulation and autoimmunity, Elsevier, North Holland, New York, p 11
12. Birch RE, Polmar SH (1981) Induction of Fc_{γ}-receptors on a subpopulation of human T-lymphocytes by adenosine and impromidine, an H_2-histamine agonist. Cell Immunol 57:455–467
13. Birch RE, Rosenthal AK, Polmar SH (1982) Pharmacological modification of immunoregulatory T-lymphocytes. II. Modulation of T-lymphocyte cell surface characteristics. Clin Exp Immunol 48:231–238
14. Birch RE, Polmar SH (1982) Pharmacological modification of immunoregulatory T-lymphocytes. I. Effect of adenosine, H_1 and H_2 histamine agonists upon T-lymphocyte regulation of B-lymphocyte differentiation in vitro. Clin Exp Immunol 48:218–230
15. Londos C, Cooper DMF, Wolff J (1980) Subclasses of external adenosine receptors. Proc Natl Acad Sci USA 77:2551–2554
16. Beer DJ, Rosenwasser LJ, Dinarello CA, Rocklin RE (1982) Cellular interactions in the generation and expression of histamine induced suppressor activity. Cell Immunol 69:101–112
17. Birch RE, Morris MN, Polmar SH (1985) Human T-lymphocytes produce immunoregulatory factors after incubation with adenosine and histamine agonists. Fed Proc 44:950
18. Polmar SH (1984) Pharmacological modifications of immunoregulatory activity of lymphocytes: facts and potential. Surv Immunol Res 3:274–279
19. Berne RM, Knabb RM, Ely SW, Rubio R (1983) Adenosine in the local regulation of blood flow: a brief overview. Fed Proc 42:3136–3142
20. Pearson JD, Gordon JL (1979) Vascular endothelial and smooth muscle cells in culture selectively release adenosine nucleotides. Nature 281:384–386

Superoxide Dismutase: Rationale of Therapeutic Use, Established Clinical Effects, and Perspectives

L. Flohé

Grünenthal GmbH, 5100 Aachen, Federal Republic of Germany

Abstract

The therapeutic effect of injected superoxide dismutase (SOD) is best explained by its enzymatic function, i.e. removal of the superoxide ion ($\cdot O_2^-$), which meets some criteria of a mediator of inflammation:

1. $\cdot O_2^-$ is released from neutrophilic and eosinophilic polymorphonucleocytes and macrophages upon stimulation e.g. by opsonized microorganisms, immune complexes, and chemotactic factors like FMLP, C 5 a and LTB_4.
2. $\cdot O_2^-$, by initiation of free radical chain reactions, leads to alteration of biomembrane permeability, to denaturation of enzymes and fragmentation of extracellular matrix molecules.
3. $\cdot O_2^-$ has been reported to generate chemotactic response of PMNs to LTB_4, FMLP and C 5 a.

Clinically, intraarticular injection of SOD in several randomized double blind trials proved to be an effective treatment of inflammatory episodes in osteoarthritis of the knee joint, and, based on clinical experience and circumstantial evidence, can be anticipated to be helpful whenever a sufficient dose of SOD can be administered locally to an inflamed tissue. Particularly impressive results have been obtained by SOD infiltration into the submucosa of the bladder in patients suffering from radiation cystitis and radiation ulcers.

Reviewing the SOD effects in pharmacological models of inflammation we feel that best responses are observed if activation of phagocytes and/or the complement system contribute substantially to the pathobiological condition. These observations and the rationale outlined above suggest that the therapeutic potential of SOD has not yet been fully evaluated. Unfortunately, only heterologous (bovine) SOD is presently approved for clinical administration. The availability of an authentic human SOD of suitable pharmaceutic quality would facilitate the unrestricted exploration of its therapeutic value.

What is Superoxide Dismutase?

Superoxide dismutases (SOD) are metalloproteins catalyzing the dismutation of superoxide radicals ($\cdot O_2^-$) [45]:

$$2\cdot O_2^- + 2H^+ \xrightarrow{SOD} H_2O_2 + O_2 \qquad (1)$$

In the cytosol of higher animals and in plants the copper- and zinc-containing SOD (Cu/Zn SOD) predominate, whereas in mitochondria and bacteria the corresponding enzymatic activities are usually associated with proteins containing iron or manganese as catalytically active transition metals (for review see [60]). However, Cu/Zn-SOD have also been detected in some bacteria [49, 61] and have been shown to be homologous to the vertebrate Cu/Zn enzymes [59], while the Fe and Mn proteins are not [60]. The predominance of SOD in aerobically living organisms suggests a crucial role of these enzymes in the defense against free radical attack on sensitive molecules, which is considered a hazard inherent in aerobic life [11, 12, 17, 60].

The best investigated SOD is Cu/Zn SOD of cattle. It is a dimeric protein with an approximate subunit size of 16300 daltons corresponding to 151 amino acid residues and one Zn and one Cu ion per subunit [60]. It is this enzymatic species which has been purified to homogeneity and approved for both veterinary use and clinical application.

Uncatalyzed, the dismutation of superoxide radicals is comparatively slow, since the negatively charged ions repel each other. $\cdot O_2^-$ would quite easily react with other constituents of the biological environment and, as a radical, initiate free radical chain reactions with hardly predictable consequences (see below).

In contrast, the reaction of SOD with $\cdot O_2^-$ takes place at the rate constant of $2 \times 10^9\ M^{-1}\ s^{-1}$ which appears to be limited by diffusion. In fact, the velocity of the reaction is not easily understood, if the probability of futile collisions between the bulky protein and the radical are taken into account and only the tiny copper ion is considered the reactive center of the enzyme. More recently, this miracle has been unraveled for the bovine Cu/Zn SOD. Getzoff et al. [18] calculated the surface charge of the enzyme and were able to demonstrate that an electrostatic field guides the negatively charged superoxide radical toward the positively charged copper ion thereby minimizing futile collisions between enzyme and substrate. The oustanding efficiency of the enzyme resulting from this "clever" mechanism of action provides the basis of its normal biological role and, if applied therapeutically, its beneficial effects under pathological situations due to unbalanced $\cdot O_2^-$ production.

Biological Sources of $\cdot O_2^-$

Schematically, $\cdot O_2^-$ is formed from molecular oxygen, O_2, by addition of a single electron, i.e., by a univalent reduction. In biological systems, $\cdot O_2^-$ was first detected as a product of xanthine oxidase [45] and other flavine-dependent dehydrogenases [35]. The mitochondrial respiratory chain, designed to reduce O_2 to water with concomitant energy conservation, can also produce some $\cdot O_2^-$ under certain circumstances [16, 36, 63]. $\cdot O_2^-$ can also be formed during microsomal drug metabolism [7, 52], and is further generated nonenzymatically by autoxidation of various natural constituents of the cell or xenobiotics. The latter processes may be amplified by redox cycling, i.e., if for example the oxidized xenobiotics are enzymatically reduced again, whereby a new autoxidation process is facilitated [33]. Another nonenzymatic source of $\cdot O_2^-$ in biological systems is aerobic irradiation of watery solutions [6].

In the context of pathogenic mechanisms of inflammation, the $\cdot O_2^-$ production by activated phagocytes, i.e., neutrophilic [1, 31] and eosinophilic [21, 53] polymorphonucleocytes (PMN) and macrophages [38], deserves special interest. Upon contact with particles marked as "foreign" by opsonization or with various soluble agents such as complement factor C5a, leukotriene B_4 (LTB_4), phorbolmyristylacetate (PMA), or formyl-methionyl-leucyl-phenylalanine (FMLP), such cells react with a more or less pronounced increase in consumption of oxygen (for review see [12, 13, 18]). This process, called "respiratory burst," is associated with reduction of O_2 to $\cdot O_2^-$, the formation of H_2O_2, and the liberation and oxidation of polyunsaturated fatty acids. In fact, it can be demonstrated that more than 90% of the extra oxygen consumption during respiratory burst is due to an enzymatic univalent reduction of oxygen at the expense of NADPH:

$$\mathrm{NADPH} + 2\,\mathrm{O_2} \xrightarrow{\text{NADPH oxidase}} \mathrm{NADP^+} + \mathrm{H^+} + 2\ \mathrm{O_2^-} \quad (2)$$

Only a minor portion of the oxygen consumed is utilized for arachidonic acid metabolism, and the observed H_2O_2 formation results exclusively from dismutation of $\cdot O_2^-$ [37].

The $\cdot O_2^-$ production by stimulated phagocytes is considered a crucial step in the host defense mechanisms operating during phagocytosis [31, 54]. Teleologically speaking, the ability of phagocytes to kill invaded microorganisms by oxygen-centered radicals is a useful phylogenetic achievement. However, the uniform response of such cells to stimuli of any kind renders the indispensable defense system a hazardous weapon of potentially self-destructive power [64].

Pathogenic Consequences of Unbalanced $\cdot O_2^-$ Production

$\cdot O_2^-$ itself belongs to the fairly stable, i.e., less reactive, free radicals and it has frequently been questioned whether it can do any harm when present in a biological system. Since many deleterious effects, however, can be blocked by SOD, it obviously contributes to pathogenic events, though it might only rarely be the ultimate toxin. At present the toxic effects of $\cdot O_2^-$ are considered to result from the initiation of free radical chains sustained and mediated by (among others) ubiquituous transition metals, H_2O_2, or other hydroperoxides.

The most aggressive oxygen-centered radical thus formed is believed to be the OH radical. For a more detailed discussion of this complicated issue we refer to recent reviews [12, 13, 27]. In brief, $\cdot O_2^-$ is the predominant initiator of free radical chains in biological systems and it is therefore justified to speak of $\cdot O_2^-$-dependent pathogenic effects, if the latter are prevented by SOD. This simplistic approach is, of course, not meant to elucidate molecular mechanisms, but rather tells us whether or not $\cdot O_2^-$ is involved at all.

With this restriction in mind, it can be stated that $\cdot O_2^-$, if not kept at minute steady-state levels, is definitely destructive for a large variety of biological structures. First of all, it can be shown that PMN known to survive for only a few hours upon activation regain their normal life span if the superoxide radicals produced in the presence of adequate stimuli are scavenged by SOD [44]. Similar observations have been made when other cell types, such as erythrocytes [9, 22, 34] or cultured myoblasts [47], were exposed to $\cdot O_2^-$-generating systems. The molecular events leading to cell death or impaired vitality are not clear. But it could be shown that $\cdot O_2^-$-dependent reactions result in biomembrane destruction accompanied by lipid peroxidation [15] and irreversible inactivation of various enzymes [47].

Beyond the deleterious effect on cells, $\cdot O_2^-$ can also attack macromulecules of the extracellular matrix. Hyaluronic acid [43], proteoglycans, and collagen [24] are depolymerized by $\cdot O_2^-$-dependent processes. These observations are particularly interesting, since the extracellular space poorly protected by SOD [43] is exposed to the superoxide radicals released from phagocytes.

Release of $\cdot O_2^-$ and other mediators from phagocytes is considered a crucial response of tissue exposed to inflammatory stimuli. Activation of a few cells, however, would not be likely to induce any relevant inflammation, if it were not amplified by further recruitment and activation of leukocytes. Again, oxygen-centered radicals appear to be intimately involved in these mechanisms. IgG, for instance, when exposed to $\cdot O_2^-$ generating systems, develops a characteristic fluorescence and forms aggregates. Such altered immunoglobulins can stimulate a renewed $\cdot O_2^-$ release from PMN [40]. Another mechanism amplifying the primary phagocyte activation would be an $\cdot O_2^-$-dependent formation of a leukotactic factor [48]. Finally, in Boyden chamber experiments the leukotactic response to established chemoattractants like LTB_4, C5a, or FMLP could be blocked by minute amounts of SOD (or catalase) added to the PMN incubation medium. The effect of SOD is restricted to directed migration; random mobility remains unaffected. This surprising observation suggests that $\cdot O_2^-$ released from the PMN surface upon contact with a chemoattractant somehow triggers a localised redox change in the membrane which tells the cell where to migrate [11].

In summary, $\cdot O_2^-$-dependent processes have been shown to result in enzyme denaturation, impairment of cellular functions, and finally cell lysis. In particular the $\cdot O_2^-$ released into the extracellular compartment by activated phagocytes may contribute to the destruction of macromolecules constituting the connective tissue matrix. $\cdot O_2^-$ may finally be involved in the amplification of a local tissue irritation by altering macromolecules, generating leukotactic activity, and mediating leukocyte recruitment by other chemoattractants. $\cdot O_2^-$ thus meets the definition of a multifunctional mediator of inflammation and, in consequence, scavenging of $\cdot O_2^-$ by SOD, if practically feasible, is considered a promising approach to complete the armamentarium for fighting inflammatory diseases.

Clinical Experience with SOD Treatment

Unfortunately, the development of SOD as an anti-inflammatory drug could not always be based on solid theoretical grounds, since its anti-inflammatory activity was discovered by serendipity [29] long before its enzymatic nature was elucidated and the biological role of $\cdot O_2^-$ became apparent. The evaluation of the therapeutic potential of SOD was further impaired by the nonavailability for clinical trials of authentic human SOD in sufficient amounts and purity. Practically all information on the clinical efficacy of SOD has been generated with the bovine enzyme. Although Cu/Zn SOD in general is a poor immunogen (apparently due to its low content of aromatic amino acids), the use of the heterologous protein in humans had to be restricted to extravascular, usually local, administration. Further, the topically applied enzyme is in most cases rapidly cleared from the site of injection. With regard to these difficulties we feel that the disorders so far successfully treated with SOD represent merely the most suitable examples, where the pharmacokinetic requirements could be met despite the inherent restrictions. The full scope of the therapeutic potential of SOD will therefore not emerge before the authentic human protein becomes available for clinical use.

For obvious reasons, systemic (i.m.) treatment of patients suffering from rheumatoid arthritis (RA) with SOD did not yield impressive results [46]. Interestingly, however, intra-articular injections of SOD in RA patients caused clear clinical improvements in controlled trials [19, 20]. But since RA is commonly a systemic disease, local SOD treatment is unfortunately not generally applicable.

In contrast, inflammatory episodes of osteoarthritis are already being treated effectively by intra-articular injections of SOD in several countries. The efficacy of this therapeutic regimen in osteoarthritis of the knee joint has been established unambiguously by three independently performed placebo-controlled double-blind trials [10, 30, 39] and confirmed by several open trials and, finally, clinical acceptance [50]. As expected, local injections of SOD also proved effective in a variety of inflammatory disorders of other joints or extra-articular tissues, whenever the site of inflammation was anatomically accessible [50].

Most impressive results were obtained when SOD was infiltrated into the bladder wall of patients suffering from radiation or interstitial cystitis [32, 42]. After several treatment courses, clinical symptoms such as micturition frequency, stranguria, and bladder capacity improved dramatically and persistently, and even radiation ulcers were cured [51, 56]. Since no alternative treatment, apart from mutilating surgery, exists in most such cases, SOD infiltration has become the treatment of choice in these indications.

Peyronie's disease, a disabling deformation of the penis, is characterized by fibrous and sometimes ossified plaques between the tunica albuginea and the corpora cavernosa. It is believed to be initiated by a vasculitis of unknown etiology, and persistent cellular infiltrations consisting of lymphocytes, macrophages, and PMN are usually observed at the borderline of the plaques [58]. Not surprisingly, this chronic inflammatory process can also be suppressed by SOD infiltrations, and even marked clinical improvements of the established disease were reported by several investigators [3, 56, 65].

Future Therapeutic Perspectives

Recently, an authentic human SOD has been cloned and expressed in yeast [14, 26], and clinical development has been scheduled. It can be anticipated that the human enzyme will also be applicable systemically at high dosages, which will allow us to explore the full therapeutic potential of SOD suggested by animal experiments.

The therapeutic animal models of inflammatory disorders in which the beneficial effects of SOD and other means to dampen free radical fluxes were reported have recently been discussed in depth [12, 13]. For the present purpose, it may suffice to summarize by saying that available data strongly suggest an involvement of $\cdot O_2^-$ in the pathogenic consequences of complement activation. In particular, C5a-dependent effects like leukocyte sticking, leukocyte recruitment, and plasma extravasation from the microcirculation appear susceptible to SOD inhibition. With regard to the ability of C5a to trigger $\cdot O_2^-$ release from PMN and possibly to mediate its cellular effects via this $\cdot O_2^-$ release, these observations are not surprising. Clinical trials with SOD in diseases presumed or known to depend on complement activation should therefore be considered. Similarly, all other noninfectious conditions associated with PMN or macrophage activation, irrespective of the responsible stimulus, might be anticipated to respond to SOD treatment.

SOD treatment, however, is also discussed for the prevention of postischemic tissue damage, i.e. a primarily noninflammatory condition. In postischemic tissue $\cdot O_2^-$ is formed abundantly, but not primarily by the NADPH oxidase according to Eq. 1. During ischemia cellular ATP is successively degraded to yield hypoxanthine, a substrate of xanthine dehydrogenase (XDH):

$$\text{hypoxanthine} + NAD^+ + OH^- \xrightarrow{\text{XDH}} \text{xanthine} + NADH \quad (3)$$

This enzyme is ubiquitously distributed and represents the physiological species responsible for purine metabolism. It is, however, easily altered by oxidation of essential thiols [55], formation of mixed disulfides [5], or proteolytically [4], whereby its specificity is dramatically changed. It now accepts oxygen instead of $NAD^{(+)}$ and can catalyze both a two-electron transition:

$$\text{hypoxanthine} + O_2 + H_2O \xrightarrow{XO} \text{xanthine} + H_2O_2 \quad (4)$$

and a one-electron transition:

$$\text{hypoxanthine} + 2O_2 + OH^- \xrightarrow{XO} \text{xanthine} + 2\cdot O_2^- + H^+ \quad (5)$$

The "pathological enzyme" thus formed (Eqs. 4 and 5) is the well-known xanthine oxidase (XO), and it has been shown convincingly that the transformation of XDH to XO takes place during ischemia [55]. Equation 5 shows the model system frequently used to generate oxygen-centered radicals in vitro [45]. This enzymatic reaction occurs in vivo, if, by reperfusion, oxygen is supplied to an ischemia-damaged tissue containing both XO and pathologically elevated amounts of substrate (hypoxanthine, xanthine).

The relevance of these mechanisms for the development of postischemic tissue damage has been amply demonstrated in animal experiments. Postischemic injury in feline intestine [23], rat skin flaps [41], dog and rabbit heart, [2, 57, 62] and rabbit kidney [28] could be effectively prevented either by pretreatment of the animals with allopurinol, an XO inhibitor, or by infusion of SOD at the time of reperfusion. In view of these findings, clinical trials in postischemic conditions, e.g., during vascular surgery or organ transplantation, appear highly rewarding. In this context SOD again deserves special consideration, since depending on the clinical situation, pretreatment of the patient with a XO inhibitor might not be appropriate.

The XO-dependent mechanism clearly operative during reperfusion might, however, not be exclusively responsible for the postischemic tissue damage. Recently, Grögaard et al. [25] demonstrated that the impaired postischemic cortical blood flow in rats could also be normalized by previous PMN depletion. This observation suggests that XO-dependent $\cdot O_2^-$ production might trigger a pathological PMN endothelium interaction, and the resulting sticking and activation of the PMN will, by means of NADPH oxidase-dependent $\cdot O_2^-$ production or other mechanisms, amplify the initial endothelial injury. This cascade of pathogenic events should, of course, be most efficiently blocked by SOD scavenging the superoxide radicals, irrespective of their source.

Both mechanisms, the postischemic XO-dependent $\cdot O_2^-$ production and the NADPH-oxidase-dependent one, might play a role in those types of shock associated with intravascular coagulation and complement activation. Not surprisingly, beneficial effects of SOD have been seen in a large variety of animal shock models [8, 64]. Even in a porcine sepsis model, lung edema, gas exchange, and survival time were improved by SOD infusion, although the bacterial count was not significantly affected [66]. Certainly, such multifactorial pathological events can probably never be successfully treated by a single drug, but SOD might be helpful in managing at least some of the shock symptoms.

This brief outlook on the clinical potential of balancing pathological free radical production is meant neither to be complete nor to ignore pathogenic contributions of other mediators of inflammation or tissue damage. My intention is rather to stimulate interest in new therapeutic approaches which will become testable in the near future.

References

1. Babior BM, Kipnes RS, Curnutte JT (1973) The production by leukocytes of superoxide, a potential bacterial agent. J Clin Invest 52:741–744
2. Bailie MB, Jolly SR, Lucchesi BR (1982) Reduction of myocardial ischemic injury by superoxide dismutase plus catalase. Fed Proc 41:1736
3. Bartsch G, Menander-Huber KB, Huber W, Marberger H (1981) Orgotein, a new drug for the treatment of Peyronies' disease. Eur J Rheumatol Inflamm 4:250–259
4. Bray RC (1975) Molybdenum iron-sulfur flavin hydroxylases and related enzymes. In: Boyer PD (ed) The enzymes XII, 3rd edn. Academic, London, pp 299–419
5. Brigelius R (1985) Mixed disulfides: biological functions and increase in oxidative stress. In: Sies H (ed) Oxidative stress. Academic, London pp 243–272
6. Czapski G (1971) Radiation chemistry of oxygenated aqueous solutions. Ann Rev Phys Chem 22:171–208
7. Esnouf MP, Green MR, Hill HAO, Irvine GB, Walter SJ (1979) Dioxygen and the vitamin K-dependent synthesis of prothrombin. In: Ciba Foundation Symposium 65 (new series). Oxygen free radicals and tissue damage. Excerpta Medica, Amsterdam, pp 187–197
8. Fantone JC, Ward PA (1982) Role of oxygen-derived free radicals and metabolites in leukocyte-dependent inflammatory reactions. Am J Pathol 107:397–418
9. Fee JA, Teitelbaum HD (1972) Evidence that superoxide dismutase plays a role in protecting red blood cells against peroxidative hemolysis. Biochem Biophys Res Commun 49:150–158
10. Flohé L, Biehl G, Hofer H, Kadrnka F, Kölbel R, Puhl W (1980) Effectiveness of superoxide dismutase in osteoarthritis of the knee joint. Results of a double blind multicenter clinical trial. In: Bannister WH, Bannister JV (eds) Biological and clinical aspects of superoxide and superoxide dismutase. Elsevier, New York, pp 424–430 (Developments in Biochemistry, vol 11 B)
11. Flohé L, Martin W, Loschen G, Günzler WA (1984) Is leukotriene B_4-induced chemotaxis mediated by superoxide? In: Life chemistry reports (supplement 2): oxidative damage and related enzymes. Harwood, Chur, pp 318–324
12. Flohé L, Giertz H, Beckmann R (1985) Free radical scavengers as anti-inflammatory drugs? In: Bonta IL, Bray MA, Parnham MJ (eds) The Pharmacology of inflammation. Elsevier, New York, pp 255–281 (Handbook of Inflammation, vol 5)
13. Flohé L, Beckmann R, Giertz H, Loschen G (1985) Oxygen-centered free radicals as mediators of inflammation. In: Sies H (ed) Oxidative stress. Academic, London, pp 403–435
14. Flohé L, Kim SMA, Ötting F, Saunders D, Schwertner E, Steffens G, Blacher R, Masiarz F, Scandella C, Hallewell R (1985) Comparison of human Cu/Zn superoxide dismutase derived from erythrocytes, recombinant E. coli and recombinant yeast (abstract). Fourth International Conference on Superoxide and Superoxide Dismutase, Rome
15. Flohé L, Zimmermann R (1974) GSH-induced high-amplitude swelling of mitochondria. In: Flohé L, Benöhr HC, Sies H, Waller HD, Wendel A (eds) Gluthathione. Thieme, Stuttgart, pp 245–255
16. Flohé L, Azzi L, Loschen G, Richter C (1977) Superoxide radicals in mitochondria. In: Michelson AM, McCord JM, Fridovich I (eds) Superoxide and superoxide dismutases. Academic, London, pp 323–334
17. Fridovich I (1978) The biology of oxygen radicals. Science 201:875–880
18. Getzoff ED, Tainer JA, Weiner PK, Kollmann PA, Richardson JS, Richardson DC (1983) Electrostatic recognition between superoxide and copper, zinc superoxide dismutase. Nature (London) 306:287–290
19. Goebel KM, Storck U (1983) Effect of intra-articular orgotein versus a corticosteroid on rheumatoid arthritis of the knees. Am J Med 74:124–128
20. Goebel KM, Storck U, Neurath F (1981) Intrasynovial orgotein therapy in rheumatoid arthritis. Lancet I:1015–1017
21. Goetzl EJ, Valone FH, Smith JA, Weller PF (1978) The modulation of migration and function of human eosinophils by immunologic reactions (abstract). International Congress of Inflammation, Bologna, p 52

22. Goldberg B, Stern A (1976) Superoxide anion as a mediator of drug-induced oxidative hemolysis. J Biol Chem 251:6468–6470
23. Granger DN, Rutili G, McCord JM (1981) Superoxide radicals in feline intestinal ischemia. Gastroenterology 81:22–29
24. Greenwald RA, Moy WW, Lazarus D (1976) Degradation of cartilage proteoglycans and collagen by superoxide radical. Arthritis Rheum 19:799
25. Grögaard B, Gerdin B, Arfors KE (1985) Involvement of neutrophils in the cortical blood flow impairment after cerebral ischemia in the rat (abstract). Fourth International Conference on Superoxide and Superoxide Dismutase, Rome
26. Hallewell RA, Tekamp-Olson P, Rosenberg S, Blacher R, Masiarz F, Scandella C (1985) Synthesis of authentic, N-acetylated human Cu/Zn SOD in yeast (abstract). Fourth International Conference on Superoxide and Superoxide Dismutase, Rome
27. Halliwell B, Gutteridge JMC (1985) Free radicals in biology and medicine. Clarendon, Oxford
28. Hansson R, Jonsson O, Lundstam S, Pettersson S, Schersten T, Waldenström J (1983) Effects of free radical scavengers on renal circulation after ischaemia in the rabbit. Clin Sci 65:605–610
29. Huber W, Schulte TL, Carson S, Goldhamer RE, Vogin EE (1968) Some chemical and pharmacological properties of a novel anti-inflammatory protein. Toxicol Appl Pharmacology 12:308
30. Huskission EC, Scott J (1981) Orgotein in osteoarthritis of the knee joint. Eur J Rheumatol Inflamm 4:212–218
31. Johnston RB, Keele BB, Misra HP, Leymeyer JE, Webb LS, Baehner RL (1975) The role of superoxide anion generation in phagocytic bactericidal activity. J Clin Invest 55:1357–1372
32. Kadrnka F (1981) Ergebnisse einer multizentrischen Orgotein-Prüfung bei Strahlen- und interstitiellen Cystitiden. Eur J Rheumatol Inflamm 4:237–243
33. Kappus H, Sies H (1981) Toxic drug effects associated with oxygen metabolism: redox cycling and lipid peroxidation. Experientia 37:1233–1241
34. Kellog EW, Fridovich I (1977) Liposome oxidation and erythrocyte lysis by enzymically generated superoxide and hydrogen peroxide. J Biol Chem 252:6721–6728
35. Knowles PF, Gibson JF, Pick FM, Bray RC (1969) Electron-spin-resonance evidence for enzymic reduction of oxygen to a free radical, the superoxide ion. Biochem J 111:53–58
36. Loschen G, Azzi A, Richter C, Flohé L (1974) Superoxide radicals as precursors of mitochondrial hydrogen peroxide. Fed Eur Biochem Soc Letters 42:68–72
37. Loschen G (1985) Superoxide formation accounts for almost all extra oxygen consumption upon stimulation of leukocytes (abstract). Fourth International Conference on Superoxide and Superoxide Dismutase, Rome
38. Lowrie DB, Aber VR (1977) Superoxide production by rabbit pulmonary alveolar macrophages. Life Sci 21:1575–1583
39. Lund-Olesen K, Menander-Huber KB (1983) Intra-articular orgotein therapy in osteoarthritis of the knee. A double-blind, placebo-controlled trial. Arzneimittelforsch. Drug Res 33:1199–1203
40. Lunec J (1984) Free-radical-mediated aggregation of human IgG stimulates neutrophils to generate superoxide radicals. Agents Actions 15:37–38
41. Manson PN, Anthenelli RM, Im MJ, Bulkley GB, Hoopes JE (1983) The role of oxygen-free radicals in ischemia tissue injury in island skin flaps. Annals of Surgery 198:87–90
42. Marberger H, Bartsch G, Huber W, Menander-Huber KB, Schulte TL (1975) Orgotein: a new drug for the treatment of radiation cystitis. Curr Ther Res Clin Exp 18:466–475
43. McCord JM (1974) Free radicals and inflammation: protection of synovial fluid by superoxide dismutase. Sci 185:529–531
44. McCord JM, Stokes SH, Wong K (1979) Superoxide radicals as a phagocyte-produced chemical mediator of inflammation. In: Weissman G, Samuellson B, Paoletti R (eds) Advances in inflammation research, vol 1. Raven, New York, pp 273–280
45. McCord JM, Fridovich I (1969) Superoxide dismutase: an enzymatic function for erythrocuprein (hemocurpein). J Biol Chem 244:6049–6055
46. Menander-Huber KB, Huber W (1977) Orgotein, the drug version of bovine Cu-Zn superoxide dismutase. II. A summary account of clinical trials in man and animals. In: Mi-

chelson AM, McCord JM, Fridovich I (eds) Superoxide and superoxide dismutase. Academics, London, pp 537–549
47. Michelson AM (1977) Toxicity of superoxide radical anions. In: Michelson AM, McCord JM, Fridovich I (eds) Superoxide and superoxide dismutases. Academic, London, pp 245–255
48. Petrone WF, Englisch DK, Wong K, McCord JM (1980) Free radicals and inflammation: superoxide-dependent activation of a neutrophil chemotactic factor in plasma. Proc Natl Acad Sci USA 77:1159–1163
49. Puget K, Lavelle F, Michelson AM (1977) Superoxide dismutases from procaryote and eucaryote bioluminescent organisms. In: Michelson AM, McCord JM, Fridovich I (eds) Superoxide and superoxide dismutases. Academic, London, pp 139–150
50. Puhl W, Sies H (1982) II. Symposium Superoxid-Dismutase. Biochemie und therapeutischer Einsatz. Perimed, Erlangen
51. Reuß K, Carl P (1982) Behandlung des Ulcus simplex vesicae und der ulzerierenden radiogenen Zystitis mit Superoxiddismutase. Urologe [Ausg A] 22:290–293
52. Richter C, Azzi A, Weser U, Wendel A (1977) The action of $Cu(tyrosine)_2$ as a superoxide dismutase model on hepatic microsomal demethylation. In: Michelson AM, McCord JM, Fridovich I (eds) Superoxide and superoxide dismutases. Academic, London, pp 375–385
53. Roos D, Eckmann CM, Yazdanbakhsh M, Hamers MN, de Boer M (1983) Excretion of superoxide by phagocytes measured with cytochrome c entrapped in resealed erythrocyte ghosts. J Biol Chem 259:1770–1775
54. Rosen H, Klebanoff SJ (1979) Bactericidal activity of a superoxide anion-generation system. A model for the polymorphonuclear leukocyte. J Exp Med 119:27–39
55. Roy RS, McCord JM (1983) Superoxide and ischemia: conversion of xanthine dehydrogenase to xanthine oxidase. In: Greenwald RA, Cohen G (eds) Oxy radicals and their scavenger systems, vol II: cellular and medical aspects. Elsevier, New York, pp 145–153
56. Schilling A, Chaussy C, Schüller J, Staehler G, Walther V (1980) Superoxyd-dismutase (SOD): erste Erfahrungen bei der Anwendung eines neuen anti-inflammatorischen Prinzips in der Behandlung der ulzerierenden Zystitis und der Induratio penis plastica (IPP). Proceedings of the German Society of Urology, p 404
57. Shlafer M, Kane P, Kirsh M (1982) Superoxide dismutase plus catalase enhances the efficacy of hypothermic cardioplegia to protect the globally ischemic, reperfused heart. J Thorac Cardiovasc Surg 83:830–839
58. Schubert GE (1984) Induratio penis plastica (IPP): pathomorphologische Gesichtspunkte. In: Weissbach L, Boedefeld EA, Widmann T (eds) IPP-Symposium Berichtsband. Brimberg, Aachen, pp 23–27
59. Steffens GJ, Bannister JV, Bannister WH, Flohé L, Günzler WA, Kim SMA, Ötting F (1983) The primary structure of Cu-Zn superoxide dismutase from *Photobacterium leiognathi:* evidence for a separate evolution of Cu-Zn superoxide dismutase in bacteria. Hoppe-Seylers Z Physiol Chem 364:675–690
60. Steinmann HM (1982) Protein chemistry and structure-function relationships. In: Oberley LW (ed) Superoxide dismutase vol 1. CRC Press, Boca Raton, pp 11–68
61. Steinman HM (1982) Copper-Zinc superoxide dismutase from *Caulobacter crescentus* CB15. J Biol Chem 257:10283–10293
62. Stewart JR, Blackwell WH, Crute SL, Loughlin V, Greenfield LJ, Hess ML (1983) Inhibition of surgically induced ischemia/reperfusion injury by oxygen free radical scavengers. J Thorac Cardiovasc Surg 86:262–272
63. Thayer WS (1977) Adriamycin stimulated superoxide formation in submitochondrial particles. Chem Biol Interact 19:265–278
64. Ward PA (1983) Role of toxic oxygen products from phagocytic cells in tissue injury. Adv Shock Res 10:27–34
65. Weissbach L, Boedefeld EA, Widmann T (eds) (1984) IPP-Symposium Berichtsband. Brimberg, Aachen
66. Welter HF, Thetter D, Siebeck M, Wiesinger H, Elster U, Jochum M (1985) 14 Versuche zur Therapie der Schocklunge mittels Superoxiddismutase (SOD) und C1-Inaktivator (C1-INA). In: Stelzner F (ed) Chirurgisches Forum 85. Springer, Berlin Heidelberg New York Tokyo, pp 63–67

Patterns of Theophylline Utilization

H. J. Wedner

Division of Immunology, Department of Medicine, Washington University School of Medicine, St. Louis, 63110, USA

Abstract

Theophylline (1,3-dimethylxanthine) is a major mainstay in the treatment of asthma in the United States. Originally introduced in 1937 and prescribed in combination with ephedrine (4:1 or 5:1) it is now clear that theophylline, or its more water soluble salts, alone is the appropriate dosage form.

Theophylline is an effective front line drug for patients with both acute and chronic asthma. It is beneficial when blood levels are maintained above 10 μg/ml and since toxicity, largely gastrointestinal, is seen at levels above 20 μg/ml the therapeutic range is generally considered to be 10–20 μg/ml. However, the metabolic rates of theophylline biotransformation vary widely and accurate dosing can only be determined by monitoring blood levels.

Theophylline or its salts are available in short acting, twice daily and once daily formulations. The longer acting forms, however, are only effective in patients with low to moderate metabolic rates. Finally a large number of factors, concomitant drug therapy and others, effect theophylline elimination and must be considered.

Introduction

Theophylline, 1,3-dimethylxanthine, has been available for the treatment of bronchospastic disorders since the late 1930s. Originally promoted as an agent for the control of hypertension, its bronchodilatory properties were actually noted by accident when theophylline was infused in an asthmatic patient with acute hypertension. Although the hypertension was not controlled it was noted that the patient's wheezing disappeared. In the mid-1940s it was suggested that theophylline was best used in combination with other agents, particularly ephedrine, and this led to the proliferation of numerous fixed drug combinations containing theophylline in a 4:1 or 5:1 ratio with ephedrine and containing phenobarbital to combat the excitatory effect of the ephedrine. In addition these combination drugs contained variably mucolytics, expectorants, and antihistaminics. It was not until 1974 that Weinberger and Bronsky [1] first demonstrated that the combination of theophylline with ephedrine offered no advantage over theophylline alone and, indeed, actually increased the toxicity of theophylline. These workers also demonstrated that adequate blood levels of theophylline were necessary for maximum benefit.

Pharmacology of Theophylline

Since the early 1970s our knowledge of the effective use of theophylline has grown markedly, as has the number of preparations of theophylline available to the physician. It is the purpose of this brief review to cover some of our knowledge of the use of theophylline.

Theophylline belongs to a large class of substituted xanthines. The methyl substituted xanthines and some of the substituted methylxanthines have been examined in great detail for their effect as bronchodilators. Of the large class of drugs that have been examined, many have been demonstrated to have smooth muscle relaxing properties. However, in the United States only 1,3-dimethylxanthine (theophylline) and various salts of theophylline and a single substituted theophylline, 7-dihydroxypropyl theophylline, dyphylline, are available. Caffeine, 1,3,7-trimethylxanthine, has been shown by at least one group to have bronchodilatory properties which occur with blood levels that can be achieved by consuming coffee or caffeine-containing soft drinks. These studies have yet to be confirmed and it is the impression of the majority of clinicians in the United States that coffee drinking or tablets which contain caffeine, ostensibly as stimulants, cannot substitute for theophylline when theophylline is in the therapeutic dose range. 3,7-dimethylxanthine, theobromine, is also a bronchodilator which is available in some European countries but is not licensed for use in the United States. There are also a large class of substituted methylxanthines and related compounds that are under intensive investigation as potential therapeutic agents and some of these are available outside the United States. The brevity of this review does not allow a discussion of these newer compounds.

Theophylline is only sparingly soluble in water. The salts of theophylline, however, are more readily soluble and many theophylline salts were prepared to increase solubility and absorption. Aminophylline, for example, is the ethylene diamine salt of theophylline and this preparation has been widely used. It is important to note that in many cases the salt makes up a significant portion of the weight of the drug and this must be taken into account when prescribing the salts of theophylline. As an example, aminophylline contains only 84% theophylline while choline theophylline is 50% theophylline. The other strategy for increasing the solubility of theophylline has been to dispense it in the form of elixirs; this was particularly true for pediatric preparations. It is now clear that it is not necessary to use either salts of theophylline or elixirs of theophylline to achieve adequate blood levels of this drug. Indeed, ethanolic solutions of theophylline serve only to increase the toxicity of the drug and therefore should be avoided.

Although direct relaxation of smooth muscle was originally proposed as the mode of action of theophylline, it is now clear that theophylline has a number of pharmacologic properties which, to a greater or lesser extent, combine to help in the treatment of bronchoconstriction. Theophylline has a direct relaxant effect on smooth muscle when the muscle is in tonic contraction but little effect on resting smooth muscle. This fact accounts for the observation that theophylline does not cause any change in the function of the normal lung. Theophylline is also a direct stimulant of the central medullary respiratory control center. This action of theophylline may be particularly important when the drug is used for the treatment of the bronchospastic component of chronic obstructive pulmonary disease. Theophylline increases diaphragmatic contractility by a direct action upon this muscle. The mechanism of the stimulation is not clear but it has been suggested that this role of theophylline may play a significant part in the overall therapeutic effect of the drug, particularly in the treatment of acute asthma. Finally, theophylline has been shown to augment or accelerate mucociliary clearance. While the contribution of this effect is not clear in the overall spectrum of theophylline action, it has been suggested that it is more important in the treatment of chronic obstructive pulmonary disease than in the treatment of asthma.

Theophylline has a number of effects that may or may not play a role in the treatment of asthma. Most notable of these is antagonism of prostaglandin action and one can speculate that if PGD_2 or $PGF_{2\alpha}$ is antagonized this might help to control the bronchospasm associated with these members of the prostaglandin group. On the other hand, antagonism of the effect of PGE_2 would be detrimental as this prostaglandin is a marked bronchodilator.

Other actions of theophylline are nontherapeutic and, indeed, play a role in the toxicity of the drug. Theophylline increases the perfusion of many organs. This action is of particular interest since it is this effect on the kidneys which may be the underlying basis for the mild diuretic action of the drug. In addition theophylline, particularly at high local concentrations, has a profound effect upon the heart and central nervous system. Cardiac effects include a mild increase in cardiac contractility and stimulation of the cardiac conduction system leading to arrhythmias, particularly of the supraventricular variety. In addition recent evidence suggests an additive effect between theophylline and β_2-adrenergic agonists. This drug interaction has been most clearly demonstrated in experimental animals but has also been suggested as playing a role in cardiac arrhythmias in asthmatic patients.

The central nervous system effects of theophylline are generally related to direct central stimulation. In addition to the stimulation of the medullary respiratory center mentioned above, theophylline also stimulates other medullary centers. This is the reason for the gastrointestinal upset which is the most prominent side-effect of the drug. At higher tissue levels it is clear that there can be direct stimulation of other parts of the brain leading to convulsions.

Theophylline has been demonstrated to have a number of cellular effects which may account for its pharmacologic action. The most studied action is inhibition of cyclic nucleotide phosphodiesterase (PDE), resulting in an increase in the intracellular levels of cyclic AMP. Elevated cyclic AMP inhibits a number of actions associated with asthma, most importantly the secretion of mast cell mediators. Elevated intracellular cAMP may also be the underlying mechanism for the direct relaxation of bronchial smooth muscle. On the other hand, there is a disparity between the test tube demonstration of the inhibition of PDE and the inhibition of PDE in vivo. For example, mast cells studied in vitro require concentrations of theophylline in excess of 1×10^{-3} molar for 50% inhibition of PDE activity, a concentration which could never be achieved in vivo. In the human chopped lung system, however, PDE activity is inhibited at more pharmacologic levels. Thus the actual role of PDE inhibition as the underlying basis for theophylline effects remains unclear.

The problems with PDE inhibition have led to the examination of other actions of theophylline. Theophylline has been demonstrated to be an inhibitor of adenosine binding to specific receptors on the mast cell [2]. Adenosine, which is released in large quantities in areas of hypoxia, has been shown to augment mast cell mediator release. This augmentation has been shown to be abrogated by prior treatment of the mast cells with theophylline. The concentration at which theophylline prevents adenosine binding correlates closely with the therapeutic dose range and this has led to speculation that this may in fact be the major action of theophylline in the treatment of asthma.

Two other actions of theophylline are worthy of mention. First, it has been shown that theophylline alters the intracellular distribution of calcium. This alteration of Ca^{2+} could inhibit mast cell mediator release and might also account for the direct relaxation of the tonically contracted smooth muscle cell. The data are not sufficient, in my judgment, to say that this is a significant part of the effect of theophylline. Second, it has been shown in in vitro systems that theophylline is able to augment the binding of cyclic AMP to intracellular binding proteins, largely cyclic AMP dependent protein kinases; this in combination with the increase in cyclic AMP, due to PDE inhibition, would serve to inhibit mast cell secretion and to relax smooth muscle. The physician could speculate that the combination of mild PDE inhibition seen at pharmacologic tissue concentrations and the increase in cyclic AMP binding makes the role of theophylline in altering cyclic AMP metabolism pivotal.

Theophylline is biotransformed largely in the liver by the cytochrome P450 system. The degradation products 3-methylxanthine, 1,3-dimethyl uric acid, and 3-methyl uric acid are excreted in the urine. In addition 10% of the drug is excreted unchanged. For this reason alteration in liver function will have profound effects on the dosing of theophylline while changes in kidney function are generally of little consequence. It is important to know that the normal biologic activity of the P450 system varies by 1000-fold and thus one cannot predict for a given patient the rate at which he or she will metabolize theophylline. It is for this reason that the starting doses which are given below refer only to the idealized "normal" individual and the actual amount of theophylline which will achieve a therapeutic dose can only be determined by frequent evaluation of the individual patient's blood levels.

Clinical Aspects

Before discussing the actual usage of theophylline I think it is important to mention the various dosage forms of theophylline. Although I will use only the term theophylline, remember that the same considerations are true for any of the salts of theophylline. Theophylline can be given intravenously, orally, and rectally. In addition in the very rare situation where necessary patients can be treated intramuscularly using the 7,*N*-dihydroxypropyl derivative of theophylline, Lufyllin, which is the only preparation which is at neutral pH in solution. Irrespective of the form of theophylline that is to be used, the pharmacologic considerations are the same. The physician should attempt to achieve a blood level which is in the therapeutic range while minimizing the side-effects of the drug. The usual therapeutic blood level is generally considered to be 10–20 μg/ml. This level has been arrived at empirically and requires some comment. It is clear that this is simply a general rule. There are many reports of patients who achieved excellent therapeutic benefit at blood levels well below 10 μg/ml and there are patients who have little or no therapeutic benefit at levels in excess of 20 μg/ml. In addition there is a definite gradation of benefit within the therapeutic range. Thus a patient who has little benefit from theophylline at a blood level of 12 μg/ml may have an excellent result if the blood level is adjusted to 18 μg/ml. As with the absolute level achieved by a given dose of the drug, the therapeutic effects of theophylline must be individualized.

With the therapeutic range of 10–20 μg/ml in mind it is also important to attempt to achieve the maximum degree of consistency in the blood level. That is with a minimum of peaks and valleys throughout the day. Clearly this can be easily achieved using intravenous preparations and indeed this may account for the observation that patients who have "therapeutic" levels as outpatients may still benefit from an i.v. infusion when they have an increase in symptoms requiring hospitalization. As a rule I generally recommend that patients who have not taken theophylline be started on i.v. theophylline using a bolus followed by a continuous infusion. The bolus is generally 5–7 mg/kg given over about 20 min. It is important that the bolus not be given too rapidly so as to avoid problems of cardiac arrhythmias in particular. The bolus is then followed by a continuous infusion of 0.9–1.2 mg/kg per hour. The actual dose should be checked frequently by measuring blood levels.

Oral preparations of theophylline are either short acting, intermediate acting, or long acting. Short-acting preparations generally must be dispensed every 6 h, the intermediate-acting forms every 12 h, and the long-acting type every 24 h. However, this depends largely upon individual metabolic rates. Thus patients who are very slow metabolizers may be able to take the short-acting form every 12 h or intermediate-acting forms once a day. In contrast a rapid metabolizer may not be able to take even the longest-acting theophylline preparation once a day. This is particularly true for children because they have elevated metabolic rates and in general the long-acting form of theophylline yield unacceptable peaks and valleys. As with the absolute dose of theophylline, the type of oral preparation used must be individualized and based upon the measurement of the blood levels.

There has been a great deal written in the U.S. literature about the real pharmacokinetics of the various and growing number of theophylline preparations. Dissolution rates, absorption rates, bioavailability, etc. have been extensively studied. While these are certainly of concern it is important not to lose sight of the fact that the range of variability in metabolic rates is much greater from patient to patient than from pill to pill. Accurate dosing with minimal variability in blood level throughout the day must still be based upon determining both the blood level and the actual therapeutic effect. Choosing the preparation with the highest bioavailability and most constant absorption rate will surely help, but this is not a substitute for accurate evaluation of the individual patient.

There are, however, some considerations which should be kept in mind when prescribing an oral preparation of theophylline. Recent studies have demonstrated that a number of theophylline preparations have altered release and absorption rates if given with meals, and that the type of meal is also important, i.e., fat vs. carbohydrate. Several preparations have exhibited the phenomena of "dumping" when given with a high fat diet. This serves to change an otherwise long-acting form into a more short-acting form. It is important that the physician be aware of the characteristics of the theophylline preparation that is being prescribed and instruct his patients accordingly. Rectal theophylline (usually aminophylline) is formulated as suppositories or enemas. The absorption of drug from suppositories is highly erratic and the use of suppositories should be discouraged. Enemas, in contrast, are effective in yielding a rapid, consistent increase in blood level. This preparation may be particularly effective in young children or adults with severe vomiting.

In addition to the formulation there are a number of other factors that must be taken into account when dispensing theophylline. Younger children have higher metabolic rates and this must be taken into account. Smokers also have elevated degradation and require more drug. It is important to note that smoking marijuana is as bad as or worse than smoking tobacco in this regard. Anything that affects liver function will have a profound effect on the metabolic rates. This includes not only primary hepatic disease but also congestive failure. Indeed, the highest levels of theophylline which have been reported are seen in patients with combined cardiac and hepatic failure. Lists of the factors that affect theophylline elimination and the means of correcting them are available and the reader is referred to these [3].

Perhaps the most important of the factors that affect theophylline dosage are drug interactions. These include drugs that will increase the metabolism of theophylline and those which will decrease the clearance rate. Within the former category phenytoin, intravenous isoproterenol, phenobarbital, and thiabendazole are important examples. In the latter category allopurinol, cimetidine, and the macrolide antibiotics erythromycin and troleandomycin are the most important. The dose of the drugs must be adjusted if the patient taking theophylline is started on one of these drugs.

One must also keep in mind that infection and immunization, particularly to influenza A, can markedly decrease the biotransformation rate of theophylline. In many cases this will necessitate a lowering of the dosage of theophylline until the infection or the effect of the immunization have been overcome. The mechanism for the effect of influenza A virus infection is not clear.

In the United States we use theophylline as a first line drug for the treatment of the asthmatic. A convenient starting dose is 20 – 28 mg/kg per 24 h divided according to the preparation used and adjusted based on blood level and patient response [3]. We have found that it is an excellent initial treatment and that many patients will have excellent results on this drug alone. One should not give up on theophylline until the blood levels have been adjusted to give the maximum benefit with a minimum of side-effects. In addition the combination of theophylline with other drugs such as β-adrenergic agonists has been demonstrated to have a synergistic effect and the addition of a small amount of one of these agents to a patient who does not seem to have complete relief on theophylline alone is very effective in many cases. There are problems with side-effects in patients treated with theophylline but these can largely be overcome by accurate titration of the blood levels. With a close watch on the dosage form and the metabolic rate of the patient based upon blood level determinations, and with adjustment of the dose when there are changes in medication or when intercurrent infection occurs, one can achieve excellent control of asthma in a large proportion of the asthmatic population.

References

1. Weinberger MM, Bronsky EA (1974) Evaluation of oral bronchodilator therapy in asthmatic children. I Ped 84:421
2. Marquardt DL, Parker CW, Sullivan TJ (1978) Potentiation of mast cell mediation release by adenosine. J Immunol 120:871
3. Wedner HJ (1984) Theophylline. In: Korenblat PE, Wedner HJ (eds) Allergy theory and practice. Grune and Stratton, Orlando, p 221

Topical Steroids: Perspectives and Retrospectives

A. M. Kligman
University of Pennsylvania, School of Medicine, Department of Dermatology, Philadelphia, PA 19104, USA

Abstract

Molecular manipulations have produced topical antiinflammatory agents of unprecedented potency, for example, clobetasole propionate. It is pointless, even dangerous, to create ever more powerful compounds.

New objectives have to be defined for obtaining maximal efficacy with the least risk. Recent efforts have focussed on the following goals:

1. Dissociation of anti-inflammatory potency from atrophogenicity. This will not soon be a reality.
2. Enhancement of efficacy by scientific formulation in accordance with pharmaceutical principals of percutaneous absorption. Diprolene (Schering, U.S.A.) is an example of the attainment of higher efficacy by optimizing the vehicle.
3. Revised schedules of application. The traditional b.i.d. or t.i.d. usage is often unnecessary, usually irrational, sometimes harmful and more costly. Recommendations regarding frequency of application should be based on the disease being treated, clearance from the skin, characteristics of the formulation and other factors.
4. Development of penetration enhancers such as dimethyl-sulfoxide but without its numerous disadvantages. The impact of Azone will be discussed.
5. Rational selection of pharmaceutical form of a specific steroid. For example, how does one choose among lotions, creams, ointments, sprays, aerosols and tapes?
6. New clinical uses for topical corticosteroids.

Introduction

Dermatologic therapeutics can be divided into two eras: B.C. and A.C., respectively before-corticosteroids and after-corticosteroids. The introduction of topical hydrocortisone 35 years ago, marked the end ot paleodermatology, a long, long period during which topical medicaments had to possess at least one of the 3 S's to qualify as efficacious, that is, they had to sting, stain, or stink.

Tars, sulfur, and permanganate are typical examples. These certainly impressed the patient if not the skin! Overnight, smelly, irritating, colored medicaments gave way to bland, white, aesthetically pleasing, and, above all, efficacious formulations [1].

The tremendous impact of corticosteroids can be instantly appreciated by noting that in the United States corticosteroids account for the great majority of topical prescriptions written by physicians [2]. The reason is obvious. All chronic inflammatory skin diseases of whatever origin are benefited to some degree. This nonspecificity of action is fundamental to their popularity and at the same time an invitation to overuse and misuse.

Since hydrocortisone, steroid chemists have brought forth molecular miracles, creating hundreds of new derivatives, following an upward path of ever-increasing potency. We seem to have reached the pinnacle of the steroid ascent with the latest agent, clobetasol propionate, so powerful that a single 15-g application to normal skin results in complete adrenal suppression in less than 12 h [3]. The market is crowded with dozens of steroid molecules and hundreds of proprietary formulations [4]. The pharmaceutical industry can rightfully boast of its prowess in creative molecular chemistry. These triumphs notwithstanding, progress always engenders new problems. We are reminded in Ecclesiastes that "he who increases knowledge, also increases sorrow." The current situation with topical corticosteroids does not warrant sadness; nonetheless, many unresolved issues remain. Irrational practices did not end with the advent of corticosteroids.

It is my intention to look at various problems with a critical eye. I announce forthwith that the following account is not a scholarly review. Rather, this is one man's perspectives and opinions. The most complete recent reviews are by Polano [5] and Miller and Munro [6].

Do We Need New Corticosteroids?

The answer is a qualified yes. The ideal compound still awaits discovery. However, there is no point in creating even more potent molecules. We are armed well enough and have reached the point of diminishing returns. The proving ground for any steroid is chronic plaque-type psoriasis. How much more can we ask for when, with b.i.d. applications of clobestasol, we can almost clear most cases in 2 weeks [7]? No other drug works so swiftly or predictably. However, there is a price to be paid for such therapeutic power, namely, the increased likelihood of adverse side effects. Some perspective is necessary on this point. Too much has been made of the hazard of adrenal suppression. Typical of this supercautious concern is the recent counseling of Parrish et al. to monitor pituitary-adrenal function whenever potent steroids are to be used for more than 2 weeks [8]! This is, of course, impractical; moreover, it is almost useless, since it will rarely affect clinical decisions. The dire fears about the systemic dangers of clobetasol propionate, which have probably delayed its entry into the U.S.A., have not been borne out in clinical practice [9]. The clinical state of the patient overrides the laboratory findings. Rarely do clinical signs of adrenal insufficiency emerge. Besides, recovery of adrenal function is usually very rapid after stopping the drug. It is a reflection of our hysterical times that bureaucrats place labeling constraints on clobetasol propionate which limit its use to 2 weeks. Of course, this warning will not be heeded by dermatologists who are actually taking care of real patients. This is the problem of defensive medicine in the United States, where testing is more important than treating. Furthermore, an important point has been lost in the safety guidelines. It is true enough that repeated applications of potent steroids to normal skin may lead to increased absorption, a result of loss of the horny layer barrier. On the contrary, in dermatitic skin, the impaired barrier function improves as the disease clears, greatly reducing absorption. Moreover, less steroid is used as the disease clears. Too many unwarranted conclusions are drawn from studies on normal skin, which, after all, is in no way comparable to diseased skin. For example, the vasoconstriction blanching test on normal skin is a very useful screening procedure for new corticosteroids. It is not sufficiently realized, however, that intensity of blanching and clinical efficacy do not always correlate [10]. With certain formulations, clinical potency, predicted from vasoconstriction tests has been over-rated.

The dangers of corticosteroids are almost all local, epitomized by the term atrophogenicity. Extreme examples, such as herniation of fat through thinned skin, are frightening but are very rare and always involve overuse [11]. The usual signs of atrophy are thinning, striae, and telangiectasia. However, there are about 20 additional types of unwanted, if unusual, side effects of which physicians are often not sufficiently aware [12]. Despite exhortations, we still see cases of severe steroid rosacea and steroid acne, induced by doctors who will not heed admonitions to avoid potent steroids on the face [13, 14]. This is an interesting predicament, because facial skin is highly permeable and disorders located there are quite responsive to lower-strength steroids. Therapy should be adjusted to region, owing to the vast anatomic differences between various sites of the integument, but few doctors actually practice regional therapeutics.

Among the exotic side reactions, recognized with difficulty, are tinea incognita (masking of fungal infection), glaucoma, cataracts, and local hypertrichosis [12]. Of all the iatrogenic mischiefs, none is more distressing than steroid addiction. This arises because of a rebound "flare", when the steroid is stopped, driving the patient back to the steroid [15]. Breaking the addiction is a formidable task.

Some critics wonder whether we have paid too high a price in side reactions for the benefits of corticosteroids [16]. It is a truism that steroids are prescribed in almost reflex fashion, often inappropriately. There is a biting joke in circulation that if the disorder fails to respond, one should then hunt for a diagnosis or refer the case! Nonetheless, the triumphs of steroid therapy far outweigh the handicaps, which are mainly due to misuse.

The ideal steroid would be highly effective and lack side effects. Only the first of these two requirements has been achieved. Nowadays, owing to market pressures, the claim is sometimes made for a new proprietary introduction that high potency has been maintained while atrophogenicity has been lessened. This is not a reality, and is not likely to become one. With every increase in potency, there is a corresponding increase in atrophogenicity. Sometimes, laboratory data are used in a questionable way to prove that a dissociation has been achieved. Thus, two recently synthesized prednisolone derivatives have been shown not to inhibit collagen synthesis while maintaining the capacity to suppress rat sponge granulomas [17], but judgement is premature until it is shown in humans that topical application clears steroid-sensitive dermatoses and that dermal atrophy does not develop. Experience indicates that the risks parallel the benefits. Dissociation is a theoretical possibility but I hold out no hope for success, since I believe it is the inherent toxicity of the steroid which mediates its therapeutic effects. Steroids are toxic to virtually all cells and suppress multiple cellular functions nonselectively. It is often said that adverse effects could be minimized by designing a steroid that the skin could rapidly metabolize. To be sure, many drugs are metabolized by skin. However, a rapidly metabolized corticosteroid would probably lose efficacy proportionately.

If I were directing the efforts of steroid chemists, I would not underwrite the search for an ideal steroid. My goals would be more mundane, such as making the ones now in our possession more efficient. Less expensive steroids would also be very welcome! I also favor a program to reduce the misuse and overuse of steroids but I doubt that educators can work such a miracle against miracle drugs.

How Do Steroids Work?

The writings on this important question are remarkably glib, pedantic, and unenlightening. The melancholy fact is that we do not know the molecular mechanisms by which corticosteroids exert their therapeutic effects. Long ago, Weissman and Thomas argued from in vitro studies that steroids, by stabilizing lysosomes, could inhibit the release of destructive hydrolases from cells [18]. This is an attractive idea, but simply does not hold for most in vivo situations [19]. This is but one of many plausible rationalizations which cannot be generalized. It is a seductive feature of in vitro studies that, by manipulating the variables, one can arrange for an outcome which fits the investigator's preferred bias. The clinical relevance of in vitro findings must always be questioned. For example, steroids can be shown to either stimulate or suppress fibroblasts in vitro, depending on the source of the cells.

It should be noted that inflammatory reactions exist which are not affected by steroids. The acute sunburn induced by ultraviolet radiation is a vivid example of this. By virtue of vasoconstriction topical corticosteroids can reduce erythema but cellular damage to the epidermis (sunburn cells) remains unaffected [10]. Likewise, there is no value, and indeed some risk, in prescribing oral steroids in high doses for severe sunburn. Still, one cannot imagine a hospitalized, blistered patient not being given this "treatment."

A special nomenclature has evolved to describe the effects of corticosteroids; they are "anti-inflammatory," "morbistatic," "antiproliferative," etc. These are phenomenologic terms that are wonderfully satisfying but tell us nothing about how steroids work. Catchy cliches arrest thought and stunt research.

It is unexpectedly difficult to explain some of the best-known effects of corticosteroids, for example, the suppression of pustules. Topical steroids prevent pustulation from croton oil. It is all too easy to assume that the mechanism is a direct effect on neutrophils, probably an inhibition of chemotaxis. This has not been demonstrated as it has for monocytes [20]. It appears that the effect of the steroid is indirect, preventing the emigration of neutrophils from small blood vessels. How this happens is also unknown. Other vasoconstrictors (adrenergic drugs) do not suppress pustules.

Receptor biochemistry has been one of the most rewarding areas of pharmacologic research, providing the theoretical basis for the developing more effective drugs of greater specificity. Corticosteroid receptors have been demonstrated in skin, raising hopes of a rational approach. Academicians like to say that steroids exert their effect on cell functions by binding to cytoplasmic receptors, which then migrate to the nucleus where they affect DNA and protein synthesis [21, 22]. This is all very neat and logical, except that there is no evidence that anti-inflammatory activity and cytosol binding are correlated or that binding is a necessary requirement for efficacy [23]. So far, steroid receptors are of purely theoretical interest. The only application so far is to provide merchandising ammunition in the commercial steroid wars.

Another notion which theorists admire is that corticosteroids exert their anti-inflammatory effects by preventing the release of phospholipase A_2 from cell membranes. Phospholipase is necessary for the generation of arachidonic acid, the starting molecule for the cascade of mediators in the cyclooxygenase and lipoxygenase pathways [20]. Thus, the very first event in the inflammatory sequence would be blocked. This is an all-encompassing theory which explains completely the ability of corticosteroids to counteract inflammatory disease. We await proof. Likewise, none of the other numerous laboratory observations adequately explain the mode of action of corticosteroids. Included here are the antimitotic effects, inhibition of DNA synthesis, immunosuppression, inhibition of release of lymphokines, etc., etc. Happily, ignorance does not prevent the effective use of this marvellous class of drugs.

It is of some comfort that another class of wonder drugs, the retinoids which have transformed dermatologic practice, are in the same predicament. Retinoids have diverse therapeutic effects, but not a single one can be satisfactorily explained at the molecular level. It is typical of medicine that revelations of therapeutic efficacy usually come first. Explanations come later! Aspirin is a good example of this sequence. It is the grandfather of all nonsteroidal anti-inflammatory drugs, but only recently has its molecular mode of action been revealed. Nonsteroidal drugs such as indomethacin and ibuprofen are all inhibitors of prostaglandin synthetase. With this knowledge, one can design in vitro tests which reliably predict efficacy, enabling rapid laboratory screening of new agents. Sooner or later, steroids will yield up their secret to modern science.

Vehicles: Old and New Perspectives

Optimizing the vehicle is an important responsibility of the pharmacologist. A potent steroid can be made feeble by formulating it in the wrong base. Rational selection of the best vehicle depends upon basic knowledge embodied in fundamental principles such as Fick's law and thermodynamics. It is important to understand diffusion constants, the effects of concentration and solubility in the vehicle on thermodynamics, partition coefficients between the vehicle and the skin, and other recondite matters. However, there are limitations in a purely laboratory approach. The clinic is the ultimate testing ground. This rule has been ignored more than once, with corrections having to be made later. For example, incorporation of fluocinoline acetonide in a vehicle containing 50%–60% propylene glycol results in maximal diffusion through skin. As expected, this correlates with greater efficacy. However, proplyene glycol in such high concentrations is a fairly strong irritant. This may be irrelevant in thick, plaque-type psoriasis. However, in atopic dermatitis and in eczemas of intertriginous areas, greater penetration of the drug is offset by irritation, and the dermatitis may actually worsen. The skin makes the final decision; one has to know the peculiarities of the different dermatoses to make the most of steroids.

A compromise makes it possible to exploit the advantageous properties of propylene glycol safely. The concentration should not be greater than 25%, and emollients should be incorporated to reduce irritation. The development of Diprolene Ointment by Schering in the United States is a striking example of how to greatly enhance the efficacy of a moderately potent steroid, betamethasone dipropionate, by using propylene glycol ingeniously. The therapeutic power of this preparation is second only to clobetasol propionate. Clinicians were quick to appreciate that this new formulation could be rapidly effective in dermatoses resistant to other potent corticosteroids in cream bases [24].

Despite its appeal, the enhancement of efficacy by pharmacologic promotion of penetration into skin is not always wise. We may use hydrocortisone as a teaching case. At a 1.0% concentration, side reactions are uncommon and rather mild [25]. In the usual cream or ointment formulations atrophogenicity its low. This has beguiled clinicians into thinking that hydrocortisone lacks this potential altogether, which is simply untrue. Intradermal injection of a hydrocortisone suspension will produce an atrophy almost equivalent to that from triamcinolone, though shorter lasting. Moreover, long-term use of hydrocortisone on an area as highly permeable as the face can certainly result in thinning and telangiectasia. The intrinsically low diffusion of hydrocortisone into skin is one of its unrecognized virtues, limiting the damage its overuse would otherwise entail. It is therefore wrong to increase the penetration of hydrocortisone by pharmacologic manipulations.

An example of this exists in the case of Dioderm cream (Dermal Labs, England) which in a concentration of 0.1% is as effective as 1.0% hydrocortisone in conventional basis [26]. This "achievement" required the presence of both propylene glycol, to help solubilize the steroid, and the anionic surfactant sodium lauryl sulfate (SLS). As a penetration enhancer SLS has no peer, greatly increasing permeability of the skin at concentrations of 1% – 3%. These levels, however, damage the barrier and are frequently irritating. Here, too, the benefits are largely cancelled out by clinical adversities. Dioderm has never caught on, at least in the U.S.A. Moreover, atrophogenicity of any steroid is potentiated on damaged, inflamed skin. Simply creating a sharp sunburn or inducing surfactant dermatitis will greatly intensify the atrophogenic effect. As in politics, one has to appreciate and calculate the trade-offs.

Modern formulators rarely appreciate that vehicles may have therapeutic effects in their own right. The vehicle is thought of merely as a device to transport the drug from the producer to the user. Typically, the vehicle is called a "placebo" or "inactive base." This is invalid and thoughtless. Our clinician forefathers, practicing in the 19th century and 1st half of the 20th, knew very well how to use "vehicles" in treating a variety of disorders. These were often pastes (Lassar's), thick greases (petrolatum), particulate creams (zinc oxide ointment), etc. The "active" ingredients in these frequently efficacious topicals would be beyond identification by today's well-trained dermatologists.

While hardly spoken about, the influence of the vehicle extends much beyond its role as a delivery device for the drug. It has beneficial effects in its own right. A venerable ointment, petrolatum, furnishes an example. Pharmacologically speaking, it is far from an optimal vehicle for corticosteroids. Release of the steroid is limited, partitioning is poor, and the drug is in suspension, rather than the theoretically desirable solution. Drugs are more readily released from emulsions. A further advantage is that the surface concentration of the drug has to increase after evaporation of the water phase. Every rational consideration favors creams over ointments. But, in fact, almost every controlled study shows that ointment formulations of steroids are therapeutically superior to creams [27]. The latter, of course, are more aesthetic, but in the treatment of disease, efficacy should override cosmetic considerations. American doctors overwhelmingly prescribe creams, catering, perhaps foolishly, to patient preferences. It is worth noting how closely glamorous cosmetic creams resemble those used as bases for topical medicaments! Europeans seem to accept ointment formulations more readily.

In view of the limitations of petrolatum in solubilizing and releasing the drug, how can we explain its therapeutic superiority, especially noteworthy in chronic dermatoses? My interpretation is that diffusional water loss is greatly increased in inflammatory hyperkeratotic eruptions such as psoriasis, owing to a poorly formed horny layer barrier. Hence, the underlying tissue tends to dry out, retarding healing. Loss of the horny layer, whether a result of topical steroids, stripping, or disease, incites an inflammatory reaction (the well known "flare" after stopping steroids). Merely covering an area denuded by stripping with an impermeable film will greatly reduce the reactive inflammation. Petrolatum is a hydrophobic substance which inhibits water loss and adds to plasticity of the horny layer, improving its barrier capacity. Moreover, petrolatum, by its very greasiness, stays in place, providing a kind of extracutaneous reservoir. Creams can be lost quickly from the site of application.

Hence one expects, and finds evidence in the literature, that petrolatum by itself is helpful in various dermatoses. Marks has come to grips with this so called "placebo effect" of ointments, emphasizing their intrinsic therapeutic possibilities [28]. These may protect dermatitic skin in multiple ways, including unexplained pharmacologic activity.

The legal requirement to perform double-blind studies to prove efficacy has repeatedly disclosed the beneficial effects of the vehicle itself. This has received too little attention. Of course, the steroid always wins handily in such a match. What is really impressive, however, is the substantial improvement achieved by the vehicle alone, particularly in steroid-sensitive dermatoses like atopic or seborrheic dermatitis. The percentage of cases achieving good to excellent improvement is sometimes startling. Mullins, in particular, has emphasized these unexpected, rarely noted, outcomes [29]. Because I am a proponent of petrolatum as a premier emollient, I conducted a study comparing 0.1% triamcinolone cream (Keralog, Squibb) to petrolatum, applied twice daily to children with atopic dermatitis. At 1 week, 9 of 13 patients had a poor result with petrolatum, while only three on triamcinolone were so rated. At the end of 3 weeks, however, 10 of 13 petrolatum patients had substantially improved, though only three were excellent, compared to nine in the triamcinolone group. By searching the record, one often finds evidence cautioning against reflex prescribing of high-potency steroids in all dermatoses. Mendelson and Bessler compared a potent fluocinonide cream to 0.5% hydrocortisone cream [30]. In atopic dermatitis, contact dermatitis, eczematous dermatitis, and seborrheic dermatitis, fluocinonide was superior in only half the cases or less! A similar comparison study by Rex, in psoriasis, showed that hydrocortisone achieved equivalence in about half the cases [31]. Such results suggest that the vehicle is also playing an important role, considering that 0.5% hydrocortisone is the weakest member of the steroid family.

Findings such as these have practical implications. For example, when should steroids be stopped? Usually, clinical clearing is the signal to terminate treatment. However, because of the skin's opacity, clinical remission may not be reliable. If one looks at biopsies from recently cleared psoriatic lesions, one will be impressed by the degree of residual changes, especially a persistent perivenular infiltrate and abnormal, dilated capillaries. The epidermis may be near normal, but a low-grade dermal inflammation persists. This suggests that steroids should not be stopped abruptly. Perhaps one should switch to a low-strength steroid for a few more weeks, staying on the lookout for relapse. Another strategy which often seems to work is to substitute b.i.d. petrolatum for a month or so, emphasizing that this will protect the recently damaged skin. Also, I have the impression, but no proof, that this delays relapse, so frequent and so frustrating in the management of this lifelong disorder.

Scheduling (Posology)

In contrast to oral or systemically administered drugs, topical therapy is embarrassingly naive and ritualistic. The frequency of application is largely based on tradition, not on scientific determinations. This situation will soon change because of increasing competition for market share in the steroid wars. Manufacturers are obliged to look more closely at such practical questions as "How often should one apply the steroid"? It seems that a majority of physicians without any thought, advise applications b.i.d. or t.i.d., more often the latter. This probably reflects the persistence of ancient rituals rooted in the magnic of numbers the number 3 being credited with special powers. The Egyptians raised this numerical superstition to a religious belief, promulgated through the priesthood.

Studies which validate t.i.d. application for any class of drugs are conspicuous by their absence. In the case of potent corticosteroids, who has shown whether t.i.d. is better than b.i.d.? Or, for that matter, whether b.i.d. is superior to o.d.? It is therefore interesting to note a recent spate of commercially inspired papers which make the claim that once daily application of high-potency steroid "A" (manufactured by the company commissioning the study) is therapeutically equivalent to t.i.d. steroid "B," a competing product. Ignoring motives, this trend is all to the good and has highlighted the fact that we have paid too little attention to treatment schedules. Typical of this new game plan is the revealing report by Cahn et al. [32]. In 109 patients with eczema, once daily 0.05% diflorasone diacetate was compared to t.i.d. 0.1% betamethasone valerate. It should not surprise anyone that both treatments were highly effective and equivalent. Of course, a more honest comparison would entail once daily vs thrice daily applications of the same steroid. This, too, has been done, with predictable results. Frederiksson et al. used halcinonide cream in psoriasis and atopic dermatitis. Except for a somewhat swifter response with t.i.d. applications, the results were equivalent for once daily application at the end of 3 weeks [33].

At last we seem to be in a fresh period in which old-fashioned rituals are giving way to properly conducted, rigorous trials. Fixed routines of application are increasingly coming under scrutiny. A new trend is alternating regimens which go under various names – pulse therapy, interval therapy, tandem therapy, etc. The basic scheme is to alternate the active steroid with the base in a specific schedule. I heartily approve of the strategy, though I think the rationale for interval therapy is based on an irrelvant concept, namely the tachyphylaxis phenomenon, discovered by De Vivier and coworkers [34, 35]. They found that with frequent applications of corticosteroids to normal skin, resistance developed to the vasoconstriction response. In mouse skin, inhibition of DNA synthesis could not be demonstrated after repeated applications. Responsiveness recurred when the steroid was stopped for a few days. However, it has not been shown that dermatitic skin becomes resistant to the anti-inflammatory action after multiple applications over a matter of days or weeks. There are various reasons for steroid resistance in chronic dermatoses, but tachyphylaxis is not one of these. Nonetheless, interval therapy seems to be effective and worthwhile, whatever the explanation [36]. The study by van Dijk et al. is typical of this new strategy. They treated 33 psoriatics with betamethasone dipropionate cream twice daily for 4 days, alternating this with the cream base b.i.d. for 3 days. This tandem therapy was equivalent to conventional b.i.d. application of the steroid.

The virtues of tandem therapy are obvious: decreased cost and decreased side effects. One may expect to see many variations on this theme. For example, the scheduling might be 2 (or 3) days on steroid, 2 (or 3) days on base. Tandem therapy should be considered in chronic dermatoses as soon as a good clinical response is obtained with conventional b.i.d. (or t.i.d.) applications. I prefer to use petrolatum as the nondrug alternative. A convenient schedule is to apply the steroid in the morning and petrolatum at night. If the response holds, alternate b.i.d. steroid for 1 day with b.i.d. petrolatum for 1 day. The next step is to alternate once daily steroid with once daily petrolatum. Ultimately, it may be possible to apply the steroid on weekends and petrolatum on weekdays. Obviously, one has to be flexible, adjusting the schedule to individual patients. One side benefit of interval therapy may be that both the physician and the patient will avoid fixed routines, encouraging the patient to become an active participant in working out the optimal schedule.

I will close with a warning against one practice which is becoming widespread, namely diluting proprietary steroids with a variety of untested lotions and creams. Unless the manufacturer specifically provides a vehicle for such dilutions it is inadvisable to risk ad hoc compounding. There may be a number of undesirable consequences of such adulterations, viz, uneven distribution of the steroid, crystallization, inadequate preservation, inactivation or transformation of the steroid, physical incompatibility. Modern corticosteroids are precisely formulated. They should not be tampered with!

References

1. Sulzberger MB, Witten VH (1952) The effect of topically applied compound F in selected dermatoses. J Invest Dermatol 19:101 – 102
2. Stoughton RB (1977) A perspective of topical corticosteroid therapy. In: Psoriasis: proceedings of the second international symposium. Farber EM, Cox AJ (eds) Yorke Medical, New York, pp 219 – 226
3. Ortega E, Burdick KH, Segre EJ (1975) Adrenal suppression by clobetasol propionate. Lancet I:1200
4. Robertson DB, Maibach HI (1983) Topical corticosteroids. Semin Dermatol 2:238 – 249
5. Polano MK (1984) Topical skin therapeutics. Churchill Livingston, New York, 1984, pp 101 – 144
6. Miller JA, Munro DD (1980) Topical corticosteroids: clinical pharmacology and therapeutic use. Drugs 19:119 – 134
7. vd Harst LC, de Jonge H, Pot F, Polano MK (1982) Comparison of two application schedules for clobetasol propionate. Acta Derm. Venereol. 62:270 – 273
8. Parrish LC, Witkowski JA, Muir JG (1985) Topical corticosteroids. Internat J Dermatol 24:435 – 436
9. Richards RN (1985) Clinical experience with 0.05% clobetasol propionate creams. J Am Acad Derm 12:891 – 892
10. Kaidbey KH, Kligman AM (1974) Assay of topical corticosteroids by suppression of experimental inflammation in humans. J Invest Dermatol 63:292 – 296
11. Sneddon IB (1970) Atrophy of the skin. Br J Dermatol 94 [Suppl]: 121 – 123
12. Kligman AM, Frosch PJ (1984) Steroid addiction. Int Soc Trop Dermatol. 18:23 – 31
13. Leyden JJ, Thew M, Kligman AM (1974) Steroid rosacea. Arch Dermatol 110:619 – 622

14. Plewig G, Kligman AM (1977) Induction of acne by topical steroids. Arch Dermatol Res 247:29–35
15. Sneddon IB (1979) Adverse effects of topical fluorinated corticosteroids in rosacea. Br Med J 1:671–675
16. Calnan CD (1976) Use and abuse of topical corticosteroids. Dermatologica [Suppl] 152:747–750
17. DePetrillo T, Lee H, Cutroneo KR (1984) Anti-inflammatory adrenal steroids that neither inhibit collagen synthesis nor cause dermal atrophy. Arch Dermatol 120:877–883
18. Weissmann G, Thomas L (1962) Studies on lysosomes. J Exp Med 116:433–450
19. Fauci AS (1979) Immuno-suppressive and anti-inflammatory activity of corticosteroids. In: Baxter JD et al. (eds) Glucosteroid hormone action. Springer, Berlin Heidelberg New York, pp 449–469
20. Snell ES (1976) Mechanisms of glucocorticoid activity a review. In: Wilson T, Marks R (eds) Mechanisms of corticosteroid activity. Churchill Livingstone, Edinburgh, pp 136–145
21. Epstein EH, Bonifas JM (1982) Glucocorticoid receptors of normal human epidermis. J Invest Dermatol 78:144–146
22. Leiferman KM (1981) Evidence for a glucosteroid receptor in human skin. Clin Res 29:604A
23. Ponec M, Kempanaar SA, DeKloet ER (1981) Corticosteroids and cultured human epidermal keratinocytes. J Invest Dermatol 76:211–214
24. Aldana GG (1981) Efficacy and tolerance of betamethasone dipropionate for resistant psoriasis and other steroid-responsive dermatoses. J Int Med Res 9:448–457
25. Kligman AM, Kaidbey KH (1978) Hydrocortisone revisited. An experimental evaluation. Cutis 22:232–244
26. Frederiksson T (1976) A topical formulation of hydrocortisone with increased activity. Dermatol Digest 18:27–29
27. Leer J (1979) The comparative efficacy of betamethasone dipropionate cream and ointment formulations in psoriasis. Cutis 23:97–101
28. Marks R (1982) Effects of emollients on inflammatory dermatoses. In: Principles of cosmetics for the dermatologist. Mosby, St. Louis, pp 334–340
29. Mullins JD (1975) Hydrocortisone: a reevaluation. Cutis 15:428–449
30. Mendelson CG, Bessler SA (1971) Clinical efficacy of fluocinonide cream. Cutis 8:557–561
31. Rex H (1973) Controlled evaluation of a new topical corticosteroid in psoriasis. Curr. Therap Res 15:833–836
32. Cahn MM et al. (1977) Comparative topical efficacy of once daily defluorasone diacetate and t.i.d. applications of betamethasone valerate applications. Curr Therap Res 22:297–302
33. Frederiksson T, Lasser A, Bleeker J (1980) Treatment of psoriasis and atopic dermatitis with halcinonide cream applied once and three times daily. Br J Dermatol 102:575–577
34. De Vivier A, Stoughton RB (1975) Tachyphylaxis to the action of topically applied corticosteroids. Arch Dermatol 111:581–585
35. De Vivier A, Phillips H, Hehir M (1982) Applications of glucosteroids. Arch Dermatol 118:305–308
36. van Dijk E et al. (1983) Intermittent topical treatment of psoriasis with betamethasone dipropionate 0.05% cream. Cutis 32:283–286

Index of Authors

Subject Index

MIX
Papier aus verantwortungsvollen Quellen
Paper from responsible sources
FSC® C105338

If you have any concerns about our products,
you can contact us on
ProductSafety@springernature.com

In case Publisher is established outside the EU,
the EU authorized representative is:
Springer Nature Customer Service Center GmbH
Europaplatz 3, 69115 Heidelberg, Germany

Printed by Libri Plureos GmbH
in Hamburg, Germany